TECHNIQUES
IN LARGE
ANIMAL
SURGERY

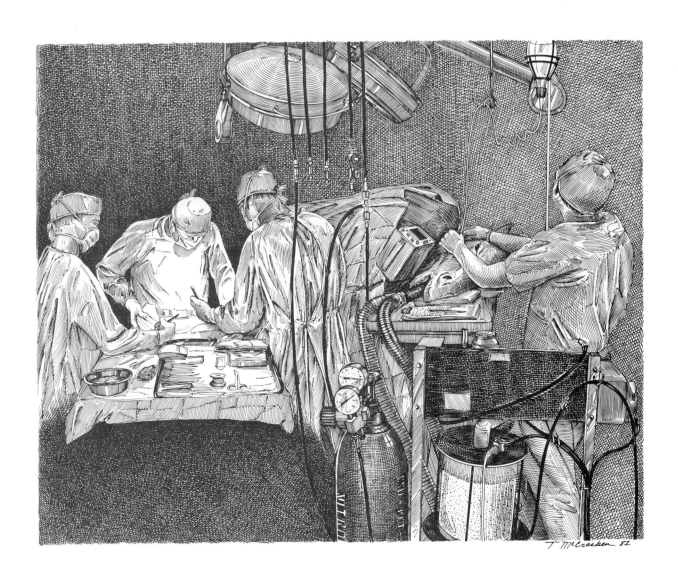

TECHNIQUES IN LARGE ANIMAL SURGERY

Second Edition

A. SIMON TURNER, B.V.Sc., M.S.

*Diplomate, American College of Veterinary Surgeons;
Professor of Surgery, Department of Clinical Sciences,
College of Veterinary Medicine and Biomedical Sciences,
Colorado State University, Fort Collins, Colorado*

C. WAYNE McILWRAITH, B.V.Sc.,
M.S., Ph.D., M.R.C.V.S.

*Diplomate, American College of Veterinary Surgeons;
Professor of Surgery, Department of Clinical Sciences,
College of Veterinary Medicine and Biomedical Sciences,
Colorado State University, Fort Collins, Colorado*

WITH CONTRIBUTIONS BY

BRUCE L. HULL, D.V.M., M.S.

*Diplomate, American College of Veterinary Surgeons;
Professor of Veterinary Clinical Sciences, College of Veterinary Medicine, The Ohio State University, Columbus,
Ohio*

ILLUSTRATIONS BY

TOM McCRACKEN, M.S.

*Assistant Professor, Department of Anatomy and
Neurobiology, Colorado State University, Fort Collins,
Colorado*

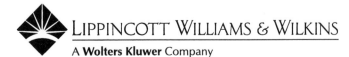

LIPPINCOTT WILLIAMS & WILKINS
A **Wolters Kluwer** Company

Philadelphia · Baltimore · New York · London
Buenos Aires · Hong Kong · Sydney · Tokyo

Lippincott Williams & Wilkins
530 Walnut Street
Philadelphia, Pa. 19106

Library of Congress Cataloging in Publication Data
Turner, A. Simon (Anthony Simon)
    Techniques in large animal surgery / A. Simon Turner,
C. Wayne McIlwraith; with contributions by Bruce L. Hull;
illustrations by Tom McCracken.
        p. cm.
    Bibliography: p.
    Includes index.
    ISBN 0-8121-1177-X
    1. Veterinary surgery.   2. Horses—Surgery.   3. Cattle—
Surgery.
    I. McIlwraith, C. Wayne.   II. Hull, Bruce L.   III. Title.
SF911.T87 1989
    636.089′7—dc19   88-13377
                                                              CIP

PRINTED IN THE UNITED STATES OF AMERICA

Print Number: 10 9 8

To our parents, Ann and Colin Turner and Kathleen and Cyril McIlwraith

PREFACE
TO THE FIRST
EDITION

The purpose of this book is to present some fundamental techniques in large animal surgery to both veterinary students and large animal practitioners. It is designed to be brief, discussing only the major steps in a particular operation, and each discussion is accompanied by appropriate illustrations. Most of the techniques presented in this book can be performed without the advantages of a fully equipped large animal hospital or teaching institution.

The book assumes a basic understanding of anatomy and physiology. Those who wish to know more about a particular technique are encouraged to consult the bibliography.

We and our colleagues at the Colorado State University Veterinary Teaching Hospital consider the procedures discussed in this book to be time honored. Some practitioners may perform certain techniques in slightly different ways. We would be happy to receive input about modifications of these techniques for future editions of this book.

All of the drawings in the book are original and based on rough sketches and photographs taken at various points during actual surgery. Occasionally, dissections were performed on cadavers.

The surgical procedures described in this text represent not only our thoughts, but suggestions from many of our colleagues as well. Their help was an important contribution to the production of this book. We are indebted to Dr. Wilbur Aanes, Professor of Surgery, Colorado State University, who unselfishly shared 30 years of his personal experience in large animal surgery with us. We are proud to be able to present in Chapter 10 of this book "Aanes' Method of Repair of Third-Degree Perineal Laceration" in the mare, a technique that he pioneered over 15 years ago. We also wish to give credit to the following faculty members at Colorado State University Veterinary Teaching Hospital who willingly gave us advice on the diagrams and manuscript of various techniques discussed in this book: Dr. Leslie Ball, Dr. Bill Bennett, Dr. Bruce Heath, Dr. Tony Knight, Dr. LaRue Johnson, Dr. Gary Rupp, Dr. Ted Stashak, Dr. Gayle Trotter, Dr. James Voss, and Dr. Mollie Wright. We also wish to express appreciation to Dr. John Baker, Purdue University, and Dr. Charles Wallace, University of Georgia, for their comments on some questions we had. Dr. McIlwraith is also grateful to Dr. John Fessler, Professor of Surgery, Purdue University, for his inspiration and training.

We are particularly grateful to Dr. Robert Kainer, Professor of Anatomy, Colorado State University, for checking the manuscript and the illustrations and advising us on nomenclature. His input impressed upon us the importance of the relationship between the dissection room and the surgery room.

The terrific amount of time and effort involved with the illustrations will be clear to the reader who cares only to leaf through the book. For these illustrations, we are indebted to Mr. Tom McCracken, Director, Office of Biomedical Media,

Colorado State University. We are thankful for his expertise, as well as his cooperation and understanding. The diagrams for "Aanes' Method of Repair of Third-Degree Perineal Laceration" were done by Mr. John Daughtery, Medical Illustrator, Colorado State University. We must also thank Kathleen Jee, who assisted with various aspects of the artwork. We would also like to thank Messrs. Al Kilminster and Charles Kerlee for taking photographs during the various surgical procedures that were used to assist with the artwork of this text.

The manuscript was typed by Mrs. Helen Mawhiney, Ms. Teresa Repphun, and Mrs. Jan Schmidt. We thank them for their patience and understanding during the many changes we made during the generation of the final manuscript.

We are grateful to the following instrument companies for allowing us to use some of the diagrams from their sales catalogs for inclusion in Chapter 3, "Surgical Instruments": Schroer Manufacturing Co., Kansas City, MO; Intermountain Veterinary Supply, Denver, CO; Miltex Instrument Co., Lake Success, NY; J. Sklar Manufacturing Co., Inc., Long Island City, NY.

The idea for this book was conceived in 1978 when one of us (AST) was approached by Mr. George Mundorff, Executive Editor, Lea & Febiger. We would like to thank him for his encouragement and guidance. We are also grateful to Mr. Kit Spahr, Jr., Veterinary Editor; Diane Ramanauskas, Copy Editor; Tom Colaiezzi, Production Manager; and Samuel A. Rondinelli, Assistant Production Manager, Lea & Febiger, for their assistance, as well as to others at the Publisher who assisted in the production of this book.

A. SIMON TURNER
C. WAYNE MCILWRAITH

Fort Collins, Colorado

PREFACE

The second edition of *Techniques in Large Animal Surgery* is in response to the acceptance of the first edition and the continued need for such a book for both veterinary students and large animal practitioners. In many instances, the techniques are time honored and require no change from 5 years ago. In other instances, however, refinements in technique as well as improved perception of indications, limitations, and complications have made changes appropriate.

A significant change is the addition of Dr. R. Bruce Hull, Professor of Veterinary Clinical Sciences, The Ohio State University, as a contributor. He has carefully analyzed the entire bovine section, and his suggested changes and additions have been incorporated into the text. In addition, two procedures, "teaser bull preparation by penile fixation" and "treatment of vaginal prolapse by fixation to the prepubic tendon," have been added. We are most grateful in having Dr. Hull's help and expertise.

Among the introductory chapters, the section on anesthesia required the most updating, and we are grateful to our colleague Dr. David Hodgson at Colorado State University for his review and advice. Two new procedures, "superior check ligament desmotomy" and "deep digital flexor tenotomy," were considered appropriate additions to this edition. We are grateful to Dr. Larry Bramlage, Ohio State University, for his comments and help with the first of these procedures. Many of the other changes in this edition are in response to the book reviews and comments on the first edition returned to Lea & Febiger. To these people, we appreciate your feedback.

A chapter on llama tooth removal was added because of the increased popularity of this species, especially in our own part of the country. Although we only discuss this one technique, it should not be inferred that other operations are unheard of in llamas. We have corrected angular limb deformities, repaired fractures, and performed gastrointestinal surgery, among other procedures, but tooth removal is the most common. Descriptions of these other procedures in llamas are beyond the scope of this book at this stage.

The need for more sophisticated equine techniques prompted us to produce the textbook *Equine Surgery: Advanced Techniques* in 1987. It is envisioned that the book will be used as a companion to this second edition, to provide a full spectrum of equine procedures, with the well-accepted format of concise text and clear illustrations.

Again, we are thankful to Mr. Tom McCracken, Assistant Professor, Department of Anatomy and Neurobiology, Colorado State University, for his talent in capturing the techniques described in his line drawings. We are also indebted to Helen Acevedo for typing our additions and Holly Lukens for copyediting. Finally, our thanks again to the excellent staff at Lea & Febiger for the production of this edition.

A. Simon Turner

Fort Collins, Colorado

C. Wayne McIlwraith

CONTENTS

TECHNIQUES
IN LARGE
ANIMAL
SURGERY

1

PRESURGICAL CONSIDERATIONS

Preoperative Evaluation of the Patient

Before a surgical procedure, a physical examination is generally indicated. This applies to both emergency and elective surgery. Packed cell volume (PCV) and total protein are measured routinely. A complete blood count (CBC) is standard in the horse. Fluid replacement should be performed if necessary. In the elective case, the surgical procedure should be postponed if the animal's physical condition or laboratory parameters are abnormal. In some animals, internal and external parasitism may have to be rectified to achieve this goal.

Exactly where to draw the line on laboratory tests is largely a matter of judgment on the part of the surgeon. Obviously, if the surgery consists of castration of several litters of piglets, then for purely economic reasons laboratory tests prior to surgery will not be performed. With equine elective surgeries, laboratory tests should consist of a PCV and total protein or a CBC. In right-sided abomasal diseases of the dairy cow, measurement of electrolytes is indicated to ascertain what needs to be replaced pre- and postoperatively. Urinalysis is used primarily in the dairy cow to evaluate the presence of ketosis, but its use in evaluation of other large animal surgery patients is seldom indicated. Measurement of blood urea nitrogen (BUN) and creatinine preoperatively in large animal species is not generally indicated unless the surgeon suspects problems with the urinary system. In the horse with colic, analysis of peritoneal fluid will sometimes be of value in making a decision if laparotomy is indeed indicated. It is rarely indicated in other instances. Chemistry panels are also considered routine when age and any other systemic problems are a consideration.

If any laboratory parameters are abnormal, the underlying causes should be investigated and efforts made to correct them. In "elective" surgery this is possible, but it may not be possible in an emergency. The owner should be made aware of any problems prior to subjecting the animal to surgery. Risks are always present in normal elective surgery, and these should be explained to the owner when they exist.

Medical records should be kept, especially for hospitalized animals; with the ever-present threat of litigation, the surgeon should adopt this policy. Obviously this will not apply to such cases as castration of several litters of piglets, but record-keeping should become an essential part of the procedure for horses and cattle in a hospital. Finally, if the animal is insured, the insurance company must be notified of any surgical procedure; otherwise the policy may be void.

Surgical Judgment

Surgical judgment cannot be learned overnight by reading a surgery textbook, nor is it necessarily attained by years of experience. The surgeon who continually makes the same mistake will probably never possess good surgical judgment. Not only should the surgeon learn from his own mistakes, but he should learn from the mistakes of others, including those documented in the surgical literature.

As part of surgical judgment, the surgeon must ask, is the surgery necessary? What would happen if the surgery was not performed? Clearly, this question cannot be asked of such procedures as castration or dehorning, but they may be applicable to a surgical procedure involving the removal of chip fracture from the carpus of a racing horse or amputation of a fractured splint bone in a horse.

If the procedure is beyond the capabilities of the surgeon, his facilities, and his technical help, then the surgeon should consider referring the case to someone who has these capabilities. Some veterinarians have a constant fear that this will mean loss of the client's business in the future, but we have found this rarely to be the case. If the surgeon explains why the case should be referred elsewhere, most clients will be grateful for such frankness and honesty. It is inexcusable to operate on a patient that could easily have been referred to a well-equipped, well-staffed hospital with specially qualified personnel and then have complications arise due to inadequate training and facilities. Clearly, the rule has exceptions, mainly the emergency patient, which may fare better by undergoing immediate surgery than being subjected to a long trailer ride to another facility.

One important question that must be considered by the large animal surgeon is that of economics. This applies especially to operations on food animal species. Would the owner be better off financially to have the animal transported to a slaughterhouse, rather than having it undergo costly surgery with the chances of a long and expensive convalescence? On the other hand, surgery may be vital even to salvage the animal for slaughter. The surgeon must not be too hasty to treat an animal with drugs if the withdrawal times of the drugs preclude the possibility of immediate slaughter and use for human consumption.

Most of the procedures described in this book can be done "on the farm." Some, such as arthrotomy for removal of chip fractures of the carpal and sesamoid bones in horses, should be done in a dust-free operating theater. If clients wish these latter procedures to be done "in the field," then they should understand the disastrous consequences of postsurgical infection. The surgeon must be the final judge of whether his facilities are suitable.

Principles of Asepsis and Antisepsis

There are three determinants of an infection in a surgical site: host defense; physiologic derangement; and bacterial contamination risk at surgery.[2]

Control methods include aseptic surgical practices as well as identification of the high-risk patient, correction of systemic imbalances prior to surgery, and the proper use of prophylactic antibiotics.[3]

We are sometimes reminded by fellow veterinarians in the field that we must teach undergraduates "how to do surgery in the real world." By this statement they mean that we must ignore aseptic draping and gloving and lower the standard to a "practical" level. This reasoning is fallacious in our opinion. Although we recognize that this ideal may be unattainable in private practice, one should always strive for the highest possible standard; otherwise, the final standard of practice may be so low that the well-being of the patient is at risk, not to mention the reputation of the veterinarian as a surgeon. For this reason, we believe that it behooves us as instructors of the undergraduate to teach the *best possible methods with regard to asepsis as well as technique.*

The extent to which the practice of asepsis or even antisepsis is carried out depends on the classification of the operation, as follows. This classification may also help the veterinarian to decide whether antibiotics are indicated, or whether postoperative infection can be anticipated.

1. *Clean surgery* is that in which the gastrointestinal, urinary, or respiratory tract is not entered. An example is arthrotomy for removal of a chip fracture of a carpal bone of a horse.

2. *Clean-contaminated surgery* is that in which the gastrointestinal, respiratory, or urinary tract is entered; however, there is no significant spillage of contaminated contents, such as with abomasopexy for displaced abomasum in the dairy cow.

3. *Contaminated-dirty surgery* is that in which gross spillage of contaminated body contents or acute inflammation occurs. Fresh traumatic wounds fall into this category.

Once the surgeon has categorized the surgical procedure, then appropriate precautions to avoid postoperative infection can be determined. In all cases, however, the surgical site is prepared properly.

Whatever category of surgery is performed, clean clothing should be worn. The wearing of surgical gloves is good policy even if to protect the operator from infectious organisms that may be present at the surgical site. Surgical gowns, gloves, and caps are recommended for clean surgical procedures, although such attire has obvious practical limitations for the large animal surgeon operating "in the field." The purpose of this book is to present guidelines, rather than to lay down hard-and-fast rules. For example, the decision between wearing caps, gowns, and gloves and wearing just gloves can only be made by the surgeon. Surgical judgment is required.

Role of Antibiotics

Antibiotics should never be used to cover flaws in surgical technique. The young surgeon is often tempted, sometimes under pressure from the client, to use antibiotics prophylactically. Again, some judgment is required, but suffice to say, antibiotics should never be a substitute for "surgical conscience." Surgical conscience consists of the following: dissection along tissue planes, gentleness in handling tissues, adequate hemostasis, selection of the best surgical approach, correct choice of suture material, closure of dead space, and short operating time.

If the surgeon decides that antibiotics are indicated, then they must be used at the correct dosage for the correct amount of time. Ample scientific literature substantiates that prophylactic antibiotics, administered in the hope of preventing infectious complications, should be given preoperatively, and at the latest, during surgery itself, to be of maximum benefit. Beyond 4 hours postsurgically, the administration of prophylactic antibiotics has little to no effect on the incidence of postoperative infection.[1] If topical antibiotics are used during surgery, they should be nonirritating to the tissues; otherwise, tissue necrosis from cellular damage will outweigh any advantageous effects of the antibiotics.

All equine surgical patients should have tetanus prophylaxis. If the immunization program is doubtful, then the horse should receive 1500 to 3000 U tetanus antitoxin. Horses on a permanent immunization program that have not had tetanus toxoid within the past 6 months should receive a booster injection.

Tetanus prophylaxis is generally not provided for food animals, but an immunization program may be considered, especially if a specific predisposition is thought to exist.

Preoperative Planning

The surgeon should be thoroughly familiar with the regional anatomy. In this book we have illustrated what we consider to be the important structures in each technique. If more detail is required, a suitable anatomy text should be consulted. Not only should the procedure be planned prior to the surgery, but also the surgeon should visit the dissection room and review local anatomy on cadavers prior to attempting surgery on a client's animal. We are fortunate in veterinary surgery to have greater access to cadavers than our counterparts in human surgery.

Preparation of the Surgical Site

For the large animal surgeon, preparation of the surgical site can present major problems, especially in the winter and spring when farms can be muddy. Preparation for surgery may have to begin with removal of dirt and manure. Some animals that have been recumbent in mud and filth for various reasons may have to be hosed off. Hair should then be removed, not just from the surgical site, but from an adequate area surrounding the surgical site.

The clipping should be done in a neat square or rectangular shape with straight edges. Surprisingly, this, along with the neatness of the final suture pattern in the skin, is how the client judges the skill of the surgeon. Clipping may be done initially with a no. 10 clipper blade, and then the finer no. 40 blade may be used. The incision site can be shaved with a straight razor in horses and cattle, but debate exists regarding the benefit of this procedure. In sheep and goats, in which the skin is supple and pliable, it is difficult to shave the edges.

Preparation of the surgical site, such as the ventral midline of a horse about to undergo an exploratory laparotomy, may have to be performed when the animal is anesthetized. If surgery is to be done with the animal standing, then an initial surgical scrub, followed by the appropriate local anesthetic technique and a final scrub, is standard procedure.

For cattle or pigs, the skin of the surgical site can be prepared for surgery with the aid of a stiff brush. For the horse, gauze sponges are recommended. Sheep may require defatting of the skin with ether prior to the actual skin scrub. The antiseptic scrub solution used is generally a matter of personal preference. We use povidone-iodine scrub (Betadine Scrub), alternated with a 70% alcohol rinse. The wound is dried between each application of alcohol. Finally, the skin is sprayed with povidone-iodine solution (Betadine Solution) and is allowed to dry.

Scrubbing of the proposed surgical site is done immediately prior to the operation. Scrubbing should commence at the proposed site of the incision and progress toward the periphery; one must be sure not to come back onto a previously scrubbed area. Some equine surgeons clip and shave the surgical site the night before the surgery and wrap the limb in a sterile, alcohol-soaked bandage until the next day. A shaving nick made the day before surgery may be a pustule on the day of surgery, however.

When aseptic surgery is to be performed, an efficient draping system is mandatory in our opinion. Generally, time taken to drape the animal properly is well spent. The draping of cattle in the standing position can be difficult, especially if the animal decides to move or becomes restless. It can be difficult to secure drapes with towel clamps in the conscious animal because only the operative site is anesthetized. If draping is not done, the surgeon must minimize contact with parts of the animal that have not been scrubbed. The tail must be tied to prevent it from flicking into the surgical field.

Several operations described in this book require the strictest of aseptic technique, and sterile plastic adhesive drapes (incise drapes) are indicated. Their purpose is to help prevent contamination of the surgical wound by immobilizing bacteria. These drapes are now available with an active antimicrobial ingredient present. Some contain iodophor*, whereas others contain polyhexamethylene biguanide.** Characteristics of sterile plastic adhesive drapes include their ability to adhere, their antimicrobial activity, and their clarity when applied to the skin. Probably, the most desirable feature is the one first mentioned. With excessive traction or manipulation, some brands of drape quickly separate from the skin surfaces, and this separation instantly defeats their purpose. Certain drapes with antimicrobial activity are superior to others.

Rubberized drapes are helpful when large amounts of fluids (such as peritoneal and amniotic fluid) are encountered during the procedure. We routinely use a sterile rubber crib sheet with a large slit cut in the middle for equine laparotomies. Rubberized drapes are also useful to isolate bowel or any other organ that is potentially contaminated, to prevent contamination of drapes.

* Ioban 3-M Company, Medical Products Division, Minnesota Mining Co., St. Paul, MN.
** Surgicide with Microcide, Surgikos, Johnson & Johnson Co., Arlington, TX.

Postoperative Infection

Prevention of postoperative infection should be the goal of the surgeon, but infection may occur despite all measures taken to prevent it. If infection occurs, the surgeon must decide whether antibiotic treatment is indicated, or whether the animal is strong enough to fight it using its own defense mechanisms. Some surgical wounds require drainage at their most ventral part, whereas others require more aggressive treatment. If, in the judgment of the surgeon, the infection appears to be serious, then a Gram stain, culture, and sensitivity testing of the offending microorganism(s) will be indicated. A Gram stain may give the surgeon a better idea of what type of organism is involved and may in turn narrow the selection of antibiotics. Sometimes in vitro sensitivities have to be ignored because the antibiotic of choice would be prohibitively expensive. This is especially true for adult cattle and horses. A broad-spectrum antibiotic should be given, if possible, as soon as practical.

References

1. Burke, J. F.: Preventing bacterial infection by coordinating antibiotic and host activity. *In* Symposium on prophylactic use of antibiotics. South Med. J., *70*:24, 1977.

2. Cristou, N. V., Nohr, C. W., and Meakins, J. L.: Assessing operative site infection in surgical patients. Arch. Surg., *122*:165, 1987.

3. Nelson, C. L.: Prevention of sepsis. Clin. Orthop., *222*:66, 1987.

2

ANESTHESIA AND FLUID THERAPY

Anesthesia

The purpose of this section is not to present an in-depth discussion of anesthesia. Details on the principles of anesthesia, recognition of stages of anesthesia, monitoring, and the pharmacology and physiology associated with anesthesia are well documented in other texts.[20,34,48] In this section, anesthetic techniques used routinely by us are presented. Many alternatives are available and personal preferences differ, but we consider these to be the best and most suitable for the individual surgical techniques presented in this textbook.

Local and Regional Anesthesia (Analgesia)

Local or infiltration anesthesia is the injection of a surgical site directly with analgesic agent. Regional anesthesia is desensitization by blocking the major nerve(s) to a given region. Both techniques permit the desensitization of the surgical site. Because they are purely analgesic techniques, the term analgesia is preferred to the term anesthesia. The two analgesic agents most commonly used are 2% lidocaine hydrochloride (Lidocaine Hydrochloride Injection 2%) and 2% mepivacaine hydrochloride (Carbocaine). Lidocaine has essentially replaced procaine hydrochloride as the standard local analgesic agent. The use of mepivacaine is increasing because of its more rapid onset, slightly longer duration, and slightly less tissue reaction.

In the ox in particular, surgical procedures are commonly performed under local or regional analgesia. In many instances, surgery is performed on the standing animal, and no sedation is used. In other instances, a combination of sedation and casting is used in conjunction with a local analgesic regimen. With the advent of safer and more efficient general anesthetic techniques in the horse, the use of local or regional analgesia in this species has decreased. Local and regional analgesic techniques that are still used routinely in individual species follow.

The principles of infiltration analgesia are simple and are similar for all species. The limits of the region to be infiltrated may be well defined by making a subcutaneous wheal. A small amount of analgesic agent is injected at an initial site with a small needle and then, if a long region of analgesia is required, a longer needle is inserted through the initial region of desensitization. Needles should always be reinserted through a region that has already been infiltrated. The skin and subcutis should be infiltrated first and then the deeper layers, such as muscle and peritoneum. Avoid the injection of significant amounts of analgesic solution into the peritoneal cavity; rapid absorption can take place, with the possibility of resultant toxicity. Infiltrating injections should be made in straight lines, and "fanning" should be avoided as much as possible because of the tissue trauma it causes.

Infiltration analgesia is commonly used for suturing wounds and for removing cutaneous lesions in all large animal species. It may also be used in the form of a "line block" for laparotomy, in which case the analgesic agent is infiltrated along the line of incision. Although convenient, the infiltration of analgesic agent into the incision line causes edema in the tissues and may affect wound healing. In this respect, regional analgesic techniques are generally considered preferable.

REGIONAL ANALGESIA IN CATTLE

The use of regional analgesia is most highly developed in the bovine species, and the following techniques are commonly practiced.

Inverted L Block. This is the simplest technique of regional analgesia for laparotomy in the ox. It may be used for either flank or paramedian laparotomies. The principles of the technique are illustrated in Figure 2-1. It is a nonspecific technique in which local analgesic agent is deposited in the form of an inverted L to create a wall of analgesia enclosing the surgical field. All nerves entering the operative field are blocked. The procedure is facilitated by the use of an 8- to 10-cm, 16- to 18-gauge needle. Up to 100 ml of local analgesic agent may be used. The vertical line of the L passes caudal to the last rib, and the horizontal line is just ventral to the transverse processes of the lumbar vertebrae. Ten to 15 minutes should be allowed for the analgesic agent to take effect.

Paravertebral Block. The thirteenth thoracic nerve (T13), the first and second lumbar nerves (L1 and L2), and the dorsolateral branch of the third lumbar nerve (L3) supply sensory and motor innervation to the skin, fascia, muscles, and peritoneum of the flank. Regional analgesia of these nerves is the basis of the paravertebral block. For practical purposes with flank laparotomy, blocking of the dorsolateral branch of L3 is not generally considered necessary and may be contraindicated because if one has miscounted the vertebrae, one may actually block L4, which has nerve fibers running to the back legs.

Various techniques for paravertebral block have been described. Walking the needle off the caudal edge of the transverse process, as illustrated in Figure 2-2, is most satisfactory. Anatomically, the nerve is most localized at its intervertebral foramen. By walking the needle off the caudal edge of the transverse process, one can deposit the analgesic solution close to the

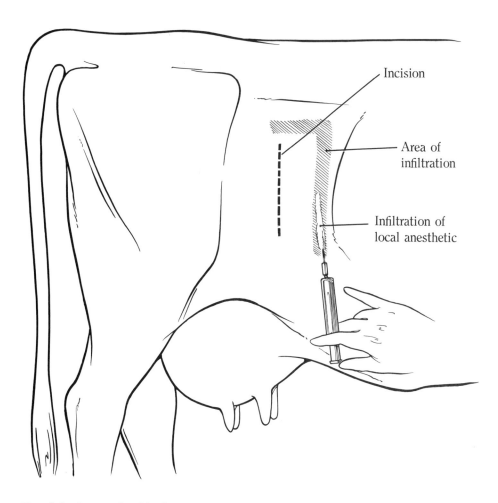

Fig. 2-1. *Inverted L block.*

foramen; therefore, one only has to block a single site rather than the dorsal and ventral branches individually. The transverse processes are used as landmarks. Remembering that the transverse processes slope forward, the transverse process of L1 is used as a landmark to block T13, and the transverse processes of L2 and L3 are similarly used to locate nerves L1 and L2, respectively. When the transverse process has been located, a line is drawn from its cranial edge to the dorsal midline. The site for injection is 3 to 4 cm from the midline (Fig. 2-2). The transverse process of L1 is difficult to locate in fat animals, in which case the site is estimated relative to the distance between the processes of L2 and L3. Local blebs are placed, and a 1-in., 16-gauge needle is inserted to act as a trocar in placing a 10-cm, 20-gauge needle. This second needle is inserted perpendicularly until the transverse process is encountered. The needle is then walked off the caudal border of the transverse process and advanced 0.75 cm; 10 ml of local analgesic solution are placed at each site. The incision site should be tested with a needle, and if the block has been properly placed, it will be effective almost immediately. In testing the block, one must remember that the distribution of the nerves is such that T13 innervates the ventral flank area, whereas L2 innervates the area close to the transverse processes.

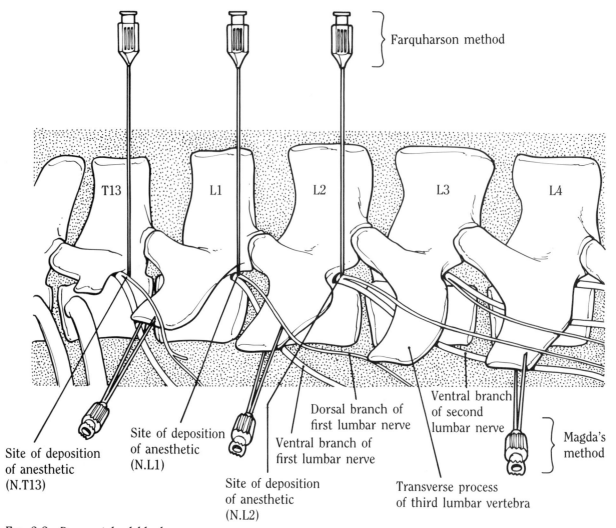

Farquharson method

T13   L1   L2   L3   L4

Dorsal branch of
first lumbar nerve

Ventral branch of
first lumbar nerve

Ventral branch
of second
lumbar nerve

Magda's
method

Site of deposition
of anesthetic
(N.T13)

Site of deposition
of anesthetic
(N.L1)

Site of deposition
of anesthetic
(N.L2)

Transverse process
of third lumbar vertebra

FIG. 2-2. *Paravertebral block.*

A temporary lateral deviation of the spine due to muscle paralysis is observed in association with paravertebral analgesia.

Another technique favored by some surgeons is that developed by Magda and modified by Cakala.[9] It uses a lateral approach to the nerves and would be more accurately described as a paralumbar rather than a paravertebral technique. The branches of T13, L1, and L2 are blocked close to the ends of the first, second, and fourth transverse processes, respectively, as illustrated in Figure 2-2. The skin is clipped and prepared at the ends of the first, second, and fourth lumbar transverse processes. An 18-gauge needle is inserted under each transverse process towards the midline, and 10 ml of solution are injected. The needle is then withdrawn a short distance and is redirected craniad and caudad while more solution is injected. In this fashion, a diffuse region ventral to the transverse process is infiltrated, to block the ventral branch of the nerve. The needle is then redirected slightly dorsal and caudal to the transverse process to block the dorsolateral branches of the nerves. About 25 ml of solution are used for each site. Because the Cakala paralumbar technique does not paralyze the lumbar muscles, lateral deviation of the spine does not occur.

Epidural Analgesia. This technique consists of the deposition of local analgesic solution between the dura mater and periosteum of the spinal canal (epidural space), which in turn desensitizes the caudal nerve roots after they emerge from the dura. Epidural analgesia can be classified into cranial (high) or caudal (low), according to the area of spread of the analgesic solution and the extent of the area in which sensory and motor paralysis develops. This paralysis, in turn, depends chiefly on the volume of solution injected and on the concentration and diffusibility of the analgesic agent. The rate of absorption of local analgesic agent from the epidural space may contribute to the analgesic effect.

Caudal epidural anesthesia implies that motor control of the hind legs is not affected. Sensory innervation is lost from the anus, vulva, perineum, and caudal aspects of the thighs. The anal sphincter relaxes, and the posterior part of the rectum balloons. Tenesmus is relieved and obstetric straining is prevented. In the ox, the injection of the analgesic agent may be made between the first and second coccygeal vertebrae or in the sacrococcygeal space, although the former site is preferable because it is a larger space and is more easily detected, especially in fat animals. To locate the space, the tail is grasped and is moved up and down; the first obvious articulation caudal to the sacrum is the first intercoccygeal space. After clipping and skin preparation, an 18-gauge, 3- to 5-cm needle (or a spinal needle) is introduced through the center of the space on the midline at a 45° angle until its point hits the floor of the spinal canal (Fig. 2-3). The needle is then retracted slightly to ensure that the end is not embedded in the intervertebral disc. If the needle is correctly placed in the epidural space, there should be no resistance to injection. The dose of analgesic solution is 0.5 to 1 ml/100 lb of 2% lidocaine or mepivacaine. Initially, the low dose of analgesic agent should be injected. After waiting 10 to 15 minutes,

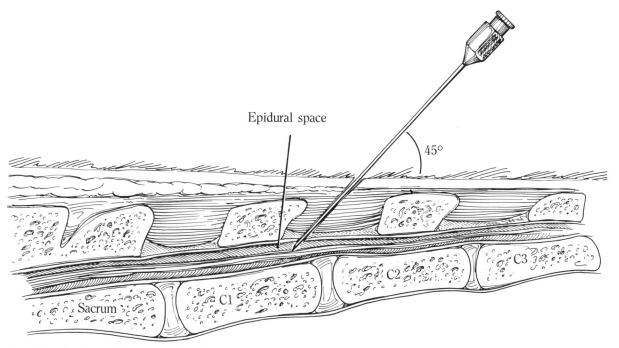

FIG. 2-3. *Bovine epidural anesthesia.*

more solution may be injected if necessary. Aspiration should be performed prior to injection to ensure that the needle is not in one of the vertebral venous sinuses. In addition, one should make sure that the bevel of the needle is pointed forward, rather than to one side, to obtain even anesthesia.

Cranial or high epidural analgesia may be used for laparotomy, pelvic limb surgery, or udder amputation, and it provides 2 to 4 hours of analgesia. The injection technique is the same as for caudal epidural analgesia, except a greater volume of analgesic agent (1 ml/10 lb of body weight) is administered. The animal will go down and should be maintained in sternal recumbency for 10 to 15 minutes to ensure the even distribution of the analgesic solution. When inducing cranial epidural analgesia in cattle, the possible development of hypotension must be considered. No signs of hypotension have been observed using volumes of 100 to 150 ml of 2% lidocaine, but they have been recorded with volumes of 150 to 200 ml.[20]

Regional Analgesia of the Eye. The main indication for analgesia of the eye in cattle is for orbital exenteration. For this purpose, the technique of local infiltration using the retrobulbar (four-point) block is convenient and satisfactory. The technique is described and illustrated under eye enucleation in Chapter 15.

An alternate technique for regional analgesia to the eye is the Peterson block. For this technique, an 11-cm, 18-gauge needle bent to a curvature of a 10-inch circle is required. A skin bleb is made at the point where the supraorbital process meets the zygomatic arch, and a puncture wound is made in this bleb with a short 14-gauge needle. The 11-cm needle is then directed mediad, with the concavity of the needle directed caudad. In this fashion, the point of the needle will pass around the cranial border of the coronoid process of the mandible, and the needle is then directed further mediad until it hits the pterygoid crest. The needle is then moved slightly rostrad and down to the pterygopalatine fossa at the foramen orbitorotundum, and 15 to 20 ml of local analgesic solution are injected. The needle is withdrawn and is directed caudad just beneath the skin, to infiltrate the subcutaneous tissues along the zygomatic arch. A small region just dorsal to the medial canthus should also be infiltrated. Although the Peterson block is preferred by some practitioners for eye analgesia, it is unpredictable, and the injection of 15 ml of local anesthetic inadvertently into the internal maxillary artery can have fatal results. The latter problem can be avoided by injecting 5 ml in one place, repositioning the needle slightly, aspirating and injecting another 5 ml, and then repeating this procedure. Placing a subcutaneous line block across (perpendicular) to the medial canthus of the eye (probably blocking a branch of the infratrochlear nerve) is also a useful adjunct in achieving complete desensitization of the eye. The retrobulbar (four-point) block has been convenient and satisfactory.

Regional Analgesia of the Horn. The cornual block is a simple technique that provides analgesia for dehorning. An imaginary line is drawn from the lateral canthus of the eye to the base of the horn along the crest dorsal to the temporal fossa; on this line, an 18-gauge, 2.5-cm needle is inserted halfway from the lateral canthus to the horn, and an injection is made under the skin and through the frontalis muscle at the lateral border of the crest. Generally, 5 ml of 2% lidocaine are sufficient, but up to 10 ml may be used in a larger animal.

In exotic breeds, especially the Simmental, it may also be necessary to block the infratrochlear nerve, which innervates the medial aspect of the horn.[6] This can be achieved by using a line block subcutaneously from the midline of the head to the facial crest across the forehead dorsal to the eye.

Intravenous Limb Anesthesia. For local analgesia of the distal limb, the technique of intravenous local analgesia is considered superior to previously used techniques of specific nerve blocks or ring blocks. The technique involves intravenous injection of local analgesic solution distal to a previously applied tourniquet.[61] The animal is cast and restrained, and the tourniquet of rubber tubing is applied distal to the carpus or hock (Fig. 2-4). A protective pad may be placed under the tourniquet. A superficial vein is detected, either the dorsal common digital vein III in the metacarpus or the cranial branch of the lateral saphenous vein in the metatarsus. After clipping and preparation of the area, an intravenous injection of 10 to 20 ml of 2% lidocaine or mepivacaine is given. It is important to avoid the use of lidocaine with epinephrine because the combination may cause vasoconstriction sufficient to prevent desensitization. Increased amounts of lidocaine may be necessary to achieve adequate analgesia of the interdigital area. The needle is withdrawn, and the injection site is massaged briefly to prevent hematoma formation. Anesthesia of the distal limb is complete in 5 minutes and persists 1 to 2 hours if the tourniquet remains in place. At the end of the operation, the tourniquet is released slowly over a period of 10 seconds, and the limb will regain normal sensation and motor function in about 5 minutes. Toxicity related to the entrance of the local anesthetic into the circulation has not been observed.[61]

REGIONAL ANALGESIA IN SHEEP AND GOATS

Surgical and manipulative procedures in sheep and goats have become important for some practices. Combinations of sedation and local analgesia frequently preclude the need for general anesthesia. Sheep are easily handled, and some procedures can be performed using local analgesia and physical restraint. On the other hand, goats have a low pain threshold and require analgesia and sedation.

Systemic toxicity is a potential complication with sheep and goats, and dosage limits should be considered. Experiments in sheep have shown that convulsions occur in adult sheep at a dose of lidocaine hydrochloride of 5.8 ± 1.8 mg/kg intravenously.[37] Subconvulsive doses of lidocaine hydrochloride often produce drowsiness, however. Above convulsive doses, hypotension occurs at 31.2 ± 2.6 mg/kg, respiratory arrest at 32.4 ± 2.8 mg/kg, and circulatory collapse at 36.7 ± 3.3 mg/kg. Such findings suggest a reasonable margin between the convulsive dose and doses causing more serious complications. If convulsions do occur, they can be controlled with an intravenous dose of 0.5 mg/kg of diazepam (Valium). The use of diluted solutions of lidocaine in local blocks of sheep and goats has been recommended.[18]

Paravertebral and epidural blocks have been used in sheep and goats.[7,18] Intravenous limb anesthesia may also be done, and analgesia of the corneal branches of the lacrimal and infratrochlear nerves is important for goat dehorning. (The technique is described and illustrated in Chapter 17.)

Indications for regional analgesia are fewer in equine species than in bovine species. Flank laparotomies are performed on standing animals, but with less frequency than in the ox. When a standing flank laparotomy is performed, an inverted L block or line block is used. Paravertebral anesthesia

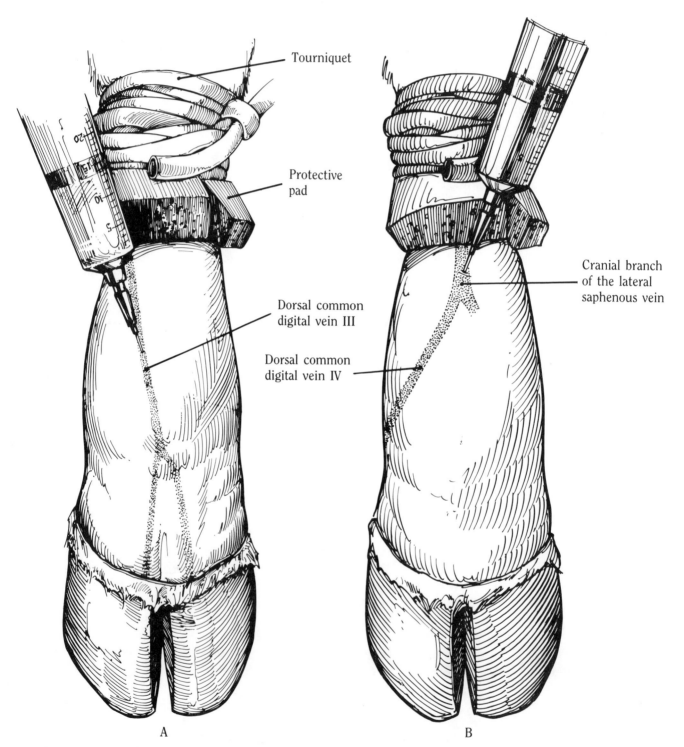

Tourniquet

Protective pad

Dorsal common digital vein III

Dorsal common digital vein IV

Cranial branch of the lateral saphenous vein

A

B

FIG. 2-4. *Intravenous limb anesthesia.* A, *Forelimb, dorsal aspect;* B, *Hindlimb, dorsal aspect.*

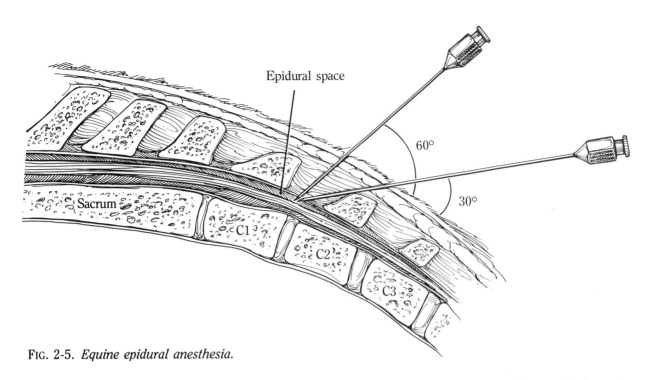

FIG. 2-5. *Equine epidural anesthesia.*

is not performed in horses. One regional analgesic technique commonly performed in the horse is the caudal epidural block. Moreover, nerve blocks and ring blocks are commonly performed in the limbs of the horse. These techniques are used mainly for the diagnosis of lameness, but they are also used when surgery is performed on the distal limb of the standing animal. As mentioned before, the majority of equine surgical procedures are performed with the patient under general anesthesia.

Epidural Analgesia. Cranial (high) epidural injection is contraindicated in the horse. Indeed, one must be careful when performing caudal (low) epidural injection; the dose of local analgesic solution should be kept to a minimum because if there is any effect on the motor control to the hind limbs, the animal will become agitated and may even fall down, with possible resulting injury. The technique for a caudal epidural injection in the horse is similar to that for the ox. Injection is through the space between the first and second coccygeal vertebrae. This site is cranial to the long tail hairs and is ascertained by moving the tail up and down. After clipping and preparing the area, a skin bleb is made to facilitate placement of the needle (an 18-gauge spinal needle is preferable). This needle may be inserted at an angle of 30° from a perpendicular line through the vertebrae, or at an angle of 60° as illustrated in Figure 2-5. We prefer the 60° angle, which enables the spinal needle to be threaded up the canal and left in place. Initially, 5 to 10 ml of 2% local analgesic are injected, the stylet is replaced, and the needle is left in place. This enables additional local analgesic to be administered if necessary and precludes overdosage in the first instance. The indications for caudal epidural analgesia for the horse are similar to those for the ox.

A method of continuous caudal epidural anesthesia using a commercial epidural catheter kit (continuous epidural tray*) has been recently described.[19]

* Continuous Epidural Tray, American Hospital Supply, McGraw Park, IL.

The kit contains a Huber-point directional needle with stylet (Tuohy spinal needle) inserted through a pilot hole at 45° to the horizontal until one encounters an abrupt reduction in resistance. The catheter is then inserted through the needle, it is advanced 2.5 to 4 cm beyond the end of the needle, and the needle is withdrawn.

Local Analgesia of the Limbs. Local nerve blocks of the limbs and intra-articular analgesic techniques have an important place in the diagnosis of lameness and are well described elsewhere.[1] These techniques are not repeated in this text.

REGIONAL ANALGESIA IN SWINE

Epidural Analgesia. This technique has been used in both young and adult pigs and in particular for cesarean section in the sow. In this instance, cranial (high) epidural analgesia has been used to effect both immobilization and analgesia, without fetal depression. Cranial, rather than caudal, epidural analgesia is commonly performed. The injection site for epidural analgesia in the pig is the lumbosacral space; this space is located at the intersection of the spine with a line drawn through the cranial borders of the ilium. An 18-gauge needle is inserted 1 to 2 cm caudal to this line in small pigs and 2.5 to 5 cm caudal to the line in larger animals. The needle is then directed ventrad and slightly caudad until it is felt to pass through the dorsal ligament of the vertebrae and into the epidural space. The needle size varies with the size of the pig: 8 cm is used for the pig weighing up to 75 kg; and 15 cm is used for pigs heavier than 75 kg. The dose is about 1 ml/5 kg to 1 ml/10 kg of 2% lidocaine for pelvic limb block; the higher dose rate is used in small pigs, and the smaller dose rate is used in large pigs. Although epidural analgesia may have advantages based on a requirement for minimal depression of the central nervous system and decreased expense, its use in swine practice has been limited by the time required to perform the technique and the temperament of the animal.

Tranquilization and Sedation

There are three general purposes for the tranquilization or sedation of large animals: (1) sedation of intractable animals for routine diagnostic and therapeutic procedures; (2) sedation for minor surgical procedures in conjunction with local anesthesia; and (3) preanesthetic medication.

TRANQUILIZATION AND SEDATION IN HORSES

The terms tranquilization and sedation in the horse imply that the animal remains standing. Agents commonly used in the horse are the phenothiazine derivatives and xylazine hydrochloride.

The two phenothiazine tranquilizers that are commonly used in the horse are promazine hydrochloride (Promazine Hydrochloride Injection) at a dose rate of 0.44 to 1.1 mg/kg intravenously or intramuscularly, and acetylpromazine maleate (Acepromazine Maleate Injectable) at a dose rate of 0.03 to 0.08 mg/kg intravenously or intramuscularly. Acetylpromazine begins to act within 15 to 20 minutes following intravenous administration, and the effects last approximately 2 to 4 hours. Promazine's effects last a similar length of time. Phenothiazine tranquilizers are commonly used alone for chemical restraint or as a premedication for general anesthesia. They should not be used after recent treatment with organophosphate anthelmintics. One other important property is their alpha-adrenergic blocking effect. These agents should not be used in cases of hypovolemic shock, except when volume replacement has been adequate and peripheral vasodilation to increase perfusion is desired.

Xylazine hydrochloride (Rompun) is a sedative that also has analgesic properties. It has become popular for restraint and sedation, as an analgesic prior to a variety of clinical procedures, and as a preanesthetic agent. In one study of 223 horses, sedation and analgesia were good to excellent in over 80% of the horses, without adverse effects from single or repeated doses.[26] With intravenous injection, maximum sedation occurred in about 3 minutes and lasted 30 to 40 minutes. The optimal dosage in this study was considered to be 1.1 mg/kg (0.5 mg/lb). The intramuscular dose rate is 2.2 mg/kg (1 mg/lb). Bradycardia and transient cardiac arrhythmias (usually partial atrioventricular block) occur when xylazine is given intravenously. These changes are not generally considered to be clinically significant, however, and can be prevented by prior administration of atropine.[30]

Although the optimum intravenous dose is 1.1 mg/kg,[26] this can be decreased to approximately 0.33 to 0.66 mg/kg for preanesthetic medication, as well as for most procedures. At 1.1 mg/kg intravenously, animal movement due to ataxia can complicate a standing procedure. Although xylazine is commonly used and its properties are generally useful and desirable, it is relatively short acting, and the horse's behavior may be unpredictable. Sudden and violent hind-limb kicking has been observed in apparently heavily sedated animals. The drug is excellent for short procedures, but it is not our choice as a sedative for longer periods of standing surgery.

A combination of acetylpromazine (0.05 mg/kg) and xylazine (0.5 mg/kg) administered intravenously also provides excellent short-term sedation in the horse.

Several sedative-analgesic mixtures may successfully provide sedation with some accompanying analgesia during standing procedures. These include (dosage for a 450-kg horse):

1. Acetylpromazine (30 mg) and pentazocine (Talwin-V) (150 mg) intravenously.

2. Acepromazine (30 mg) and meperidine hydrochloride (Demerol) (250 mg) intravenously.

More recently, combinations of xylazine and analgesics have been used, including:

1. Xylazine (0.66 mg/kg) and morphine sulfate (0.66 mg/kg) intravenously.[31,40]

2. Xylazine (1.1 mg/kg) and butorphanol tartrate (Torbugesic) (0.1 mg/kg).[44] The dose is lower than initially described.[44]

Chloral hydrate may also be given to effect for sedation in the standing animal. The foregoing chemical restraining regimens are for normal, healthy animals.

TRANQUILIZATION AND SEDATION IN CATTLE

Surgical and other procedures are commonly performed when the bovine patient is standing, without any accompanying sedation. In this situation, the animals are commonly restrained in a chute or crush. Sedation in the bovine patient generally implies that the animal will be placed in recumbency and secured with ropes or restrained on a tilt table. Phenothiazine tranquilizers are rarely used in cattle. In contrast to the effects of this drug in the horse, xylazine in cattle causes recumbency at the low intramuscular dose of 0.11 to 0.22 mg/kg (0.05 to 0.1 mg/lb) and is a satisfactory casting agent for simple procedures such as hoof trimming. It can also be used in combination with local analgesia for certain surgical procedures if the nature of the animal or the procedure precludes the animal's standing during surgery with local analgesia. If xylazine is used intravenously, the dose rate is 0.055 to 0.11 mg/kg (0.025 to 0.05 mg/lb). Gastrointestinal side effects (manifested as diarrhea) have been noted with xylazine.[32] These effects have been observed in large bulls and are possibly related to the increased amount of drug administered to these heavy animals. Note that xylazine is not approved for use in cattle. Tranquilization can be achieved with acetylpromazine at 0.05-0.2 mg/kg intramuscularly or 0.05 mg/kg (maximum 25 mg) intravenously.[59]

Chloral hydrate may be used effectively to cast a bovine patient into recumbency. A good example of an indication for this method is paramedian abomasopexy. Chloral hydrate (7% solution) is administered intravenously until the patient becomes recumbent. The ox is then fixed on its back with ropes, and local analgesic infiltration of the surgical site is performed. With this type of analgesia, the animal generally will not need any more sedation and will rise as soon as released at the completion of surgery. Chloral hydrate may also be given orally as a sedative in cattle. Used orally, it is administered at a dose of 1 oz/500 lb, and because of its caustic properties, it must be given in gelatin capsules or by stomach tube.

General Anesthesia

General anesthesia should be used whenever it is considered the optimal technique. Many surgical procedures have either been cancelled or performed under compromised circumstances because of reluctance to anesthetize the patient. General anesthesia offers the ultimate in restraint and, therefore, the ideal situation for aseptic surgery, proper handling of tissues, and hemostasis. General anesthesia should never be done casually, however, and the operator should be experienced in performing general anesthesia before electing to use the technique.

A thorough preanesthetic evaluation of the patient should be made, followed by appropriate preoperative preparation. The preanesthetic patient evaluation should include a history, clinical examination, and a complete blood count (CBC) or at least a packed cell volume (PCV)/total protein determination. Complete serum chemistry profiles are indicated in certain situations. The patient should be carefully monitored during the procedure and throughout postoperative recovery.

GENERAL ANESTHESIA IN HORSES

Premedication. Acetylpromazine or xylazine is routinely used as a preanesthetic agent. Acetylpromazine is less expensive and longer acting. Xylazine takes effect faster following intravenous injection. Preanesthetic tranquilizers are not generally administered to foals because of inadequate development of the microsomal enzyme system in the liver and the consequent slow metabolism of these drugs. Anesthetic induction without premedication is also practiced in a compromised animal, such as a patient with an acute abdominal disorder. If pain in a colic patient makes induction of anesthesia impossible, it is preferable to administer an analgesic agent rather than a phenothiazine tranquilizer. Hypotension, tachycardia, and persistent penile paralysis are potential side effects of the phenothiazine tranquilizers.[29] Xylazine produces transient hypertension followed by hypotension, decreases in heart rate and cardiac output, increases in peripheral resistance, and decreases in respiratory rate.

Anticholinergic drugs such as atropine are not used as preanesthetic agents. The advantages do not outweigh the disadvantages, which include postoperative ileus and increased myocardial oxygen consumption.[12,29]

Induction of Anesthesia. Several alternate regimens are available for the intravenous induction of anesthesia in the horse. The methods that we discuss currently receive the most use.

The thiobarbiturates have been used widely in practice as routine agents for anesthetic induction. Both thiopental sodium (Pentothal) and thiamylal sodium (Surital) are commonly used.

Following tranquilization of the patient, either drug is administered by rapid intravenous injection. A 5 to 10% solution is used with both drugs at a dose rate of 6.6 to 8.8 mg/kg (3.0 to 4.0 mg/lb). Although these techniques of rapid induction are convenient for the single-handed practitioner and are popular and valid methods of anesthetic induction, they do produce some profound physiologic effects. The drugs are myocardial depressants, which cause marked drops in perfusion pressure and cardiac output. The patient may also have a period of initial apnea. Such physiologic changes may lead to cardiac arrhythmias. As sole anesthetic agents, the barbiturates are useful only for short procedures. When anesthetic maintenance is required, halothane is administered at the appropriate concentration to maintain the required depth of anesthesia. This practice, in turn, may exacerbate the hypotension already caused by the barbiturate.

Acidosis potentiates the action of the barbiturates, and decreased doses must be administered to acidotic patients. Preferably, a barbiturate should not be used as a single induction agent in any toxic animal. Indeed, their use as a sole induction agent in any animal has been largely replaced by the combinations of agents described in the following paragraphs.

Guaifenesin, used alone or in combination with thiobarbiturates or ketamine, has become a common induction agent.[13,29] The drug is a muscle relaxant that acts at the level of the internuncial neurons and provides a calm state similar to sleep. Because it is centrally acting, guaifenesin provides some analgesia. It has minimal depressant effects on the respiratory and cardiac systems, and induction is smooth, without involuntary movements of the forelimbs (dog paddling). The drug is administered as a 5% solution in 5% dextrose or as a 10% solution in sterile distilled water.[14,15]

Guaifenesin has been used alone as a casting agent,[46] but it is not an anesthetic. It is now used generally in combination with a short-acting thiobarbiturate or ketamine. With the guaifenesin-barbiturate combination, two methods of administration can be used. In the first method, 2 to 3 g of thiamylal sodium (depending on the size of the horse) are added to a liter of guaifenesin solution immediately prior to use. The solution is administered to effect by rapid intravenous administration (600 to 800 ml of a 5% solution are required to induce anesthesia in a 450-kg horse). Most unsatisfactory reports from practitioners can be related to slow administration of the drug. The solution should be administered through a wide-bore (10- to 12-gauge) needle or pumped through a catheter. The patient also needs to be supported during administration of the anesthetic solution. Because the drug is given to effect, the required depth of anesthesia for intubation is achieved, and the transition to an inhalation agent is generally more convenient than with the thiobarbiturates. The combination also may be administered by giving the guaifenesin solution intravenously until the horse becomes slightly ataxic, then administering a 2-g dose of thiobarbiturate intravenously as a bolus.[14] The advantage of this method is a quieter, smoother induction because of the bolus effect of the barbiturate.

Recovery from guaifenesin and thiobarbiturate anesthesia is generally smooth. If guaifenesin is used beyond induction to maintain anesthesia, an excess of three times the therapeutic dose (110 mg/kg or 1.0 ml/lb of a 5% solution) may be administered to horses without toxicity. This is feasible, provided the drug is administered in increments required to maintain anesthesia and not as a bolus dose. Recovery times may be prolonged, however.

A popular short-term anesthetic regimen in the horse is the combination of xylazine and ketamine hydrochloride (Ketalar). Xylazine is administered intravenously at a dose of 1.1 mg/kg, followed 3 to 5 minutes later by intravenous ketamine hydrochloride at a dose of 2.2 mg/kg. The disadvantage of large-volume administration through a catheter or needle (as is necessary with guaifenesin) is eliminated. Induction of anesthesia is usually smooth if sufficient time is allowed for the xylazine to achieve its maximum sedative effect. The duration of anesthesia is short (12 to 15 minutes), but is satisfactory for short procedures or anesthetic induction. The disadvantages of the xylazine-ketamine regimen include increased cost and the inability to control the duration of anesthesia by repeatedly administering the same agent. Convulsions, muscle tremors, and spasms have been reported with repeated doses of ketamine; therefore, it is contraindicated. Convulsions or tremors seen occasionally during induction of anesthesia are usually associated with insufficient amounts of xylazine or with the administration of ketamine before the xylazine has taken full effect. Improved induction has been reported using premedication with diazepam administered at a dose rate of 0.22 mg/kg (0.1 mg/lb) 20 minutes prior to the administration of xylazine.[8] Note that with the xylazine-ketamine combination, active palpebral, corneal, and swallowing reflexes are maintained; nevertheless, it is possible to pass an endotracheal tube and to initiate inhalation anesthesia. The degree of anesthesia obtained with this induction regimen is variable, however, and the progression to inhalation anesthesia can be more time consuming and difficult. The cardiopulmonary effects are only acceptable with the quoted dosage regimens.[39] For these reasons, we prefer the next regimen described.

The combination of guaifenesin and ketamine works well and is excellent for debilitated patients. It provides a relatively nonexcitable induction of anesthesia with little cardiopulmonary depression.[14] Guaifenesin is given as a 5% or 10% solution intravenously until ataxia or a slight buckling of the legs occurs. Ketamine is then administered as a bolus (1.8 to 2.2 mg/kg).

Additional guaifenesin can then be administered after induction of anesthesia as necessary.

The use of succinylcholine is dangerous for casting horses, and death may result.[14] This drug is not an anesthetic agent.

The safest and most satisfactory way of inducing anesthesia in foals is by "masking down" with halothane. The mask is applied, and initially, oxygen alone (6 to 7 L/min) is administered. The vaporizer is then set at 0.5 to 1% to introduce the foal to the smell of halothane, and the concentration is gradually increased to 4% until anesthesia is induced. The foal is then intubated and placed on a maintenance plane of anesthesia.

Maintenance of Anesthesia. Although the maintenance of anesthesia with intravenous agents is not ideal, it may be the only method available to the practitioner. Intravenously maintained anesthesia has the advantages of minimal equipment requirements and economy; however, lengthy maintenance on any of the injectable regimens is associated with a prolonged, and sometimes stormy, recovery. Because excretion of the anesthetic agent is slower than with an inhalation agent, the plane of anesthesia cannot be reduced quickly, particularly in debilitated or young animals. In general, any period of intravenously maintained anesthesia should last no longer than an hour.

If large doses of thiobarbiturates are used to maintain anesthesia, recovery will be prolonged. We recommend limiting the total dose of thiamylal sodium to 5 g for any horse. Guaifenesin and thiamylal are preferred over thiamylal alone for maintenance of anesthesia. Recovery may still be prolonged, but it is generally calm and quiet.

Inhalation anesthesia is the preferred method of maintaining general anesthesia in the horse, especially when procedures involve a total anesthetic time of longer than an hour. The combination most commonly used is that of halothane and oxygen.

Halothane provides rapid induction and recovery, adequate muscle relaxation, and easy monitoring of anesthetic depth. Enflurane and isoflurane have been evaluated in the horse,[4,50,52,54] and their effectiveness has been established. Neither drug is used routinely. Respiratory depression and unpleasant recoveries are reasons that enflurane is not a desirable alternative to halothane. Isoflurane has been used in clinical cases. A smooth, rapid recovery (compared to halothane) is seen as an advantage.[4] Expense is a precluding factor to its routine use.

When halothane is used, the halothane-vaporizer setting may range from 1.5 to 3%, and the oxygen flow rate may be around 4 to 6 L/min for a 450-kg horse.

The use of a halothane and nitrous oxide combination has been suggested in the past. Such practice is not now recommended, based on concerns with ventilation and oxygen delivery and the risk of hypoxia.

Ventilatory compromise is of concern in anesthetized, recumbent horses. The causes include pharmacologic depression of the respiratory control center, decreased lung volume, inadequate thoracic expansion or diaphragmatic excursions, and mismatched distribution of ventilation and perfusion in recumbency.[21,27,35,36,48,51] Hypercarbia and hypoxemia develop unless ventilation is assisted. Controlled ventilation is the most effective means of maintaining normal blood gas levels, but it has detrimental cardiovascular effects. Assisted ventilation reduces arterial carbon dioxide levels and raises oxygen levels, when compared to spontaneous ventilation, with less cardiovascular depression than during controlled ventilation.[25] Hypoxemia is another potential problem in the recovery period.[36] Only oxygen supplementation through a demand valve seems sufficient to maintain arterial blood gas tensions similar to those in awake horses.[36]

Details on inhalation anesthetic machines, equipment, techniques, and monitoring are available in other texts.[20,34,42,48,49]

Careful clinical monitoring of the patient during anesthesia is important, including measurement of reflexes and physical monitoring of the cardiovascular system.[29] More definitive monitoring of the cardiovascular system is accomplished by direct or indirect blood pressure measurements and electrocardiograms (ECG). For performance of short procedures in "the field," monitoring equipment is minimal. For longer procedures in a hospital situation, however, the measurement of arterial blood pressure (using arterial catheterization and a pressure transducer or indirect measurement with the Doppler system over the coccygeal artery), in addition to the normal monitoring of vital signs, is desirable. ECG monitoring is also useful.

Patients in hypotensive states that do not respond to intravenous fluids require the use of vasoactive agents. Dopamine, dobutamine, and ephedrine are practical and effective drugs used to increase blood pressure.[29,38,60] Clinical experience in anesthetized horses indicates that dopamine or dobutamine is superior to ephedrine in time-to-peak response, improvement of blood pressure, and increases in cardiac output. Atrial and ventricular arrhythmias occur at higher doses (75 mg/kg/min) of dopamine and dobutamine, but they are easily controlled by reducing the rate of administration. Cardiac arrhythmias are mainly observed after ephedrine administration.[38]

Positioning of the patient is important when procedures of over 30 minutes are performed in a hospital situation. Faulty positioning of the hind limbs can lead to peroneal or femoral nerve paresis.[23] In addition, failure to support the upper pelvic limb when the horse is in lateral recumbency can lead to venous occlusion and subsequent rhabdomyolysis. The recumbent thoracic limb should be pulled craniad to relieve pressure between the rib cage, brachial plexus, and vessels along the humerus; otherwise, rhabdomyolysis or nerve paresis may result. The routine use of a waterbed or air mattress is recommended when placing anesthetized animals on an operating table for periods of longer than 30 minutes. Hypotension during anesthesia is a significant contributor to postanesthetic myopathy in horses anesthetized with halothane.[16]

GENERAL ANESTHESIA IN CATTLE

Most surgical procedures in cattle can be performed with physical restraint (and sedation in some instances) and local anesthesia. In some situations, however, these conditions are less than optimal, and the use of general anesthesia is definitely indicated. The fear of administering general anesthesia is generally greater when dealing with a bovine patient. Although there are special problems, general anesthesia can be carried out safely on the bovine patient with the appropriate techniques and experience.

Premedication. Feed should be withheld from all patients before general anesthesia unless the urgency of the problem precludes it. Adult cattle should be kept from ingesting roughage for 48 hours, grain and concentrates for 24 hours, and water for 12 hours. This precaution decreases the likelihood of bloating and regurgitation of ruminal contents, which are 2 special hazards with bovine general anesthesia, by decreasing the amount of ingesta within the rumen. Regurgitation is less of a problem in younger cattle. Their feed should be withheld for 12 to 24 hours and water withheld overnight if possible.[2]

Premedication with tranquilizers is not routine prior to the induction of general anesthesia in cattle. Quiet cattle have little need for tranquilization, and wilder patients are not easily controlled with tranquilizers. In addition, few tranquilizers are approved for use in food animals. The surgeon must assume responsibility when using these drugs. If acetylpromazine is used as preanesthetic premedication, the dose should be low (0.05 mg/kg).

Induction of Anesthesia. Several intravenous agents can be used to induce anesthesia in cattle. Chloral hydrate, given slowly as a 7% solution to effect (approximately 20 to 30 ml/45 kg or 100 lb), may be used, but it is preferred as a sedative to achieve recumbency rather than as an induction agent. Thiamylal sodium has been extensively used to induce anesthesia in cattle. It is effective at the recommended dose of 4 to 8 mg/kg and gives deeper, more prolonged initial anesthesia with less apnea than thiopental sodium. Thiopental sodium has also been used effectively, however. The dose is 6 to 12 mg/kg. Guaifenesin, with 2 g of a thiobarbiturate, may be used in the same manner as in the horse, but it is not approved for use in food animals.[42] This regimen has the advantage of being effective when administered more slowly than thiobarbiturates alone, thus allowing induction of anesthesia to the desired depth.[55]

The use of ketamine (2 mg/kg) as an intravenous bolus following premedication with atropine and xylazine has been reported as an effective induction regimen.[55] Jaw relaxation is not as effective as with guaifenesin and thiobarbiturates, but endotracheal intubation can be performed.[53] The same authors have conducted clinical trials with the use of 5% guaifenesin solution containing 1 mg/ml of ketamine and 0.1 mg/ml of xylazine and have found it to be safe and effective for general anesthesia in cattle, sheep, and goats. Initially 0.55 mg/kg of the solution is given rapidly, and then a 2.2-ml/kg/hr maintenance level is used.

The use of an intramuscularly administered regimen of xylazine (0.04 mg/lb) and ketamine (2.0 mg/lb) provides satisfactory anesthesia for short surgical procedures in calves and small ruminants. The xylazine and ketamine can be mixed and given in the same syringe, or they can be given separately. About 30 to 40 minutes of anesthesia can be expected from this combination. If anesthesia becomes too light, the ketamine can be repeated at a half-dose (0.5 mg/kg).[43]

On induction of anesthesia, a mouth speculum is immediately inserted, and an endotracheal tube is introduced. To avoid the aspiration of regurgitated rumen contents, intubation should be performed even if anesthesia is to be maintained by an intravenous agent. Endotracheal intubation in cattle can be accomplished digitally by direct visualization of the larynx or by blind passage of the tube into the pharynx coupled with external manipulation of the larynx.[28] In adult cattle, digital intubation can be performed by placing a speculum to hold the patient's mouth open and by directing the tube into the larynx with one's hand cupped over the end of the tube. Blind intubation can also be performed by extending the animal's head, elevating the larynx by external manipulation, and passing the tube into the trachea. In calves and smaller cattle, the use of a laryngoscope is beneficial.

Although intubation can be performed after sedation with xylazine, the incidence of regurgitation is lower if surgical anesthesia is induced before endotracheal intubation is performed.[59] Regurgitation while an endotracheal tube is in place is of minor concern, provided the pharynx is cleared and drained and the nasal cavity is flushed before extubation.[59]

Induction of anesthesia in young animals may be performed with a combination of halothane and oxygen.

Maintenance of Anesthesia. As in horses, inhalation anesthesia is the preferred method for maintaining general anesthesia in cattle because the depth of anesthesia is easily controlled and recovery time is rapid. A halothane-oxygen mixture is the maintenance anesthetic of choice. When halothane is used for induction, the concentration is often initially 5% to complete induction. Anesthesia is generally maintained by an oxygen flow of 4 to 5 L/min and 1 to 3% halothane for adult cattle. Calves can generally be maintained at a halothane concentration of 1 to 1.5%.[42]

As with horses, halothane is considered to cause cardiopulmonary depression in a dose-dependent manner. It has been recently shown, however, that a guaifenesin and thiobarbiturate induction and a halothane maintenance regimen would cause bulls to be hypertensive, despite a decrease in cardiac output.[47]

Clinical monitoring during bovine anesthesia with halothane includes careful attention to the cardiovascular and respiratory parameters and to the eyes.[28] Rotation of the eyeball is a reliable means of monitoring anesthetic depth, as well as progression of recovery from halothane anesthesia.[55,58] As the anesthesia deepens, the eyeball rotates ventrad and mediad. As depth of anesthesia further increases, the cornea is completely hidden by the lower eyelid (this is plane 2 to 3 of surgical anesthesia). A further increase in the depth of anesthesia causes the eye to rotate dorsad to a central position between the palpebral folds. This point denotes deep surgical anesthesia. Palpebral reflexes dull progressively, but the corneal reflex should remain strong. During recovery, eyeball rotation occurs in reverse order to that observed during induction of anesthesia. Cardiovascular monitoring is performed as with the horse. The recovery of cattle from general anesthesia is usually smooth. As the animal recovers, it should be supported in sternal recumbency to reduce the chances of inhaling rumenal contents or developing bloat.

GENERAL ANESTHESIA IN SHEEP AND GOATS

General anesthesia in sheep and goats is basically the same as in bovine patients.

Premedication. For general anesthesia, a routine preoperative examination should be performed. Feed should be withheld for 24 hours and water for 12 hours to minimize regurgitation. Xylazine may be used as a sedative, as in the bovine patient, but it is not approved in the United States for use in sheep and goats. The dose rate for xylazine is 0.05 to 0.11 mg/kg (0.025 to 0.05 mg/lb) intravenously and 0.11 to 0.22 mg/kg (0.05 to 0.1

mg/lb) intramuscularly. Atropine is not generally used. Atropine will reduce saliva in volume and render it more viscous; this may facilitate visualization of the laryngeal opening for intubation. The intramuscular dose requirements are higher than for monogastric animals—0.4 to 0.7 mg/kg as a premedicant followed by repeated doses of 0.2 mg/kg every 15 to 30 minutes during surgery.[17]

Induction of Anesthesia. Both thiopental sodium and thiamylal sodium may be used for induction of general anesthesia at dose rates of 10 to 16 mg/kg and 8 to 14 mg/kg intravenously to effect, respectively. Recovery problems are not as great as in cattle, and additional increments may be used to maintain anesthesia. The use of thiamylal sodium and guaifenesin has been described.[17] The use of xylazine at 0.22 mg/kg (0.1 mg/lb) and ketamine at 11 mg/kg (5 mg/lb) intramuscularly to induce anesthesia in goats has been described.[33] The drugs may be administered sequentially or together; their combination induces anesthesia for 40 to 45 minutes. In addition, anesthesia can be safely extended to 2.5 to 3 hours by supplemental increments of either ketamine or a mixture of xylazine and ketamine.

The use of acetylpromazine intravenously (0.55 mg/kg) followed by ketamine by slow intravenous injection 10 minutes later (22 mg/kg) has been reported as an anesthetic agent in sheep.[56] In this situation, anesthesia may also be maintained with increments of 6.6 mg/kg (3 mg/lb) of ketamine given intramuscularly as needed. Ketamine can be used as a sole anesthetic agent in sheep and goats, but it does not provide adequate muscle relaxation, and opisthotonos, trembling, and jaw champing may be seen.[17]

Anesthesia may also be induced in both sheep and goats with a combination of halothane and oxygen administered by mask.

Maintenance of Anesthesia. Inhalation anesthesia is again the method of choice for maintenance of anesthesia in sheep and goats. Halothane and methoxyflurane both work satisfactorily. The longer recovery time with methoxyflurane is not as critical in these species as it is in the equine and bovine species. Anesthesia is maintained with 1 to 2% halothane. Oxygen flow rates of 11 ml/kg/min (5 ml/lb/min) or greater are used during anesthesia.

Injectable anesthetic regimens are available, and their effects in sheep and goats seem more satisfactory than in equine and bovine species. The use of inhalation anesthesia is still the optimal method, however. Local analgesic techniques are preferable to general anesthesia for cesarean section in the ewe.[11]

Various reflexes are used to judge the depth of anesthesia in sheep and goats, but none are reliable enough to be used as the sole assessment of anesthetic depth. Jaw tone should be used cautiously because some exists at deep levels of anesthesia. Swallowing movements signify lightening of anesthesia. Eye rotation is not a useful method of assessing anesthetic depth as it is in cattle.[17] Pupillary dilation is evident during light anesthetic planes and may also be evident during deep anesthesia.

GENERAL ANESTHESIA IN SWINE

Because most procedures performed on swine on the farm are of relatively short duration, they lend themselves to the use of injectable agents, and the indications for inhalation anesthesia in swine are few. Because of the physical features and temperament of swine, however, induction of any form of general anesthesia is often difficult. Accessible superficial veins are few, intubation is generally more difficult than in other species, and swine are prone to malignant hyperthermia.[3]

Premedication. Preanesthetic tranquilization is certainly indicated in swine to ease the induction of general anesthesia. Tranquilization or sedation is also used for restraint during minor procedures. Patients vary in response time and degree of sedation following administration of tranquilizers. Acetylpromazine may be used at the rate of 0.11 to 0.22 mg/kg intramuscularly. The total dose of acetylpromazine in any pig should not exceed 15 mg.[5] Xylazine is not an effective tranquilizer for swine.[5] The use of the combination of droperidol and fentanyl (Innovar-Vet) provides sedation that is reasonably dependable.[45] The intramuscular dose is 1 ml/9 kg to 1 ml/14 kg. Maximal effect occurs in 20 minutes. An inducing dose of intravenous thiobarbiturate can be reduced by one-third to half when droperidol-fentanyl is used as a preanesthetic agent. The drug may also be administered prior to inducing anesthesia with an inhalation anesthetic and has also been effectively used in combination with epidural anesthesia. Diazepam administered intramuscularly at a dose of 5.5 to 8.5 mg/kg has been used in miniature swine and is an excellent sedative and preanesthetic agent.[41] Prior to the use of droperidol-fentanyl or the induction of general anesthesia, the patient should be given atropine sulfate to reduce salivation and to minimize bradycardia associated with vagal stimulation. A dose of 0.40 mg/kg is administered subcutaneously, intramuscularly, or intravenously.

The butyrophenone derivative azaparone (Stresnil) is now available and has been approved for swine in the United States. It may be the tranquilizer of choice; it is certainly the most predictable. The preanesthetic or sedative dose is 1.25 to 2.5 mg/kg, administered intramuscularly.[5]

Induction of Anesthesia. Thiamylal or thiopental sodium may be used in 2.5 to 5% solutions to induce anesthesia. The anesthetic dose is 6.6 to 11 mg/kg. Surgical anesthesia from a single dose lasts 15 to 30 minutes.[45] Additional doses increase anesthetic risk proportionately and should be administered with caution.

In a comparative study of anesthetic regimens, the use of thiamylal sodium following acetylpromazine premedication was the most effective in producing a motionless animal for shorter procedures.[10] A technique of intratesticular anesthesia with pentobarbital sodium (45 mg/kg body weight) is useful for castration of boars. The anesthetic agent is administered using a 4-cm, 16-gauge needle inserted below the epididymis in the upper third of the testis at an angle of 30° from the perpendicular. Satisfactory anesthesia is usually obtained within 10 minutes.[24]

Ketamine hydrochloride has been used to induce anesthesia in swine.[57] Excitement during the recovery period can occur, however, if the ketamine is not supplemented with thiobarbiturates or inhalation agents.[57] Ketamine in combination with droperidol-fentanyl has been successfully used for various surgical procedures in pigs weighing less than 45 kg.[5] The patient is given atropine (0.4 mg/kg) and droperidol-fentanyl (1 ml/14.6 kg) intramuscularly. With the onset of sedation (10 to 15 minutes), ketamine is administered intramuscularly at the rate of 11 mg/kg. Surgical anesthesia is induced in 5 to 10 minutes and lasts 30 to 45 minutes. To prolong anesthesia, supplemental ketamine may be given intramuscularly at the rate of 2.2 to 6.6 mg/kg or intravenously to effect. Pentobarbital sodium is effective for controlling reactions that may occur during recovery.

Guaifenesin (5% solution in 5% dextrose) containing 1 mg/ml of ketamine and 1 mg/ml of xylazine has been used to induce and maintain anesthesia in mature swine.[55] It is administered through the central ear vein using a 16- to 18-gauge catheter. This combination of drugs is initially given rapidly at a dose of 0.5 to 1.0 mg/kg to induce anesthesia. This infusion may be continued at a rate of 2 ml/kg/hr to maintain anesthesia for up to 2.5 hours.[55] Recovery is rapid once the infusion is discontinued.

Halothane, administered by face mask, may also be used to induce anesthesia in pigs.[42]

Maintenance of Anesthesia. Some of the regimens just outlined are sufficient to provide a total anesthetic course for most procedures. For long term anesthesia, however, the use of inhalation agents for maintenance is preferable and becomes necessary as more sophisticated procedures are performed.

Endotracheal intubation can be difficult in swine. The larynx in the pig is long and mobile, and there is a middle ventricle in the floor of the larynx near the base of the epiglottis. The arch of the cricoid cartilage is on an oblique angle with the trachea. Laryngeal spasm is easily induced. A laryngoscope is used for intubation of swine, and a malleable metal-rod stylet is placed inside the lumen of the endotracheal tube with the tip slightly curved to facilitate the maneuvers necessary to place the tube in the trachea. A topical anesthetic should be sprayed on the larynx to prevent laryngospasm. A technique for nasal intubation has also been described.[42] Nasal intubation works well, but one disadvantage is the lack of protection against regurgitation and aspiration, because the trachea is not intubated. Anesthesia in pigs may be maintained by mask, but this technique uses excess halothane if leaks are present between the mask and the animal's snout and is not in the best interest of the operators' health.

Both halothane and methoxyflurane may be used for anesthesia maintenance. Nitrous oxide may be administered as 25 to 40% of the total gas flow with 1 to 2% halothane or with 1 to 1.5% methoxyflurane.[42] Halothane is one of several anesthetic agents capable of triggering hyperthermia in stress-prone pigs. Pigs should be carefully monitored for body temperature. A rapid rise in temperature to 41°C (106°F) or above accompanied by tachypnea, hyperventilation, muscular rigidity, blotchy cyanosis, and tachycardia is an indication for cessation of anesthesia.[3]

Ocular reflexes are usually of no value in monitoring anesthesia in pigs. The lack of superficial arteries makes it difficult to monitor anesthesia on the basis of pulse strength. Heart rate should range from 80 to 150/min in normal swine under anesthesia, and the respiratory rate should be 10 to 25/min. The depth of anesthesia can also be judged by the degree of muscle relaxation and muscle fasciculations in response to the surgical stimulus.[42]

References

1. Adams, O. R.: Lameness in Horses, 3rd Ed. Philadelphia, Lea & Febiger, 1974.

2. Ames, K. N., and Reibold, T. W.: Anesthesia in cattle. *In* Proceedings of the 11th Annual Convention of the American Association of Bovine Practitioners in 1978: 1979, p. 75.

3. Anderson, I.: Anaesthesia in the pig. Aust. Vet. J., *49*:474, 1973.

4. Auer, J. A., et al.: Recovery from anaesthesia in ponies: a comparative study of the effects of isoflurane, enflurane, methoxyflurane and halothane. Equine Vet. J., *10*:18, 1978.

5. Benson, G. J., and Thurmon, J. C.: Anesthesia of swine under field conditions. J. Am. Vet. Med. Assoc., *174*:594, 1979.

6. Benson, G. J., and Thurmon, J. C.: Regional analgesia of food animals. *In* Current Veterinary Therapy: Food Animal Practice. Vol. 2. Edited by J. L. Howard. Philadelphia, W. B. Saunders, 1986, p. 71.

7. Brock, K. A., and Heard, D. J.: Field anesthesia techniques in small ruminants. Part 1. Local analgesia. Compend. Contin. Educ., *7*:5407, 1985.

8. Butera, T. S., et al.: Diazepam/xylazine/ketamine combination for short-term anesthesia. VM/SAC, *74*:490, 1978.

9. Cakala, S.: A technique for the paravertebral lumbar block in cattle. Cornell Vet., *51*:64, 1961.

10. Cantor, G. H., Brunson, D. B., and Reibold, T. W.: A comparison of four short-acting anesthetic combinations for swine. VM/SAC, *76*:716, 1981.

11. Copland, M.D.: Anaesthesia for caesarean section in the ewe: a comparison of local and general anesthesia and the relationship between maternal and foetal values. N. Z. Vet. J., *24*:233, 1976.

12. Ducharme, N. G., and Fubini, S. L.: Gastrointestinal complications associated with use of atropine in horses. J. Am. Vet. Med. Assoc., *182*:229, 1983.

13. Funk, K. A.: Glyceryl guaiacolate: some effects and indications in horses. Equine Vet. J., *5*:15, 1973.

14. Geiser, D. R.: Practical equine injectable anesthesia. J. Am. Vet. Med. Assoc., *182*:574, 1983.

15. Grandy, J. L., and McDonell, W. N.: Evaluation of concentrated solutions of guaifenesin for equine anesthesia. J. Am. Vet. Med. Assoc., *176*:619, 1980.

16. Grandy, J. L., et al.: Arterial hypotension and the development of postanesthetic myopathy in halothane-anesthetized horses. Am. J. Vet. Res., *48*:192, 1987.

17. Gray, P. R., and McDonell, W.: Anesthesia in goats and sheep. Part II. General anesthesia. Compend. Contin. Educ., *8*:S127, 1986.

18. Gray, P. R., and McDonell, N. N.: Anesthesia in goats and sheep. Part I. Local analgesia. Compend. Contin. Educ., *8*:S33, 1986.

19. Green, E. M., and Cooper, R. C.: Continuous caudal epidural anesthesia in the horse. J. Am. Vet. Med. Assoc., *184*:971-974, 1984.

20. Hall, L. W.: Wright's Veterinary Anaesthesia and Analgesia, 7th Ed. Philadelphia, Lea & Febiger, 1971.

21. Hall, L. W., Gillespie, J. R., and Tyler, W. S.: Alveolar-arterial oxygen tension differences in anesthetized horses. Br. J. Anaesth., *40*:560, 1968.

22. Heath, R. B.: Inhalation anesthesia. *In* Proceedings of the American Association of Equine Practitioners in 1976:1977, p. 335.

23. Heath, R. B., et al.: Protecting and positioning the equine surgical patient. VM/SAC, *68*:1241, 1972.

24. Henny, D. P.: Anaesthesia of boars by intratesticular injection. Aust. Vet. J., *44*:418, 1968.

25. Hodgson, D. S., et al.: Effects of spontaneous, assisted and controlled ventilatory modes in halothane-anesthetized geldings. Am. J. Vet. Res., *47*:992, 1986.

26. Hoffman, P. E.: Clinical evaluation of xylazine as a chemical restraint agent, sedative and analgesic in horses. J. Am. Vet. Med. Assoc., *164*:42, 1974.

27. Hornof, W. J., et al.: Effects of lateral recumbency on regional lung function in anesthetized horses. Am. J. Vet. Res., *47*:277, 1986.

28. Hubbell, J. A. E., Hull, B. L., and Muir, W. W.: Perianesthetic considerations in cattle. Compend. Contin. Educ., *8*:F92, 1986.

29. Hubbell, J. A. E., et al.: Perianesthetic considerations in the horse. Compend. Contin. Educ., *6*:S401, 1984.

30. Kerr, D. D., et al.: Sedative and other effects of xylazine given intravenously to horses. Am. J. Vet. Res., *33*:526, 1972.

31. Klein, L. V., and Baetjar, C.: Preliminary report: xylazine and morphine sedation in horses. Vet. Anesth., *2*:2-C, 1974.

32. Knight, A. P.: Xylazine. J. Am. Vet. Med. Assoc., *176*:454, 1980.

33. Kumar, A., Thurmon, J. C., and Hardenbrook, J. H.: Clinical studies of ketamine HCl and xylazine HCl in domestic goats. VM/SAC, *72*:1707, 1976.

34. Lumb, W. V., and Jones, E. W.: Veterinary Anesthesia, 2nd Ed. Philadelphia, Lea & Febiger, 1984.

35. McDonell, W. N., Hall, L. W., and Jeffcott, L. B.: Radiographic evidence of impaired pulmonary function in laterally recumbent anesthetized horses. Equine Vet. J., *11*:24, 1979.

36. Mason, D. E., Muir, W. W., and Wade, A.: Arterial blood gas tensions in the horse during recovery from anesthesia. J. Am. Vet. Med. Assoc., *190*:989, 1987.

37. Morishima, O. H., et al.: Toxicity of lidocaine in adult, newborn and fetal sheep. Anesthesiology, *55*:7, 1981.

38. Muir, W. W., and Bednarski, R. M.: Equine cardiopulmonary resuscitation. Part II. Compend. Contin. Educ., *5*:S287, 1983.

39. Muir, W. W., Skarda, R. T., and Milne, D. W.: Evaluation of xylazine and ketamine hydrochloride for anesthesia in horses. Am. J. Vet. Res., *38*:195, 1977.

40. Muir, W. W., Skarda, R. T., and Sheehan, W. C.: Hemodynamic and respiratory effects of xylazine-morphine sulfate in horses. Am. J. Vet. Res., *40*:1417, 1979.

41. Ragan, H. A., and Gillis, M. F.: Restraint, venipuncture, endotracheal intubation and anesthesia of miniature swine. Lab. Anim. Sci., *25*:409, 1975.

42. Reibold, T. W., Goble, D. O., and Geiser, D. R.: Principles and Techniques of Large Animal Anesthesia. East Lansing, Michigan State University Press, 1978.

43. Rings, D. M., and Muir, W. W.: Cardiopulmonary effects of intramuscular xylazine-ketamine in calves. Can. J. Comp. Med., *467*:386, 1982.

44. Robertson, J. T., and Muir, W. W.: A new analgesic drug combination in the horse. Am. J. Vet. Res., *44*:1667, 1983.

45. Runnels, L. J.: Practical anesthesia and analgesia for porcine surgery. *In* Proceedings of the American Association of Swine Practitioners in 1976:1976, p. 80.

46. Schatzmann, U., et al.: An investigation of the action and haemolytic effect of glyceryl guaicolate in the horse. Equine Vet. J., *10*:224, 1978.

47. Sembrad, S. D., Trim, C. M., and Hardee, G. E.: Hypertension in bulls and steers anesthetized with guaifenesin-theobarbiturate-halothane combination. Am. J. Vet. Res., *47*:1577, 1986.

48. Soma, L. R.: Equine anesthesia: causes of reduced oxygen and increased carbon dioxide tensions. Compend. Contin. Educ., *2*:S57, 1980.

49. Soma, L. R.: Textbook of Veterinary Anesthesia. Baltimore, Williams & Wilkins, 1971.

50. Steffey, E. P.: Enflurane and isoflurane anesthesia: a summary of laboratory and clinical investigations in horses. J. Am. Vet. Med. Assoc., *172*:367, 1978.

51. Steffey, E. P., et al.: Body position and mode of ventilation influences arterial pH, oxygen and carbon dioxide tensions in halothane-anesthetized horses. Am. J. Vet. Res., *38*:379, 1977.

52. Steffey, E. P., et al.: Enflurane, halothane and isoflurane potency in horses. Am. J. Vet. Res., *38*:1037, 1977.

53. Tadmor, A., Marcus, S., and Eting, E.: The use of ketamine hydrochloride for endotracheal intubation in cattle. Aust. Vet. J., *55*:537, 1979.

54. Taylor, P. M., and Hall, L. W.: Clinical anaesthesia in the horse: comparison of enflurane and isoflurane. Equine Vet. J., *17*:51, 1985.

55. Thurmon, J. C., and Benson, G. J.: Anesthesia in ruminants and swine. *In* Current Veterinary Therapy: Food Animal Practice. Vol. 2. Edited by J. L. Howard. Philadelphia, W. B. Saunders, 1986, p. 51.

56. Thurmon, J. C., Kumar, A., and Link, R. P.: Evaluation of ketamine hydrochloride as an anesthetic in sheep. J. Am. Vet. Med. Assoc., *162*:293, 1973.

57. Thurmon, J. C., Nelson, D. R., and Christy, D. J.: Ketamine anesthesia in swine. J. Am. Vet. Med. Assoc., *160*:1325, 1972.

58. Thurmon, J. C., Romack, F. E., and Garner, H. E.: Excursion of the bovine eyeball during gaseous anesthesia. VM/SAC, *63*: 967, 1968.

59. Trim, C.M.: Sedation and general anesthesia in ruminants. Calif. Vet., *4*:29, 1981.

60. Trim, C. M., Moore, J. N., and White, N. A.: Cardiopulmonary effects of dopamine hydrochloride in anaesthetized horses. Equine Vet. J., *17*:41, 1985.

61. Weaver, A. D.: Intravenous local anesthesia of the lower limbs in cattle. J. Am. Vet. Med. Assoc., *160*:55, 1972.

Fluid Therapy

The need for fluid therapy in the physiologically compromised patient is well recognized. The horse undergoing exploratory laparotomy for acute abdominal crisis is often in a state of impending or fulminant shock. Similarly, the bovine patient with abomasal torsion often has major fluid volume and electrolyte deficits.

In the majority of the procedures in this textbook, the patients are systemically healthy and do not have fluid imbalances prior to surgery; however, such animals do need attention with respect to intravenous fluid therapy while they are under anesthesia. The purposes of fluid therapy for normal animals during anesthesia are to maintain adequate renal perfusion, to provide fluids for the patient's maintenance requirements, to maintain normal acid-base balance, and to maintain an intravenous route for emergency medication if needed.[13]

Two basic approaches are available in fluid management of the surgical patient: the first approach is to adopt a standard protocol devised to meet likely or anticipated deficits; the second approach is to acquire clinical and laboratory data on an individual patient and to administer the appropriate fluids to meet the patient's specific requirements. The first approach is simple and particularly convenient for the practitioner in the field, where it is not possible to obtain laboratory data instantly. In addition, this approach is satisfactory for fluid administration during routine elective surgery. For the patient with a systemic illness, however, such as an acute abdominal crisis in the horse or ox, it is desirable to obtain as accurate an assessment of the patient's fluid volume, acid-base balance, and electrolyte status as possible.

Diagnosis of Fluid Volume Deficits

The degree of dehydration or fluid volume deficit may be estimated by knowing the duration of the problem and evaluating various clinical signs including skin elasticity, pulse rate and character, character of the mucous membranes, temperature of the extremities, and nature and position of the eyes (these parameters are defined in Table 2-1). Skin elasticity is estimated by picking up skin on the side of the neck and pinching it: if the skin flattens out in 1 to 2 seconds, it has normal elasticity; if the skin takes longer than 6 to 8 seconds to flatten, severe dehydration is present. In dehydration, the mucous membranes change from moist and warm to sticky and dry, and then to cold and cyanotic. Volume deficits also increase the capillary refill time from its normal 1 to 3 seconds.

A severe hypovolemic situation, such as fulminant endotoxic shock, presents a sequence of obvious clinical signs. These include a weak, irregular pulse and color changes in the mucous membranes (brick red in the vasodilatory phase of septic shock, progressing through the cyanotic "muddy" appearance in the vasoconstricted phase). Capillary refill time is greater than 3 seconds, and the extremities are cold. Although these signs do not

TABLE 2-1. *Assessment of degrees of clinical dehydration.*

	Mild	Moderate	Severe*
Skin	Elasticity	Decreased elasticity	No elasticity
Eyes	Slightly sunken, bright	Slightly sunken, duller than normal	Deeply sunken, dry cornea
Mouth	Moist, warm	Sticky or dry	Dry, cold, cyanotic
Body weight decrease estimated (%)	4 to 6%	8%	10%
Fluid deficit (450-kg animal)	18 to 27 L	36 L	45 L

* Will see more dramatic clinical signs in acute hypovolemic shock.

give a quantitative estimate of the volume deficit, they do indicate an urgent need for rapid infusion of intravenous fluids. The quantity of fluids given is based on the patient's response to therapy, rather than on any previous calculations.

It is possible to estimate the approximate fluid volume deficit by using clinical signs (Table 2-1). Under a state of moderate dehydration, the fluid deficit is considered to be 4 to 6% of body weight. If signs of severe dehydration are observed, one generally considers that a fluid deficit is at least 10% of the body weight. This means that, in a 450-kg cow, a fluid volume deficit of 45 L exists.

A simple laboratory estimate of the degree of hypovolemia may be obtained by simultaneous measurement of the packed cell volume (PCV) and total plasma protein (TPP). The use of PCV has been criticized because of its wide normal range (in the horse, the normal range is 32 to 52%) and its tendency to undergo changes associated with splenic contraction or hemorrhage, thus confusing attempts to estimate intravascular volume. When the PCV is considered in conjunction with the TPP, however, it is a valuable tool. The range of normal TPP values is more limited. Under certain conditions, such as peritonitis, protein loss can occur, and again, both PCV and TPP need to be evaluated simultaneously and serially.

The use of PCV and TPP estimations is particularly valuable as a monitoring aid during volume replacement. If TPP remains at a normal level while PCV decreases, or if TPP and PCV concurrently decrease, this generally signifies that volume replacement is proceeding satisfactorily. A continued increase in PCV and TPP despite intensive fluid therapy is a poor sign, signifying a continued decrease in intravascular volume, associated with persistent pooling of fluid peripherally. A decreasing TPP accompanied by an increasing PCV usually signifies that the intravascular volume is not increasing and that protein is being lost from the vascular system.

Admittedly, the foregoing parameters actually provide an estimate of intravascular hydration, and acute loss from the interstitial or intracellular compartments may not be recognized initially. Equilibration between compartments takes place, however, and with sequential monitoring, most disadvantages in the use of PCV and TPP are eliminated.

Other laboratory tests thought to have advantages in the evaluation of fluid deficits include the estimation of serum sodium or plasma osmolality.[10,12]

Serum sodium estimation helps to characterize the nature of the fluid loss, but in most clinical situations, the clinician can decide whether the fluid loss is hypotonic, isotonic, or hypertonic based on the clinical problem. In addition, serum sodium estimation generally is not immediately available to the clinician. An accurate method of assessing volume deficits is through estimation of plasma osmolality.[10] Unfortunately, this test is not routinely available in clinical institutions, let alone in practice.

The practical methods available for assessing volume deficits in the surgical patient include the surgeon's clinical assessments and knowledge of the pathophysiology of the disease, estimation of the PCV and TPP, and probably most important, serial evaluation of the response to replacement therapy by both clinical examination and PCV and TPP estimation.

Diagnosis of Acid-Base Imbalance

Acid-base physiology is complex, and consequently, discussions on the cause, diagnosis, and treatment of acid-base imbalance are frequently confusing. The following is a simplified (and one hopes practical) summary of the identification of acid-base imbalance. Although some accuracy may be compromised because of simplification, it is of little significance to the animal.

The two methods currently used in veterinary medicine to evaluate acid-base status are the blood-gas analyzer, which provides simple, accurate measurements of pH, P_{CO_2} and P_{O_2}, and the Harleco CO_2 apparatus, which measures total carbon dioxide.[8] The use of both is presented.

The pH represents the net effect of the influences of respiratory and metabolic mechanisms. The magnitude of the respiratory component is identified by the P_{CO_2}. A P_{CO_2} greater than 45 mm Hg generally indicates respiratory acidosis, whereas a P_{CO_2} less than 35 mm Hg indicates respiratory alkalosis. The magnitude of the metabolic component is identified by either the bicarbonate concentration (HCO_3^-) or the base deficit/excess.[11]

The bicarbonate concentration can be misleading as a quantitative estimate of the metabolic component, because a primary change in carbon dioxide concentration directly causes a change in bicarbonate concentration that is not due to any change in the metabolic component. In addition, because of the presence of other buffer systems, the bicarbonate system is not responsible for buffering all of a given acid or base load. Base deficit/excess is a more accurate measure of quantitative changes in the metabolic component. Base deficit/excess is defined as the titratable acid or base, respectively, when titrating to a pH of 7.4 under standard conditions of P_{CO_2} (40 mm Hg), temperature (38°C), and complete hemoglobin saturation.[14] The base deficit/excess is estimated by aligning the measured values of pH and P_{CO_2} on a nomogram or is computed directly by the blood-gas machine. A base deficit less than -4 mEq/L indicates metabolic acidosis, whereas a base excess greater than $+4$ mEq/L indicates metabolic alkalosis.[11]

Despite the theoretic deficiencies in using bicarbonate levels as the measure of the metabolic component, the difference is negligible in most practical clinical situations. When P_{CO_2} is within normal range, the bicarbonate deficit (actual HCO_3^- − normal HCO_3^-) approximates the base deficit. It is commonly assumed in clinical practice that these two values are the same.

If this approximation is accepted, then the bicarbonate may be read off a nomogram in the same fashion as the base deficit.

To identify a respiratory-derived acid-base imbalance, arterial blood samples are necessary. In most presurgical and postsurgical patients, any acid-base problems have a primary metabolic component, and it is not usually necessary to obtain arterial samples. In large animals, most acid-base imbalances with a primary respiratory origin occur during anesthesia, when arterial blood samples may be conveniently obtained. Treatment of respiratory acidosis involves proper ventilation. Respiratory alkalosis is generally iatrogenic or compensatory.

In evaluating metabolically derived acid-base imbalance, venous blood samples are satisfactory. Normal values for venous blood gases are listed in Table 2-2. Severe metabolic acidosis is treated with an infusion of sodium bicarbonate. The following is an example of a calculation of the amount of bicarbonate needed using the blood-gas data from a patient with severe metabolic acidosis.

pH	7.113
Pco_2	43.8 mm Hg
HCO_3^-	11.9 mEq/L
TCO_2	12.9 mEq/L
Base deficit	13.6 mEq/L

Using the base deficit, the patient's bicarbonate deficit is calculated by the equation:

$$\frac{\text{Base deficit} \times \text{body weight (kg)} \times .3}{\text{Equivalent weight of } HCO_3^-}$$

$$= \frac{13.6 \times 450 \times .3}{12}$$

$$= 153 \text{ g bicarbonate}$$

The bicarbonate deficit may also be calculated from the bicarbonate level using the formula shown on page 37.

TABLE 2-2. *Normal values used in the evaluation of fluid balance in large animals.*

	Horse	Ox	Sheep	Swine
PCV (%)	32–52	24–46	24–50	32–50
Total protein (g/dl)	6–8	6–8	6–7.5	6–7
Electrolytes				
Sodium (mEq/L)	128–140	130–147	139–150	135–150
Potassium (mEq/L)	2.8–4.3	4.3–5.0	3.9–5.4	4.4–6.7
Chloride (mEq/L)	99–109	97–111	95–103	94–106
Blood gases (venous)				
pH	7.32–7.44	7.31–7.53	7.32–7.53	
PCO_2 (mm Hg)	38–46	35–44	36–40	
HCO_3 (mEq/L)	24–27	25–35	20–25	18–27
TCO_2 (mM/L)	24–32	21.2–32.2	21–28	

$$\frac{(\text{Measured bicarbonate level} - \text{normal bicarbonate level}) \times BW \times .3}{12}$$

$$= \frac{(11.9 - 25) \times 450 \times .3}{12}$$

$$= \frac{13.1 \times 450 \times .3}{12}$$

$$= 147 \text{ g bicarbonate}$$

This example demonstrates the general approximation between using base deficit and bicarbonate levels.

The factor 0.3 is an approximation of the volume of distribution of the bicarbonate, which is mostly accounted for by the extracellular fluid compartment. Higher factors have been used by some (up to 0.6, which approximates the volume of distribution of total body water), but these factors are not recommended because of the long time required for complete equilibration with the intracellular space and the possible overadministration of bicarbonate. This is discussed in the section on treatment of fluid imbalances.

If a blood-gas machine is not available, the measurement of total carbon dioxide determined by the Harleco CO_2 apparatus is a suitable alternative and gives a reliable measure of the bicarbonate excess or deficit.[8] The addition of acid to serum or plasma results in the liberation of free carbon dioxide, which is almost completely bicarbonate in origin:

$$\text{Total } CO_2 = \text{Dissolved } CO_2(P_{CO_2} \times 0.03) + HCO_3^-$$

and

$$\frac{HCO_3^-}{CO_2} = \frac{20}{1}$$

The bicarbonate, therefore, can be estimated by the following formula:

$$HCO_3^- = TCO_2 - \text{Dissolved } CO_2$$

$$= TCO_2 - 1.2 \text{ mEq/L}$$

This method is a convenient and economical way for the practitioner to plan and to monitor therapy for metabolic acidosis and to avoid overcorrection or undercorrection of the base deficit.

Although the situation of metabolic acidosis has been used to demonstrate the calculation of imbalances, clinical cases of metabolic alkalosis are identified in a similar manner. The bicarbonate excess is calculated from the base excess or bicarbonate levels using the same formula. If specific therapy is required, physiologic saline solution is administered, and the acid-base status is monitored until it returns to normal.

More recently, it has been recognized that blood gases alone will not enable one to detect the presence or severity of metabolic acidosis in horses with previous alkalinizing therapy or mixed acid-base disturbances. The measurement of the anion gap allows detection of these cases.

$$\text{Anion gap} = Na^+ - (Cl^- + HCO_3^-)$$

An increased anion gap is a reflection of a metabolic acidosis and could be found in the presence of a relatively normal blood-gas picture in, for example, a horse with L-lactic acidosis previously administered sodium bicarbonate or in mixed acid-base disturbance, such as in a horse with anterior enteritis and metabolic acidosis due to L-lactic acidosis and metabolic alkalosis due to gastric reflux.[9]

Diagnosis of Electrolyte Abnormalities

The electrolytes of principal concern in the fluid management of surgical patients are sodium, potassium, and chloride ions. The levels of these electrolytes are not evaluated routinely in every patient in which the need for fluid therapy is anticipated. In specific situations, however, evaluation of the status of these electrolytes is important. Sodium ion is an important electrolyte, and its concentration is intimately associated with fluid content in the body. Sodium and water are lost together (an isotonic loss) in surgical patients, and sodium ion is a routine component in replacement fluids; therefore, specific abnormalities in sodium are not of common concern unless there is a specific loss or gain of sodium. Hypernatremia may become a clinical problem in the patient that has received intensive fluid therapy and in which the addition of sodium bicarbonate to the balanced electrolyte solution has caused an excessive administration of sodium ion. This situation should be monitored in such patients.

A hyperkalemic state may occur during metabolic acidosis because of the redistribution of body potassium. Intracellular potassium moves out of the cells into the extracellular fluid as excess hydrogen ions move into the cells. Hyperkalemia usually is not a clinical problem in the nonanesthetized animal, except when the renal threshold is exceeded and potassium is lost from the body, resulting in a state of hypokalemia when the acidosis has been corrected. For this reason, potassium levels should be evaluated once acidosis has been corrected and equilibration of intracellular and extracellular potassium and hydrogen ions has recurred. Serum potassium levels under 3 mEq/L in the horse are indicative of significant hypokalemia.[4] Severe deficits of potassium also occur with diarrhea in horses. Thus, hypokalemia may be a clinical problem prior to surgery in a patient with such a history.

Calculation of the overall body deficit in potassium is difficult because the actual volume of distribution for the ion is uncertain. For convenience, an arbitrary volume of distribution of 40% of the body weight is used. In a 450-kg horse, for example, the potassium "space" may be considered $450 \times .4 = 180$ L. If a patient has a potassium level of 2.0 mEq/L, it is considered to have a deficiency of $180 \times (4 - 2) = 360$ mEq (normal potassium level is 4.0 mEq/L). The equivalent weight of potassium is 14. The patient is therefore deficient $360/14 = 26$ g potassium. If hyponatremia is encountered, a factor of 0.3 is used for the sodium "space."

Decreases in chloride levels are observed in cattle with abomasal torsion. A significant correlation has been observed between postsurgical outcome and the presurgical serum chloride concentration.[15] Serum concentrations of sodium and potassium also decrease, but less dramatically.

Fluid Therapy in the Anesthetized Patient Undergoing Elective Surgery

In general, there are four essential principles of fluid therapy: the replacement of existing deficits, the fulfillment of maintenance requirements, the replacement of anticipated additional losses, and the monitoring of the patient's response to therapy. The routine surgical patient has no deficit at the time of anesthetic induction, but fluid should be administered during anesthesia in anticipation of maintenance requirements and metabolic changes during anesthesia.

A polyionic, isotonic solution with an alkalinizing effect should be administered during anesthesia. Lactated Ringer's solution, for example, is appropriate for this purpose (Table 2-3). In the uncompromised patient, metabolism of lactate by the liver yields a bicarbonate equivalent; the acetate and gluconate in Normosol-R are metabolized by the muscle to yield a bicarbonate equivalent. An extracellular replacement fluid made at the Veterinary Teaching Hospital at Colorado State University contains sodium, potassium, chloride ions, and acetate as a bicarbonate precursor (composition in Table 2-3). Acetate, rather than lactate, is used mainly for convenience, because it is available in a powder.

Fluids should always be administered intravenously, using an indwelling catheter or needles at least 5 cm in length and properly threaded in the vein. If intravenous catheters are used, an aseptic preparation should be made before insertion, and every precaution should be taken to avoid phlebitis. A rate of administration of 4.4 to 6.6 ml/kg/hr is sufficient to maintain the patient's hydration in elective cases;[13] however, the patient should be monitored continually to ensure that such maintenance therapy is adequate.

If a patient becomes compromised during surgery, the fluid therapy regimen should be changed immediately to satisfy any specific requirements.

TABLE 2-3. *Composition of intravenous fluids (mEq/L).*

Polyionic Replacement Solutions	Na^+	K^+	Ca^{++}	Mg^{++}	Cl^-	Bicarbonate Precursor
Ringer's solution	147.5	4	4.5		156	
Lactated Ringer's solution	130	4	3		109	28 (lactate)
Normosol-R	140	5		3	98	50 (acetate, gluconate)
Polysol	140	10	5	3	103	55 (acetate)
Extracellular replacement fluid	140	5			115	30 (acetate)
Physiologic saline solution	154				154	
5% Bicarbonate	600					600
Lactated Ringer's solution + 5 g/L $NaHCO_3$	190	4	3		109	87

Fluid Therapy in the Compromised Patient, According to Requirements

Fluid therapy in the compromised patient should be directed specifically at the volume deficits, acid-base imbalances, and electrolyte changes. At the same time, intensive monitoring is required to ensure that the therapy is satisfactory and to recognize developing needs.

Volume replacement is usually the most important and urgent requirement in the compromised large animal patient. Polyionic replacement fluids of the alkalinizing type are used, except in case of metabolic alkalosis. Because the rate of administration varies with the state of the animal, formulas for administration rate have little value in the compromised patient. Fluids are generally given rapidly, and the administration rate is dictated by changes in the clinical signs and the PCV and TPP. Rapid volume replacement is particularly urgent in shock patients, to maintain circulating blood volume. Untoward sequelae of overzealous volume replacement are rare unless the animal is recumbent or has a low TPP or kidney failure. The usual error in volume replacement in large animals is the administration of an inadequate volume of fluids or slow administration of the volume.

When monitoring massive fluid replacement, a continued decrease in TPP without evidence that the volume deficit is being replaced indicates a vital protein loss. A TPP of less than 4 g/dl is an indication for plasma administration. Plasma expanders such as dextran preparations are not used routinely; they are costly, and adverse reactions have been reported.

The specific treatment of metabolic acidosis is not so straightforward. In the past, any base deficit was treated immediately with sodium bicarbonate (often in bolus form with priority over volume replacement), and it was generally considered better to give too much than too little. Based on more recent information, this practice requires modification for several reasons. The first is that metabolic acidosis in the large animal surgical patient usually occurs secondary to hypovolemia and inadequate peripheral tissue perfusion. Rectification of the primary problems usually corrects any accompanying acidosis (at least mild acidosis) and makes the specific administration of sodium bicarbonate unnecessary. In addition, as volume and tissue perfusion are restored, the acetate, gluconate, or lactate in the polyionic replacement fluids acts as a source of bicarbonate (Table 2-3).

Opinions vary on the value of the lactate in lactated Ringer's solution as a bicarbonate source in the compromised patient. The conversion of lactate to bicarbonate requires a functioning liver and adequate perfusion to provide oxygen; consequently, immediate provision of bicarbonate by lactate cannot be anticipated in the patient in shock. As perfusion is restored, exogenously administered lactate does not accumulate, but acts as a bicarbonate source. In addition, the liver can still metabolize lactate when the blood flow to the organ is 20% of normal and oxygen saturation is 50%.[7] The other criticism of giving lactated solutions for the treatment of patients in shock has been that lactic acidosis already exists in these patients. Although lactate will not be converted to bicarbonate in these patients while they are in shock, there is no evidence that its presence causes any harm. Exogenous lactate, given in lactated Ringer's solution, does not increase blood lactate levels in normal or shock patients.[3]

For more severely compromised patients in which conversion of the bicarbonate precursors to bicarbonate is not anticipated, specific administration of bicarbonate is appropriate. Bicarbonate supplementation is certainly indicated when the base deficit is 10 mEq/L or greater. The amount administered is based on calculation of the deficit, as described previously. It is important to avoid overadministration. In the past, practitioners considered sodium bicarbonate a benign drug because excess bicarbonate could be excreted by the kidneys or converted to carbon dioxide and eliminated by the lungs.[5] Several potential hazards have been suggested, however: hypernatremia leading to hyperosmolality; iatrogenic alkalosis, which could interfere with neuromuscular function; and paradoxic acidosis of cerebrospinal fluid (CSF).[5] The last condition has been recognized in dogs and man.[1,2] The problem is best demonstrated by this equation:

$$HCO_3^- + H^+ \rightleftharpoons H_2CO_3 \rightleftharpoons H_2O + CO_2$$

Overadministration of sodium bicarbonate drives this reaction to the right, producing increased carbon dioxide. The carbon dioxide could potentially diffuse across the blood-brain barrier in preference to bicarbonate. The increased carbon dioxide in the CSF could cause the same reaction to be driven to the left, increasing hydrogen in the CSF and thereby leading to acidosis. The significance of this problem in large animals has yet to be substantiated, however.

Supplementary bicarbonate may be added to the polyionic replacement solution (if it does not contain calcium) or administered separately. If prolonged bicarbonate therapy is necessary, it may be desirable to give sodium bicarbonate in isotonic solution with sterile water or to substitute 5% dextrose solution for some of the sodium-containing replacement fluid, to minimize the development of hypernatremia.

If a patient has metabolic alkalosis (typically a cow with an abomasal disorder), physiologic saline solution is administered. This will replace lost volume and restore depleted chloride levels, which are the cause of the alkalosis. At the same time, surgical correction of the abomasal problem with cessation of chloride sequestration is an equally important part of the therapy. In man, the use of sodium chloride is not satisfactory for the treatment of severe cases of metabolic alkalosis.[17] If kidney function is decreased, hypernatremia becomes a problem; dilute hydrochloric acid, administered until the base excess is corrected, improves this condition.[17] This treatment may be appropriate in severe cases in animals.

In the patient with a recognized potassium deficit, potassium may be added to the intravenous fluids at a rate of up to 10 mEq/L,[16] with a total maximum of less than 100 mEq.[6] Higher rates (20 to 25 mEq/L) are used in the dog and man, but caution is advised when treating the horse. Correct levels of potassium may be achieved by the addition of 0.75 g of potassium chloride per liter of fluid. Administering this additional potassium intravenously is safe for horses with adequate renal function. In most cases, hypokalemia is recognized when the animal's condition is stabilized following a hypovolemic, acidotic crisis. In most of these cases, potassium replacement can be accomplished satisfactorily by administering 30 g of potassium chloride by stomach tube and repeating if necessary. Treatment of the other major electrolyte imbalances, hypochloremia and hypernatremia, has been already discussed.

The best indication of any fluid therapy protocol is the clinical response of the animal to the therapy. These observations should be accompanied by routine PCV and TPP estimations, acid-base status (blood gases or total carbon dioxide), and electrolyte assessment as appropriate. The animal's fluid status is dynamic, and the interval between measurement of these parameters depends on the individual clinical case. Because of the marked variability between cases and the need for continued monitoring, we have avoided quoting rates of administration.

Fluid Administration in the Compromised Patient Without Preliminary Data

In certain field situations, the practitioner must initiate fluid therapy when the only preliminary data are those noted in the clinical examination. This practice is appropriate, but certain guidelines need to be followed. If volume replacement therapy is prolonged, PCV and TPP should be evaluated as soon as possible. If acid-base data are not available, 50 to 100 g of bicarbonate may be given empirically along with other fluids in the case of the horse. Such empiric administration is not recommended in an anesthetized horse, however, because bicarbonate administration increases carbon dioxide production in a horse that is usually hypoventilating. Surgical conditions in cattle almost always result in metabolic alkalosis. Metabolic acidosis is only usually seen in adult cattle when they are terminally ill and can no longer maintain circulation. Therefore, in cattle, either saline solution or straight Ringer's solution should be used when acid-base information is unavailable. Electrolyte determination should be made before specific electrolyte disturbances are treated.

When performing volume replacement based on clinical examination alone, the clinician needs to have some concept of the volume of fluid necessary. Twelve to 20 L of fluid per hour have been given to horses in shock. When frequent or excessive urination occurs, the rate of the infusion should be decreased. After the initial rapid administration of fluids, the usual recommended flow rate is 3 to 5 L/hr.[4] A 450-kg horse needs 27 L of water per day for maintenance alone.[6]

References

1. Berenyi, K. J., Wolk, M., and Killip, T.: Cerebrospinal fluid acidosis complicating therapy of experimental cardiopulmonary arrest. Circulation, *52*:319, 1975.

2. Bishop, R. L., and Weisfeldt, M. L.: Sodium bicarbonate administration during cardiac arrest. J. Am. Med. Assoc., *235*:506, 1976.

3. Brasmer, T. H.: Fluid therapy in shock. J. Am. Vet. Med. Assoc., *174*:475, 1979.

4. Carlson, G. P.: Fluid therapy in horses with acute diarrhea. Vet. Clin. North Am. (Large Anim. Pract.), *1*:313, 1979.

5. Coffman, J.: Acid:base balance. VM/SAC, *75*:489, 1980.

6. Donawick, W. J.: Metabolic management of the horse with acute abdominal crisis. J. S. Afr. Vet. Assoc., *46*:107, 1975.

7. Garner, H. E., et al.: Postoperative care of equine abdominal crises. Vet. Anesth., *4*:40, 1977.

8. Gentry, P. A., and Black, W. D.: Evaluation of Harleco CO_2 apparatus: comparison with the Van Slyke method. J. Am. Vet. Med. Assoc., *167*:156, 1975.

9. Gossett, K. A., French, D. D., and Cleghorn, B.: Laboratory evaluation of metabolic acidosis. *In* Proceedings of the Second Equine Colic Research Symposium. Athens, GA, University of Georgia, 1986, p. 161.

10. Green, R. A.: Perspectives in clinical osmometry. Vet. Clin. North Am. (Small Anim. Pract.), *8*:287, 1978.

11. Haskins, S. C.: An overview of acid-base physiology. J. Am. Vet. Med. Assoc., *170*:423, 1977.

12. Kohn, C. W.: Preoperative management of the equine patient with an abdominal crisis. Vet. Clin. North Am. (Large Anim. Pract.) *1*:289, 1979.

13. Reibold, T. W., Goble, D. O., and Geiser, D. R.: Principles and Techniques of Large-Animal Anesthesia. East Lansing, Michigan State University Press, 1978.

14. Siggaard-Anderson, O.: Blood acid-base alignment nomogram: scales for pH, pCO_2, base excess of whole blood of different hemoglobin concentrations, plasma bicarbonate, and plasma total CO_2. Scand. J. Clin. Lab. Invest., *15*:211, 1963.

15. Smith, D. F.: Right-side torsion of the abomasum in dairy cows: classification of severity and evaluation of outcome. J. Am. Vet. Med. Assoc., *173*:108, 1978.

16. Waterman, A.: A review of the diagnosis and treatment of fluid and electrolyte disorders in the horse. Equine Vet. J., *9*:43, 1977.

17. Williams, D. B., and Lyons, J. H.: Treatment of severe metabolic alkalosis with intravenous infusion of hydrochloric acid. Surg. Gynecol. Obstet., *150*:315, 1980.

3

SURGICAL INSTRUMENTS

The purpose of this chapter is to familiarize the inexperienced surgeon with some general instruments commonly used in veterinary surgical practice. When different techniques are discussed, reference is made to various instruments used for special procedures in large animal practice. This chapter serves as a reference for these instruments, which are illustrated at the end of the chapter. In learning this plethora of instruments, it helps to handle them and to use them in situations such as laboratories and practical sessions whenever possible. Some instruments shown in this chapter are used only occasionally; others, such as scalpels, hemostats, and needle holders, are used every day in any surgical procedure.

Use of Surgical Instruments

The most important aspect of instrumentation is knowing which instrument to use at which time; this is essential to good surgical technique. It ensures that the particular surgical procedure is undertaken with minimal trauma to the tissues, is performed in the minimal amount of time, and, ultimately, results in the least harm to the patient.

Scalpel

The scalpel is used for the sharp division of tissue with minimal damage to nearby structures. Today, scalpels come with a variety of blade configurations, each designed for a specific purpose. The blades are disposable, thereby avoiding the need to sharpen them. Scalpel handles come in different sizes; no. 3 and no. 4 are generally adequate for most large animal surgical procedures. For work in deep cavities, such as rectovaginal fistula repair and urine-pooling operations, longer-handled scalpels are essential.

The scalpel must be held so it is under complete control. It is grasped between the thumb and the third and fourth fingers, with the index finger placed over the back. To cut, make a smooth sweep with the rounded portion of the blade, or "belly," rather than the point. The amount of pressure applied varies, but the aim is to produce a bold, single, full-thickness skin incision with a single sweep of the scalpel blade. The skin of the bovine flank, for example, is tough, and the neophyte surgeon usually does not apply enough pressure when making an incision in this area; the skin in the inguinal area of the horse, on the other hand, is thin, and a light stroke over the tissues with the middle of the blade is adequate.

Figure 3-1*A* shows the stroke made with nos. 10, 20, 21, and 22 scalpel blades. The handle should be at an angle of 30 to 40° to the surface incised. Figure 3-1*B* depicts the pencil grip with nos. 10, 20, 21, and 22 scalpel blades. The pencil grip is used for nos. 11 and 15 blades when more precise incisions are required (Fig. 3-2*A*). Figure 3-2*B* shows the incorrect use of a no. 15 blade. The bistoury blade (no. 12) has a hook shape and is used for lancing abscesses. The bayonet tip blade (no. 11) can also be used for lancing abscesses and for severing ligaments.

When the scalpel blade becomes dull, the blade is removed carefully by grasping the blade with a needle holder or hemostat (Fig. 3-3). The proximal end of the blade is then bent slightly to clear the blade from the hub of the handle. Then the blade is pushed up over the end of the scalpel handle. The reverse process is used to replace a scalpel blade. Although the blade may be too dull for a particular surgical procedure, the blade is still sharp enough to cause serious injury if care is not taken while removing it from the scalpel handle. The spent blade should be discarded appropriately.

To remove the new scalpel from its packet, the ends of the packet are grasped by the operating room nurse or nonscrubbed assistant and peeled open, exposing the end of the blade. The blade is carefully plucked out of the packet, contacting only the blade itself, to avoid a break in aseptic technique (Fig. 3-4). Various types of scalpel blades and scalpel handles are illustrated on page 52.

Scissors

A variety of scissors are available and are used for such procedures as cutting tissues or dissecting between tissue planes. Generally speaking, scissors used for tissue are light and are made with precision in mind. They must be kept sharp or they will crush tissues rather than cut them. Mayo or Metzenbaum scissors are used for most tissues. They are available with curved or straight blades. Straight scissors are used for working close to the surface of the wound, whereas the curved scissors are used for working deeper in the wound. Scissors are also classified according to the shape of the tips, for example, sharp/sharp, sharp/blunt, and blunt/blunt. Some scissors are designed to cut wire. The heel of the wire-cutting scissors is used for this purpose. Various types of scissors are illustrated on pages 52 and 53.

The scissors are grasped by placing the thumb and ring finger through the rings and setting the index finger against the blades. The index finger provides control of the tips of the scissors. The scissors must be kept near the last joint of the finger, and the fingers must not be allowed to slip through the rings of the handle (Fig. 3-5). The end of the blade is used for cutting; however, when tough structures are encountered, the heel of the blade is used. The scissors should not be closed unless the surgeon can see the tips of the blades; otherwise, vital structures may be endangered. For blunt dissection, insert the closed tips of the scissors into the tissue, and then open the points. Scissors used for tissue work should not be used

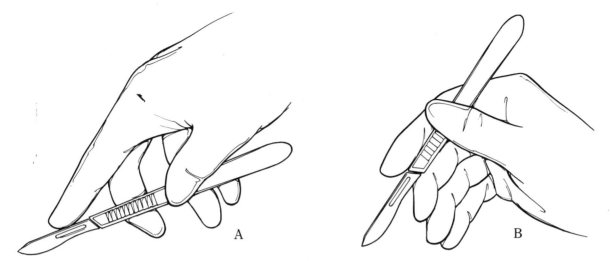

FIG. 3-1. *Use of nos. 10, 20, 21, and 22 blades. A, stroke; B, pencil grip.*

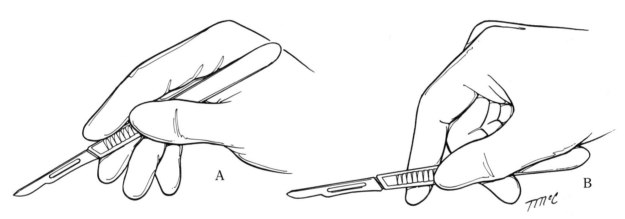

FIG. 3-2. A, *pencil grip for nos. 11 and 15 blades.* B, *incorrect use of no. 15 blade.*

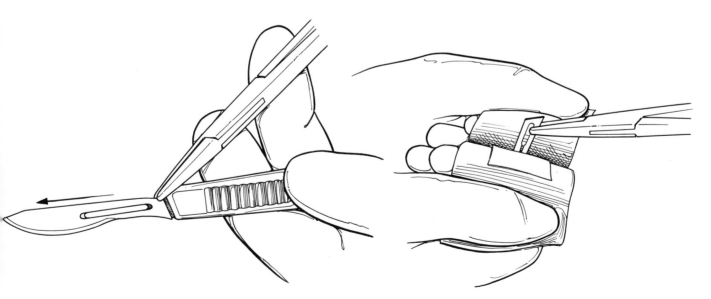

FIG. 3-3. *Removing the used scalpel blade.*

FIG. 3-4. *Aseptic technique for handling new blade.*

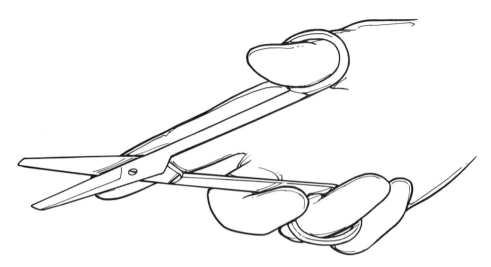

FIG. 3-5. *Correct way to hold scissors.*

for cutting suture material; one of the various types of suture scissors should be used instead.

Bandage scissors are an essential part of large animal surgery instrumentation, especially in equine limb surgery, in which the areas to be treated are commonly under bandage, and much of one's day may be spent changing bandages on horses' limbs. Some bandage scissors have slightly angled blades, and the lower blade has a small "button" tip on it to protect structures under the bandage. If bandage scissors are used against soiled or contaminated wounds, they must be sterilized after use to prevent transfer of infection to another wound or another patient.

Needle Holders (Needle Drivers)

During a large portion of an operation, the surgeon uses needle holders. The type of needle holder depends on individual tastes. Some needle holders, such as Olsen-Hegar or Gillies, have suture-cutting scissors incorporated into the jaws, to enable the surgeon to cut suture without reaching for suture-cutting scissors. These needle holders are useful in large animal practice where the surgeon is commonly on his own. Care must be taken to avoid cutting the suture accidentally during the procedure. There are many variations of width and serrations in the heads of the needle holders.

The needle holder is held as the surgeon would hold scissors, that is, with thumb and the ring finger in the rings of the handles. The needles used with needle holders are curved; straight needles are held by hand only and are usually reserved for the skin and bowel. With the needle holder, the needle should be driven through the tissues in an arc-like motion, following the curve of the needle. The needle holder is then removed and is reapplied to the protruding point of the needle, which is extracted from the tissue. The needle should be grasped by its thicker portion, rather than by the tip, because the tip may be easily bent or broken.

Some needle holders, such as Mathieu, have a ratchet on the handle that releases when additional pressure is applied to the spring handles. These are time-saving, but if the tissues resist passage of the needle, a firm grip cannot be applied to a needle without causing the needle holder to unsnap. Various types of needle holders are illustrated on pages 53 and 54.

Thumb Forceps

Thumb forceps are used for grasping and holding tissues. They are held between the thumb and the middle and index fingers. It is common for the inexperienced surgeon to hold thumb forceps incorrectly, like a scalpel handle, especially toward the end of the operation when fatigue is setting in. Thumb forceps are usually held in the left hand while the right hand holds the scalpel or needle holder. Thumb forceps with teeth bite into tissue and prevent the instrument from slipping. Some surgeons consider these forceps too traumatic for use on hollow organs or blood vessels and reserve them for skin. Thumb forceps are illustrated on page 54.

Grasping Forceps

A variety of forceps used for larger portions of tissue maintain their hold with the use of a ratchet device on the handle. Allis tissue forceps have opposing edges with short teeth. They may be used for grasping tissues such as fascia and tendon, but they should not be used on skin edges or viscera. Vulsellum forceps are useful for grasping the uterine walls of the various large animal species, to stabilize the walls during closure. Sponge forceps are used in the inguinal approach for cryptorchidism, to grasp the vaginal process. Towelholding forceps (clamps) are useful for grasping skin edges, as well as for holding drapes in position.

Hemostatic Forceps

Hemostatic forceps are used to clamp the ends of blood vessels and thereby to establish hemostasis. They vary not only in size, but in the shape and direction of the serrations. Halsted mosquito forceps are used for clamping small vessels.

When larger vessels are encountered, Kelly forceps may be more suitable. The amount of tissue crushed should be kept to a minimum. Hemostatic forceps are frequently used in conjunction with electrocautery. When ligating bleeding points, the tips of the instruments should be elevated to facilitate passage of the ligature. Curved hemostats should be affixed with the curved jaws pointing upward. If a scrubbed assistant is present during an operation, he should pass the instruments by slapping them handles first into the hands of the surgeon (Fig. 3-6).

It is not within the scope of this chapter to describe the applications of more than a few forceps. A variety of the forceps used in large animal practice are shown on pages 62 and 63.

Retractors

Retractors are used to maintain exposure at various surgical sites. Handheld retractors are held by an assistant. If the surgeon does not have the luxury of an assistant, as is often the case in large animal practice, then self-retaining retractors can be used. Self-retaining retractors anchor themselves

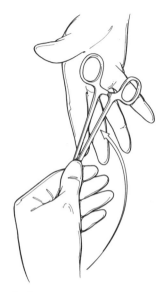

Fig. 3-6. *Passing hemostatic forceps.*

against the wound edges by maintaining fixed pressure on the retractor arms. When abdominal or thoracic retractors are used, moist sponges or towels are placed between the retractor blades and the tissues to minimize trauma to the wound edges. Examples of handheld retractors are United States Army retractors, malleable retractors, Volkmann retractors, Jansen retractors, and Senn retractors. Among the self-retaining retractors, Weitlaner retractors and Gelpi retractors are useful for small incisions, such as laryngotomy and arthrotomy incisions in the horse. The large Balfour retractors are predominantly used in laparotomy incisions. Occasionally, if thoracotomy is indicated, Finochietto rib retractors are the instrument of choice. Retractors are illustrated on pages 56 to 58.

Standard Set of Instruments

Listed below is a standard set of instruments routinely used by us. Such a set of instruments suffices for most basic procedures. In the remainder of the text, only instruments needed in addition to these are listed as each individual procedure is described. Instruments in this standard set are:

16 Towel forceps
 4 Curved mosquito hemostats
 4 Straight mosquito hemostats
 2 Curved Kelly forceps
 2 Straight Kelly forceps
 2 Allis tissue forceps
 1 Curved Mayo scissors
 1 Straight Mayo scissors
 1 S/S operating scissors (sharp/sharp)
 1 Curved Metzenbaum scissors
 1 Straight Metzenbaum scissors
 2 Needle holders (1 Mayo-Hegar, 1 Snowden-Pencer)

2 Right-angle forceps
1 Curved 6″ Ochsner forceps
1 Straight 6″ Ochsner forceps
1 No. 3 scalpel handle
1 No. 4 scalpel handle
3 3″ × 4″ thumb tissue forceps
2 1″ × 2″ Adson tissue forceps
1 Sponge forceps (curved or straight)
1 Grooved director
1 Saline bowl
4 Towels
Sponges in inverted bowl

Preparation of Instruments

The classification of the surgical procedure as clean, clean-contaminated, contaminated-dirty may influence how the surgeon prepares the surgical instruments. To illustrate, we obviously do not advocate that the instruments used to castrate piglets all be individually wrapped and sterilized. Yet for some of the *clean* surgical procedures described in this book, the use of instruments that have been "cold" sterilized may be construed as malpractice.

As part of overall planning, all the necessary instruments for the particular procedure should be obtained and prepared prior to the operation. In most cases, the surgeon must attend to his own needs for instruments and so must be able to anticipate the necessity for particular instruments.

Autoclaving, a sterilization technique using moist heat from steam, is the method of choice for preparing instruments for aseptic surgery. Once the packs are open, it is the surgeon's responsibility to be sure that the autoclaving process has reached all the instruments by observing the indicator system used to ensure sterility.

Gas sterilization with ethylene oxide gas is used for instruments that would be damaged by the heat of autoclaving. Materials that have been sterilized with ethylene oxide must be aerated for 1 to 7 days, depending on the material; otherwise, residual gas may diffuse from the goods and may irritate living tissues.

Cold (chemical) sterilization is commonly used by large animal surgeons in practice for preparation of instruments. The instruments are soaked in one of the commercially available solutions for whatever time and at whatever concentration recommended by the manufacturer. Some of these solutions can be irritating to tissues, so care must be taken not to transfer excessive amounts of the solution into the surgical site. This method of instrument sterilization or disinfection is recommended for multiple surgical procedures, such as dehorning and castration.

Boiling the instruments is also a popular method used by the large animal surgeon. Boiling can be used for contaminated and dirty surgery. In an emergency, it can be used for clean-contaminated surgery, but it is not recommended for clean surgery. The boiling process also dulls sharpened instruments, although with disposable scalpel blades, this problem is not serious.

General Surgical Instruments

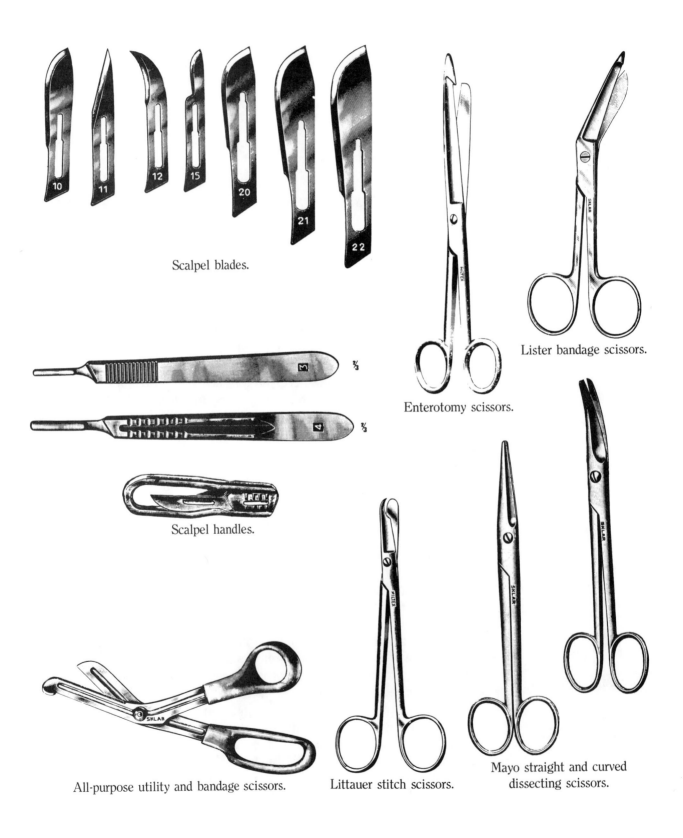

Scalpel blades.

Scalpel handles.

Enterotomy scissors.

Lister bandage scissors.

All-purpose utility and bandage scissors.

Littauer stitch scissors.

Mayo straight and curved dissecting scissors.

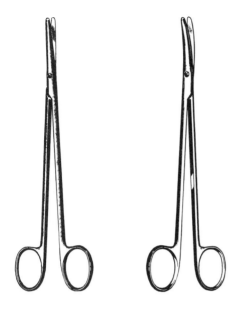

Metzenbaum straight and curved scissors.

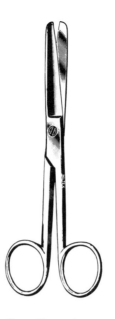

Operating scissors
with blunt/blunt
points.

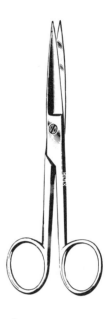

Operating scissors
with sharp/sharp
points.

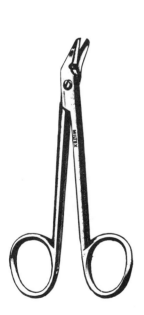

Wire-cutting scissors.

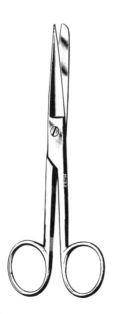

Operating scissors with
sharp/blunt points.

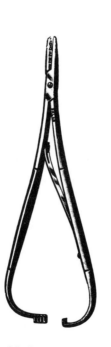

Mathieu needle
holder.

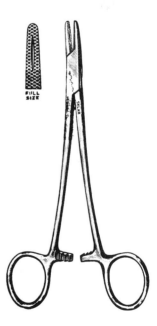

Mayo-Hegar needle holder.

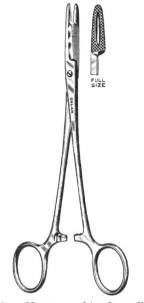

Olsen-Hegar combined needle
holder and scissors.

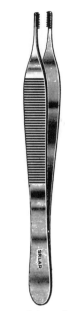

Brown-Adson forceps.

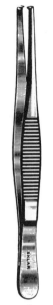

Tissue forceps.

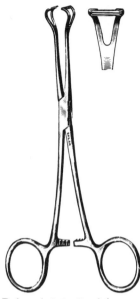

Babcock intestinal forceps.

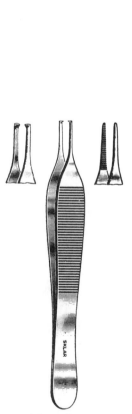

Adson forceps.

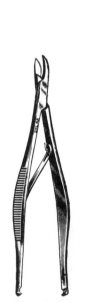

Michel clip
applying-and-removing
forceps.

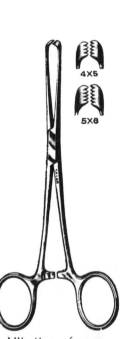

Allis tissue forceps.

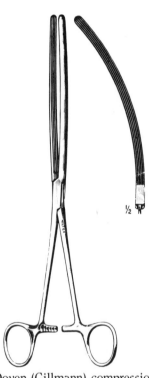

Doyen (Gillmann) compression
forceps.

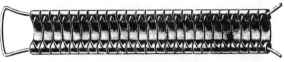

Michel clips.

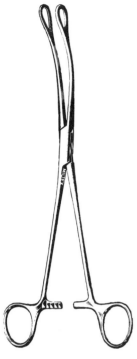

Foerster curved sponge
forceps.

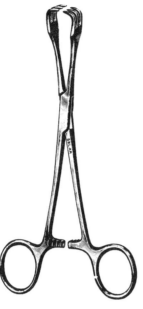

Lahey traction forceps.

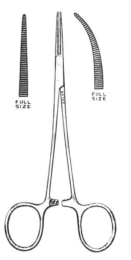

Crile straight and curved
hemostatic forceps.

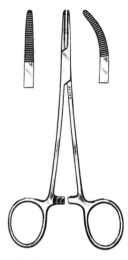

Kelly straight and
curved forceps.

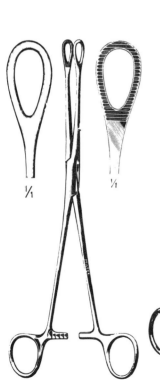

Foerster straight sponge
forceps.

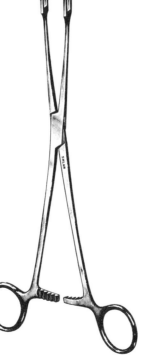

Vulsellum forceps.

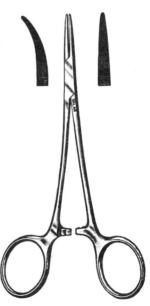

Halsted mosquito straight
and curved forceps.

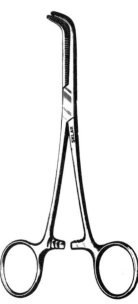

Mixter curved hemostatic
forceps.

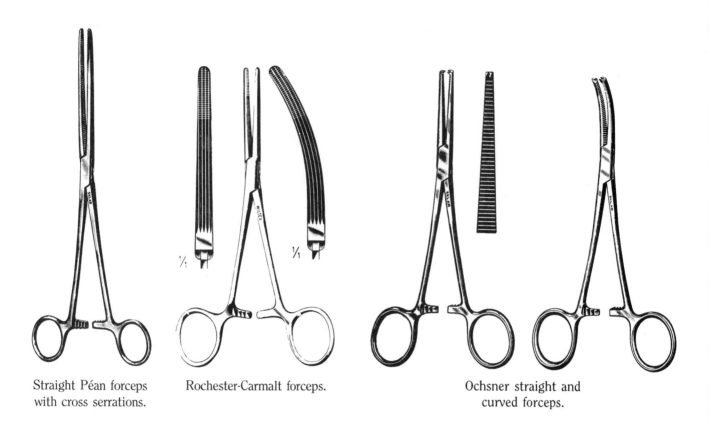

Straight Péan forceps
with cross serrations.

Rochester-Carmalt forceps.

Ochsner straight and
curved forceps.

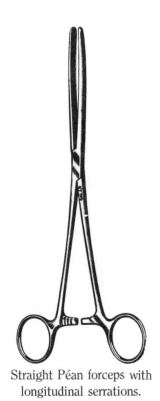

Straight Péan forceps with
longitudinal serrations.

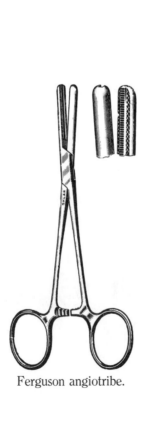

Ferguson angiotribe.

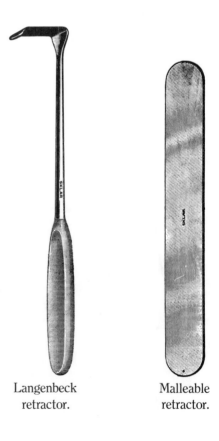

Langenbeck
retractor.

Malleable
retractor.

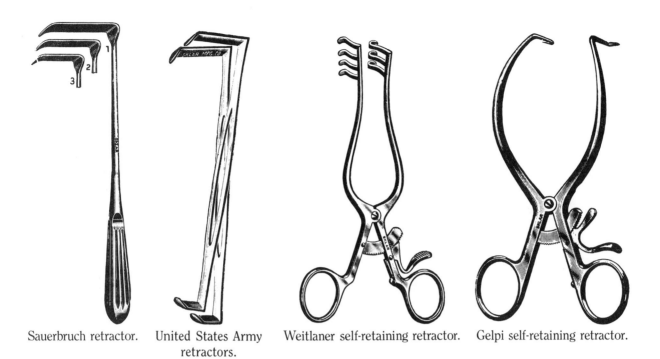

Sauerbruch retractor.   United States Army   Weitlaner self-retaining retractor.   Gelpi self-retaining retractor.
                            retractors.

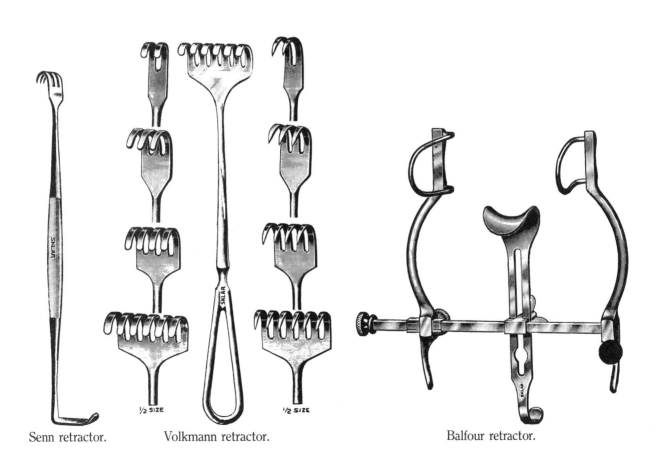

Senn retractor.   Volkmann retractor.   Balfour retractor.

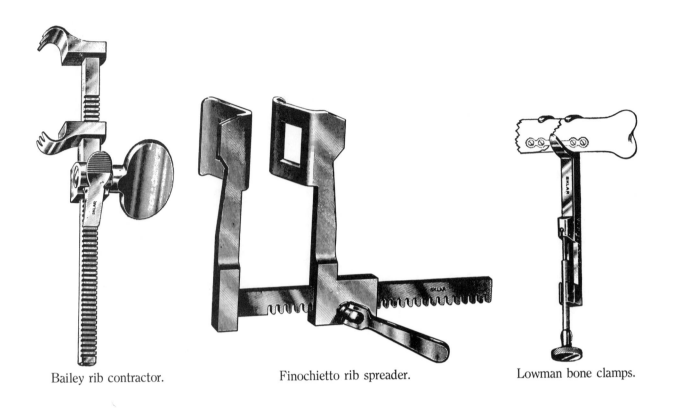

Bailey rib contractor.

Finochietto rib spreader.

Lowman bone clamps.

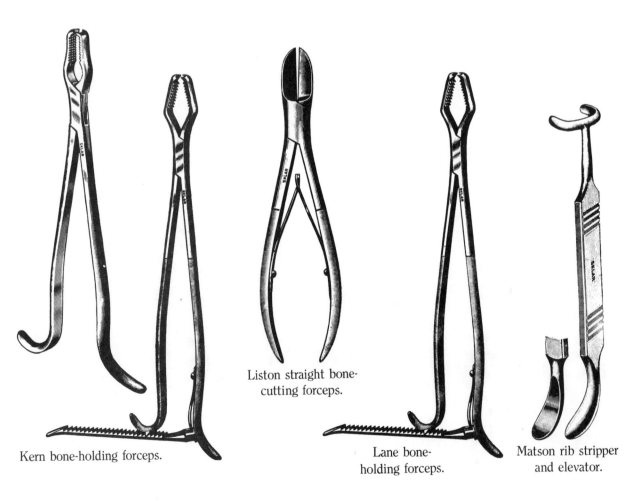

Kern bone-holding forceps.

Liston straight bone-cutting forceps.

Lane bone-holding forceps.

Matson rib stripper and elevator.

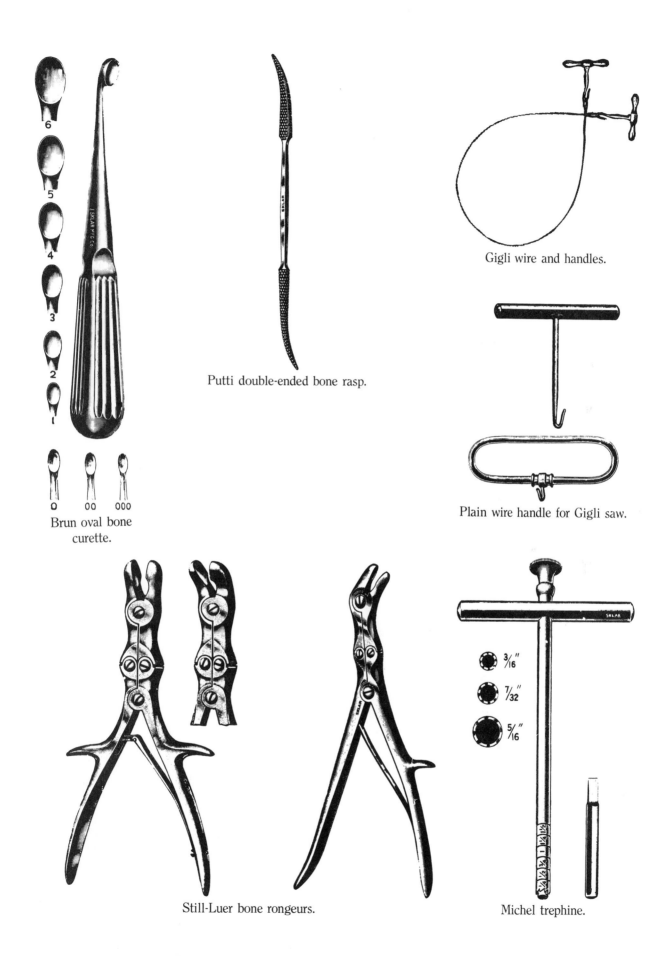

Brun oval bone
curette.

Putti double-ended bone rasp.

Gigli wire and handles.

Plain wire handle for Gigli saw.

Still-Luer bone rongeurs.

Michel trephine.

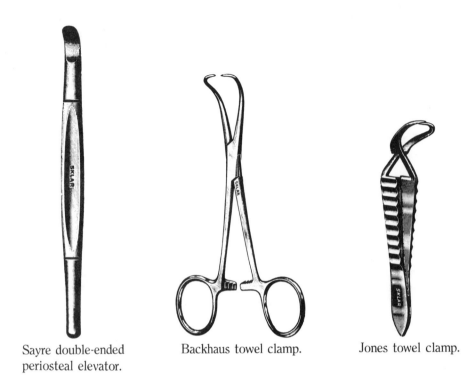

Sayre double-ended
periosteal elevator.

Backhaus towel clamp.

Jones towel clamp.

Castrating knife with
hook blade.

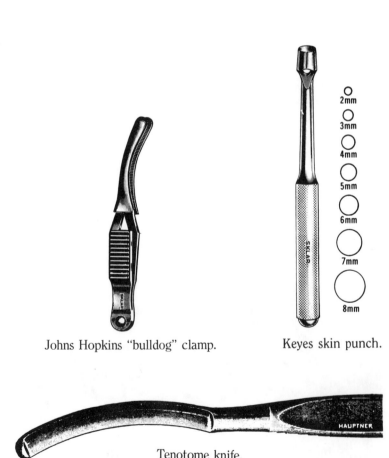

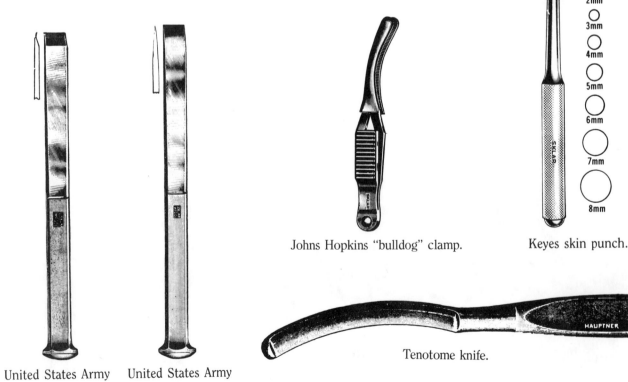

Johns Hopkins "bulldog" clamp.

Keyes skin punch.

2mm
3mm
4mm
5mm
6mm
7mm
8mm

United States Army
chisel.

United States Army
osteotome.

Tenotome knife.

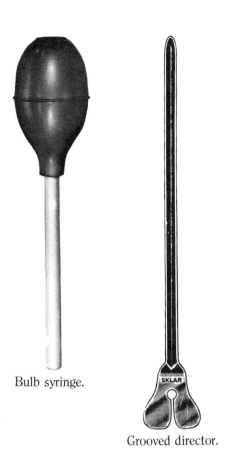

Bulb syringe.

Grooved director.

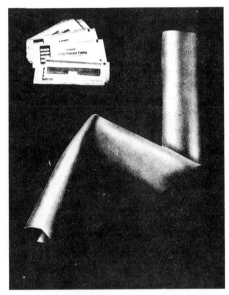

Penrose tubing.

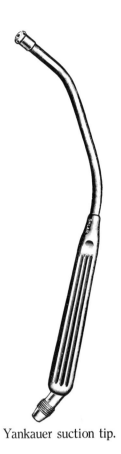

Yankauer suction tip.

Instruments Used Specifically in Large Animal Surgery

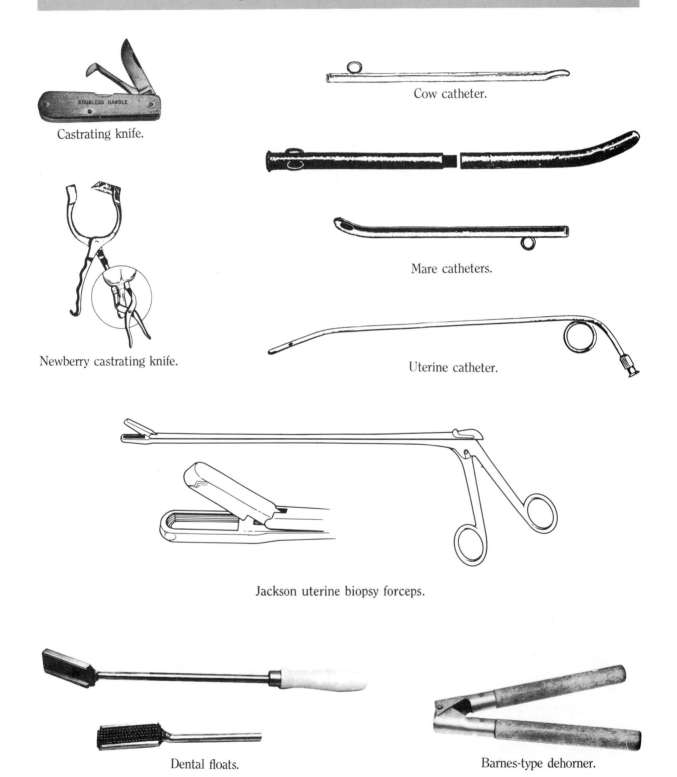

Castrating knife.

Cow catheter.

Newberry castrating knife.

Mare catheters.

Uterine catheter.

Jackson uterine biopsy forceps.

Dental floats.

Barnes-type dehorner.

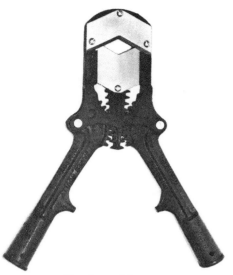

Keystone dehorner.

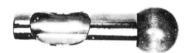

Tube dehorner.

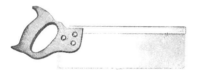

Dehorning saw.

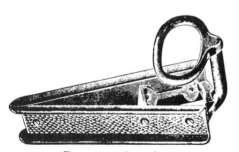

Bayer mouth wedge.

Straight dental punch.

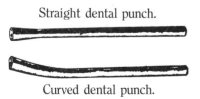

Curved dental punch.

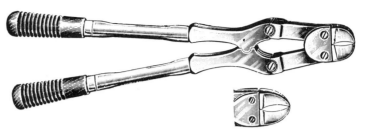

Equine molar cutter.

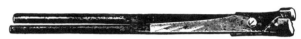

Equine molar forceps.

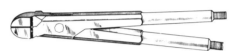

Closed, drop-jaw molar cutter.

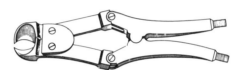

Drop-jaw multiple molar cutter.

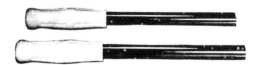

Interchangeable steel handles for foregoing dental instruments.

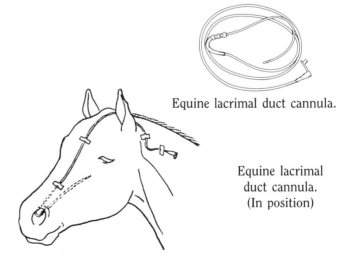

Equine lacrimal duct cannula.

Equine lacrimal
duct cannula.
(In position)

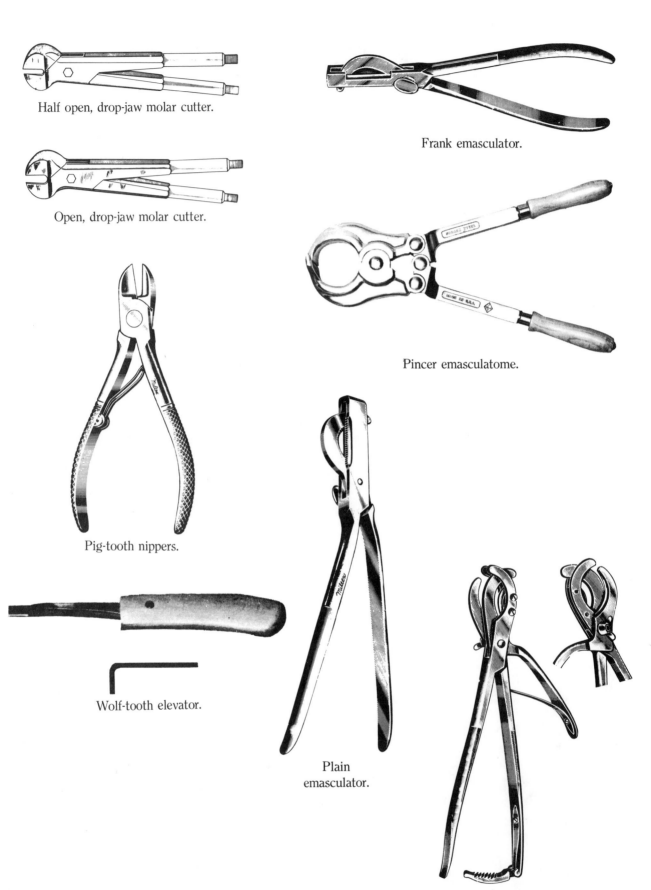

Half open, drop-jaw molar cutter.

Open, drop-jaw molar cutter.

Frank emasculator.

Pincer emasculatome.

Pig-tooth nippers.

Wolf-tooth elevator.

Plain
emasculator.

Reimer emasculator.

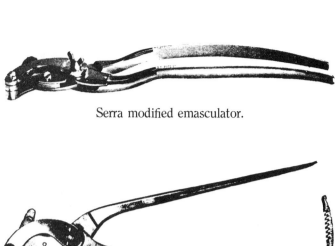

Serra modified emasculator.

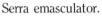

Serra emasculator.

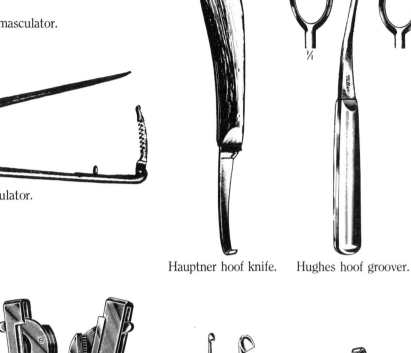

Hauptner hoof knife.   Hughes hoof groover.

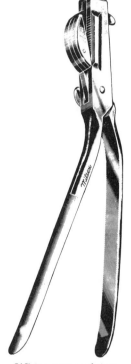

White emasculator.

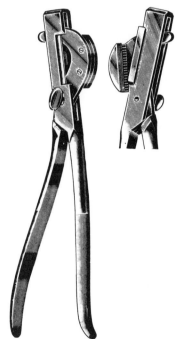

White modified emasculator.

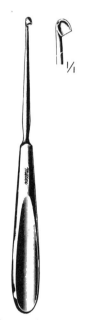

Hughes nail-hole curette.

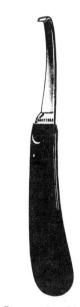

German hoof knife.

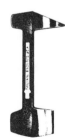

Clinch cutter (hoof buffer).

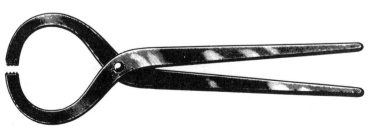

Large hoof tester.

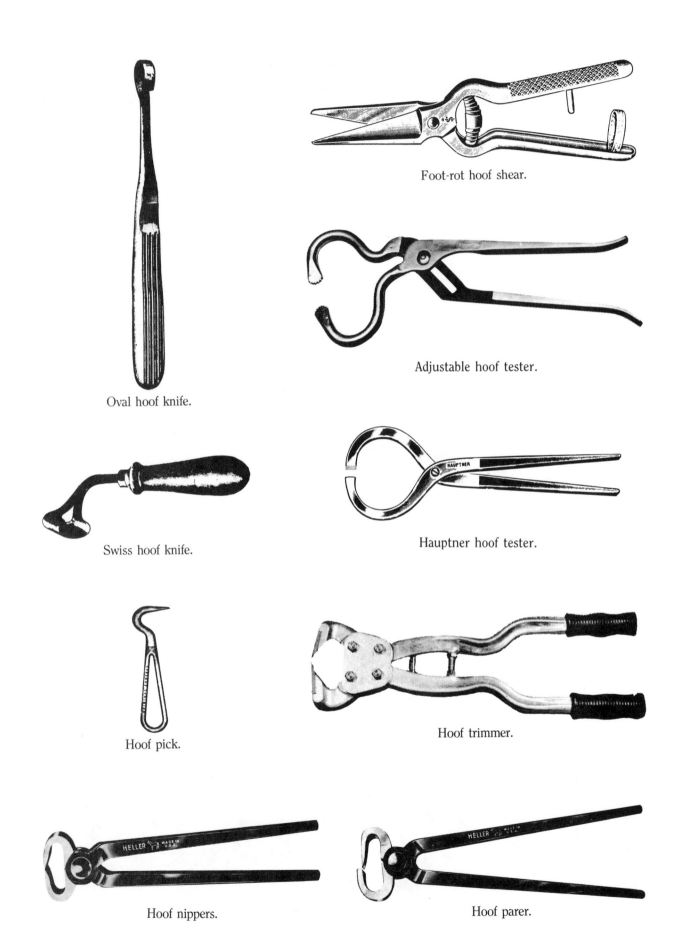

Foot-rot hoof shear.

Oval hoof knife.

Adjustable hoof tester.

Swiss hoof knife.

Hauptner hoof tester.

Hoof pick.

Hoof trimmer.

Hoof nippers.

Hoof parer.

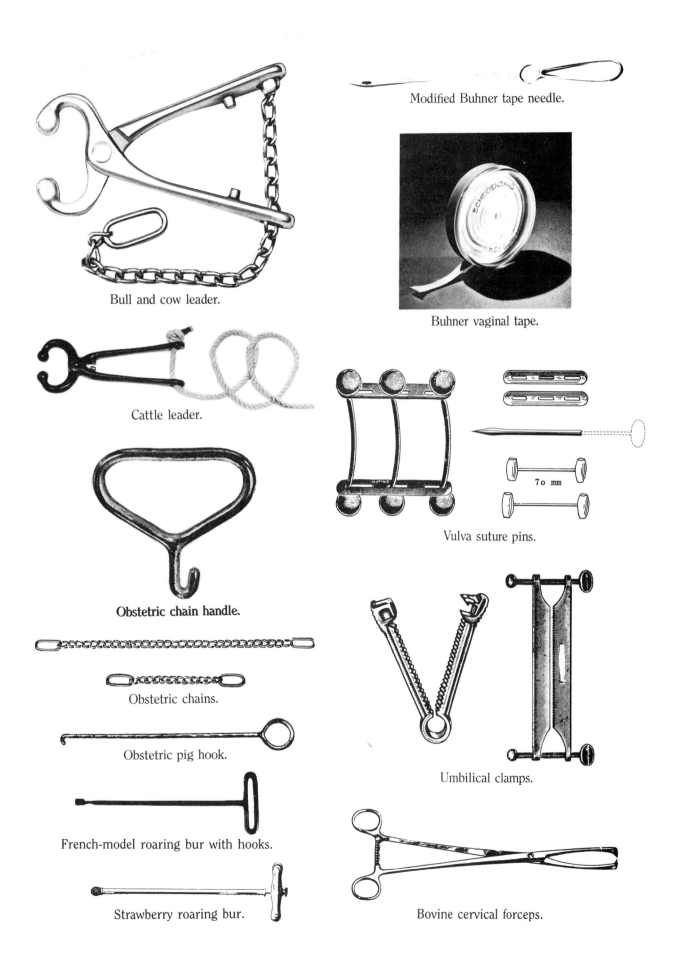

Bull and cow leader.

Modified Buhner tape needle.

Buhner vaginal tape.

Cattle leader.

Vulva suture pins.

Obstetric chain handle.

Obstetric chains.

Obstetric pig hook.

Umbilical clamps.

French-model roaring bur with hooks.

Strawberry roaring bur.

Bovine cervical forceps.

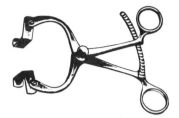

Hobday's roaring retractor.

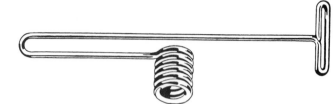

Equine speculum by Schoupe.

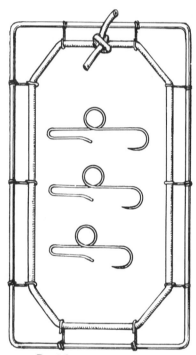

Danish rumenotomy set.

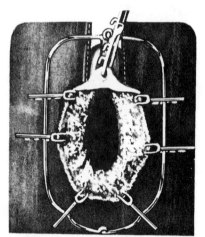

Weingart's rumenotomy set.

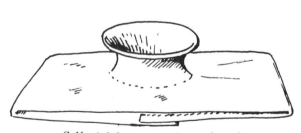

Self-retaining rumenotomy shroud.

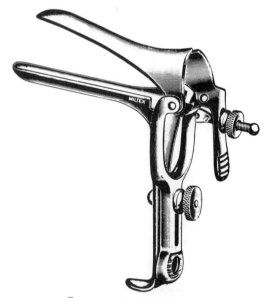

Graves vaginal speculum.

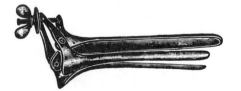

Thoroughbred vaginal speculum.

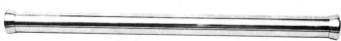

Frick cattle speculum.

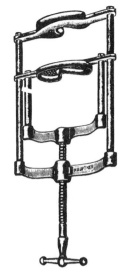

Hauptner's Guenther mouth
speculum.

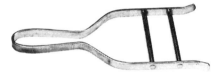

Heavy-swine mouth speculum.

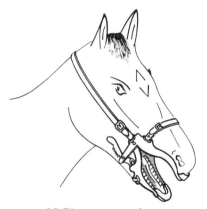

McPherson speculum.

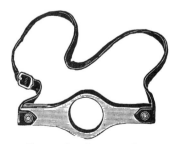

Stomach-tube speculum.

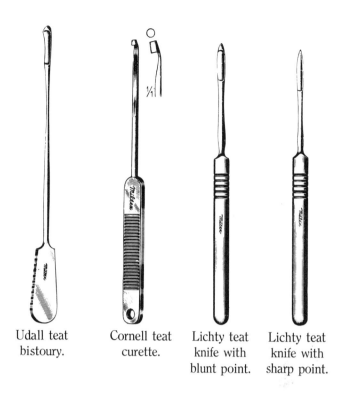

Udall teat
bistoury.

Cornell teat
curette.

Lichty teat
knife with
blunt point.

Lichty teat
knife with
sharp point.

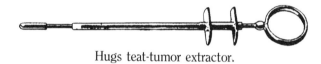

Hugs teat-tumor extractor.

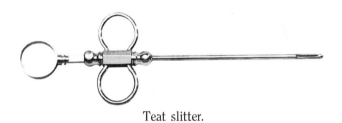

Teat slitter.

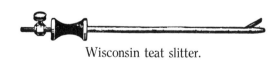

Wisconsin teat slitter.

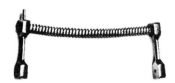

Canine mouth gag (for llama tooth extraction).

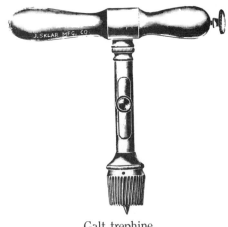

Galt trephine.

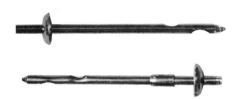

Dr. Larson's plastic teat tube.

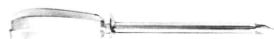

Milking tubes.

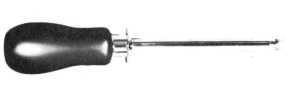

Trocar and cannulas.

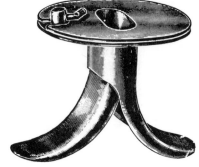

Trachea tube.

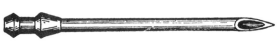

Bleeding trocar.

Tracheotomy tube.

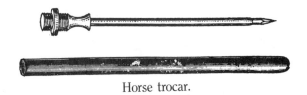

Horse trocar.

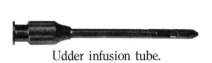

Udder infusion tube.

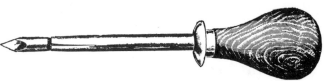

Wood-handle cattle trocar.

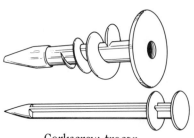

Corkscrew trocar.

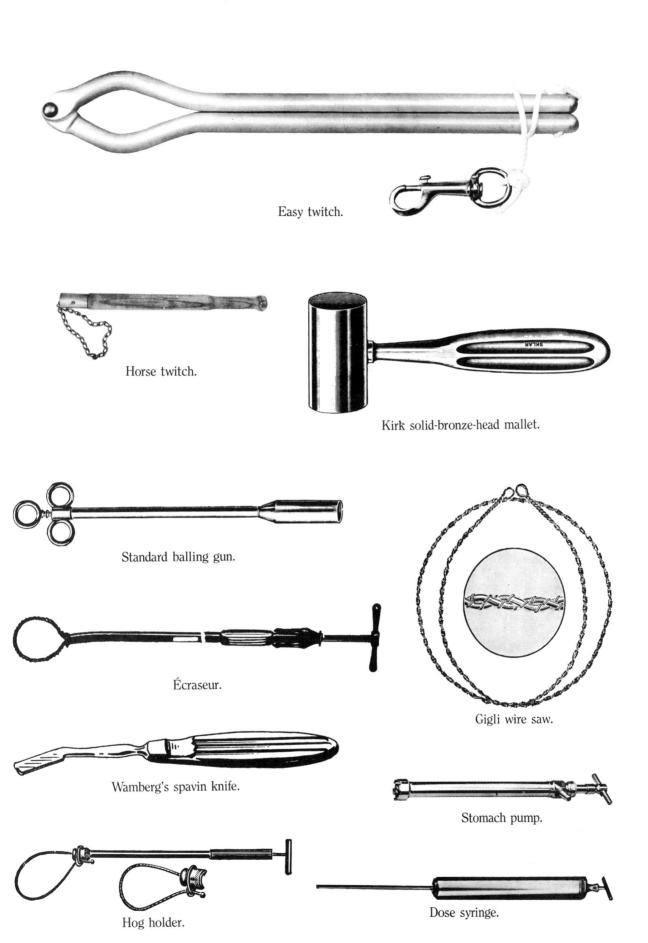

Easy twitch.

Horse twitch.

Kirk solid-bronze-head mallet.

Standard balling gun.

Écraseur.

Gigli wire saw.

Wamberg's spavin knife.

Stomach pump.

Hog holder.

Dose syringe.

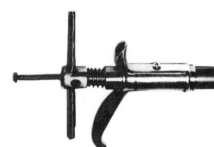

Kimberling-Rupp spaying device.

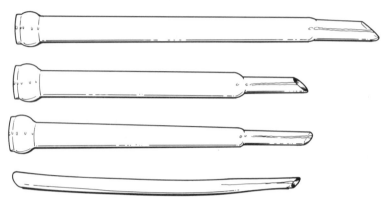

Cole pattern endotracheal tubes.

Equipment Used for Fluid Therapy in Large Animal Surgery

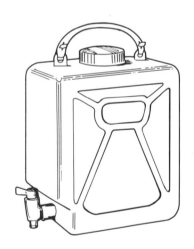

Carboy, rectangular, with spigot.

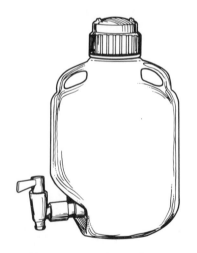

Carboy, screwneck, with spigot.

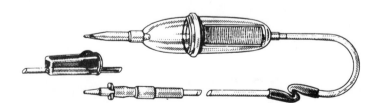

Disposable blood transfusion and infusion set.

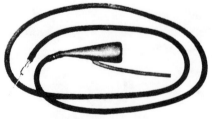

Intravenous set.

4

SUTURE
MATERIALS
AND NEEDLES

Suture Materials

Sutures and ligatures are fundamental to any surgical technique because they maintain approximation of tissues as the wound heals. All sutures should maintain their strength until the wound has healed. The ideal suture material should elicit minimal tissue reaction, not create a situation favorable for bacterial growth, and it should be nonelectrolytic, noncapillary, non-allergenic, and noncarcinogenic. It should be comfortable for the surgeon to handle and should hold knots securely without cutting or fraying. In large animal surgery, suture materials must also be economical to use. This point is often overlooked by new graduates who are eager to "try out" new suture materials without considering their cost. Needless to say, the ideal suture material has not been found and probably never will be; therefore, the surgeon must be familiar with the advantages and disadvantages of the various materials, and the selection of sutures should be based on scientific reasons, rather than on habit or tradition.

It is not the purpose of this chapter to present all the suture materials available, but rather, to discuss the salient features of those commonly encountered in large animal practice. We have found that good surgeons, whether oriented to large or small animal practice, use a small variety of suture material. They learn the limitations, indications, and contraindications of these sutures, so they are able to adapt them to differing situations. Above all, they learn that, in most situations, the surgical technique is more important than the suture material.

Clinical Application of Sutures

The selection of suture type and size is determined by the purpose of the suture, as well as by its biologic properties in the various tissues. Unfortunately, there is a paucity of information on the reaction of different suture materials to the various tissues of large animal species. Therefore, much of the information presented here is extrapolated from studies of small animals, laboratory animals, and man. Veterinary surgeons deal with larger, more uncooperative patients than do their counterparts in human surgery; this often necessitates the use of a suture of greater durability and strength.[7] The surgeon must take into account the rate of healing of the particular tissue because wounds of different tissues achieve maximal strength at different times. For example, visceral wounds heal rapidly, as do superficial wounds around the head. The surgeon must also consider whether infection or drainage will be likely. Catgut, for example, disappears more rapidly in the face of infection because of an increase in the local phagocytic activity. On the other hand, a braided synthetic material must be used under aseptic conditions (uncommon in much of large animal surgery), because once infection occurs, the material will become a nidus and will actually harbor bacteria. If strength is required for a long period of time, as during the healing of a fascial wound, for example, then the use of a braided synthetic may be a calculated risk. The presence of crystalloids is also a factor in choosing a suture material; for example, a nonabsorbable suture used in the bladder wall represents a foreign body conducive to urinary calculus formation. An absorbable suture would be a better choice, but even some absorbable sutures initiate stone formation in certain species.[6] Other factors influencing the choice of suture are the surgeon's training, experience, judgment, and habits.

Once the surgeon has chosen what he believes to be the best type of suture material, he must consider the size of the suture. The holding power of the tissue is the factor that usually determines the size of the suture material. Although all sutures enhance the development of infection, larger sutures retard wound healing and create a foreign-body reaction that is greater than the reaction caused by sutures with a smaller diameter.

The number of sutures placed in a wound is another consideration. As each new suture is placed in a wound, the stress on the other sutures decreases. In regard to wound healing, it is better to increase the number of sutures than to increase the size of the suture.[11] Sutures that are placed too far apart lead to poor apposition of the wound edges and contribute to dehiscence.[11,16] Generally speaking, sutures should be as far from each other as the sutures are wide (tension sutures for secondary support are an exception); however, in thicker-skinned areas, the spacing between the sutures may be increased.[16] The sutures must bite the correct amount of tissue and should not be placed too tightly. Too much tension with sutures delays wound healing by causing ischemia at the wound edges. If the bite in the tissue is too small, the suture will cut through the tissues, and dehiscence may occur.

Knotting the suture is the next important consideration. The knot is the weakest point of a suture loop and actually decreases the strength of the suture material. Variations in knot type are more important than variations in suture material and thread dimensions.[17] Good-quality knots are essential to any surgical procedure; unfortunately, a surgeon's performance decreases with time because of boredom or fatigue.[10] The reader is referred to Chapter 5, "Knots and Ligatures."

Absorbable Sutures

Suture materials have traditionally been divided into two categories: absorbable and nonabsorbable sutures. Suture materials can also be subdivided into multifilament and monofilament sutures. Absorbable sutures begin to be digested or hydrolyzed by the patient during healing of the wound and continue to disappear when the wound has healed.

SURGICAL GUT (CATGUT)

Catgut is one of the most frequently used suture materials in veterinary surgery, and it is especially popular with large animal surgeons. It consists mainly of collagen obtained from the submucosa of sheep intestine or from the serosa of beef intestine. It is packaged in at least 85% alcohol, is sterilized with gamma irradiation, and cannot be resterilized once the package is open.

Catgut may be plain or chromic. Plain catgut loses its strength so rapidly that its use in certain regions may be contraindicated. Chromic catgut is produced by exposure to basic chromium salts. This process increases the intermolecular bonding and results in greater strength, decreased reaction in tissues, and slower absorption. Catgut is further classified according to the degree of chromicization: type A (plain) is untreated; type B has mild treatment; type C has medium treatment; and type D (extra chromic catgut) has prolonged treatment.

The subject's reaction to catgut is variable, but in general, plain catgut loses its strength in 3 to 7 days. Catgut is gradually digested by acid proteases from inflammatory cells and may be used when a suture is needed for only a week or two and absorption is desirable. The rate of absorption varies, depending on where the catgut is implanted and, to some extent, on the size of the suture. It is rapidly absorbed if it is implanted in regions with a greater blood supply. Similarly, it is absorbed rapidly if exposed to gastric juices or other organ enzymes. Catgut may be used in the presence of infection; however, the increased environment for enzyme digestion causes it to be absorbed rapidly.

Catgut handles well and possesses some elasticity. Three throws are required for knotting, and, when wet, the knot-holding ability decreases. The ends should be left slightly longer than other types of suture material, to minimize the chances of untying. Despite the advent of synthetic absorbable sutures, catgut is still a popular suture material in large animal surgery and will remain so even if for purely economic reasons.

COLLAGEN

Collagen is a suture material related to catgut. It is produced from the flexor tendons of steers, is smoother and more uniform than catgut, and has less tendency to fray. It is occasionally used in ophthalmic surgery.

POLYGLYCOLIC ACID AND POLYGLACTIN 910

In our experience, the synthetic absorbable suture materials, polyglycolic acid (Dexon) and polyglactin 910 (Vicryl), have, with few exceptions, replaced catgut. Both these materials have become increasingly popular in large and small animal surgery, yet reports in the literature of their use in veterinary medicine are scarce.[7]

These materials are both polymers that are extruded as filaments. Polyglycolic acid is a polymer of glycolic acid (hydroacetic acid), whereas polyglactin 910 is a polymer containing glycolic acid and lactic acid in a ratio of 90 to 10. Both compounds differ from catgut in their reaction in tissues. They are invaded by macrophages, yet their disappearance is independent of the local cellular reaction. Both compounds are hydrolyzed into natural body metabolites, rather than absorbed by an enzymatic process. The breaking strength of polyglycolic acid and polyglactin 910 diminishes more or less in a straight line, when compared to the almost exponential decline of the strength of catgut in tissues. This characteristic disappearance pattern was the main reason for the introduction of these synthetic materials, because they are more consistent and reliable in this regard than catgut. Because neither of these suture materials contains protein, they are both nonantigenic.[5] Unlike catgut, they do not swell when wet. These materials have a low coefficient of friction, and it is necessary to use a surgeon's knot with multiple throws to prevent slippage or untying of the knots. Both polyglycolic acid and polyglactin 910 handle much like silk. One disadvantage of these suture materials is that they tend to drag through tissues and cut soft organs; this property has prompted the manufacturers to coat them with an absorbable lubricant to make them smoother, to decrease pulling, and to improve overall handling.[1,4]

Polyglactin 910 is now coated with equal parts of a copolymer of glycolide and lactide (polyglactin 370) and calcium stereate (coated Vicryl). Polyglycolic acid is now constructed of filaments finer than the original suture, to provide better handling and smoother passage through the tissues (Dexon-S). The newer designs of the suture materials have not altered their reactivity or other biologic properties. We have used both coated Vicryl and Dexon-S, but we cannot tell what effect this has had on the eventual outcome of the case. Tissue drag can be considered an advantage in some situations, however, because the suture will not slide out of the tissue when the surgeon is placing continuous suture patterns. Polyglycolic acid has been used successfully for closure of skin wounds in man as well as in large and small animals.[7,9]

POLYDIOXANONE

Polydioxanone (PDS) is a synthetic monofilament suture material that has become recently available. It is a polymer of paradioxanone. Like polyglycolic acid and polyglactin 910, it is degraded by hydrolysis in a predictable manner, although more slowly. It also causes the same tissue reaction as these other suture materials. Because it is a monofilament, it is theoretically better in an infected wound because it is less likely to harbor bacteria.[3,8] It also has less tissue drag; however, polyglycolic acid and polyglactin 910 are now made in a smoother form to minimize these problems. We and our colleagues have used PDS in the horse. We do not like the "memory" of this suture, however, and suture extrusion has also occurred. (See Page 77 for further discussion of "memory.") We are also aware of breakage and dehiscence when no. 2 PDS is used.

Nonabsorbable Sutures

Nonabsorbable sutures retain their tensile strength for longer than 60 days and may remain in situ indefinitely, even though they may be altered slightly.

SILK

Silk, a continuous protein filament produced by silkworms, is the traditional nonabsorbable suture. It is braided, dyed, and coated with wax or silicone. Silk is popular in human surgery despite the availability of synthetic materials that are biologically superior. In our practice, its use is minimal; it is popular with some veterinary surgeons, however, and its superb handling quality the standard for the producers of the synthetic suture materials. It has good knot-holding properties as well. Silk possesses capillary action, which means it should not be used in the presence of infection because it will provide a refuge for bacteria and will result in a nidus of infection. Although grouped as a nonabsorbable suture, silk loses its strength slowly and disappears several years later. Its use in large animal practice is confined mainly to skin closure and ophthalmologic procedures. It is used by some surgeons for closure of joint capsules following arthrotomy in the horse, and it is still an excellent material for anastomosis of blood vessels (rare in large animal practice), although the newer synthetic sutures are becoming popular for this purpose.

COTTON

The most common application of cotton in large animal practice is as umbilical tape. Cotton is the twisted yarn from the filament of the cotton plant. It handles well, but produces more tissue reaction than silk. Cotton potentiates infection because it harbors bacteria, and the fistulation that may result resolves only when the offending suture material has been removed. Nevertheless, cotton is a useful, economical suture material in a variety of situations, especially those involving food animals. It has been used as a suture in the perineal region for prolapses of the uterus, vagina, and rectum.

NYLON

Nylon (Dermalon, Ethilon) is a long-chain polymer available in monofilament and multifilament forms. It is most commonly used in the monofilament form. Nylon is a stiff suture that should be stretched out following its removal from the manufacturer's packet. This property is called "memory," and it is defined as the suture's ability to resist bending forces and to return to its original configuration. As a result, nylon and, to a lesser extent, polypropylene are difficult to knot securely. The additional throws required for security produce a bulky knot. Nylon is relatively inert when implanted in tissues; a thin connective tissue capsule is produced around the suture, and this characteristic is one of its major advantages when it is used as a buried suture. Nylon loses a slight amount of strength initially, after which no appreciable diminution in strength is noted. Because there are no interstices to harbor bacteria, the monofilament form of nylon fares better than multifilament sutures in the presence of infection.

Nylon is available in multifilament forms (Nurolon). Braiding this suture gives it some roughness to provide better knot retention and better handling characteristics than the monofilament form.

POLYPROPYLENE AND POLYETHYLENE

Polypropylene (Prolene) and polyethylene are polyolefins that are usually available in monofilament form. They are probably the most desirable of the monofilament sutures: they have greater knot security than nylon and are better to handle. Nevertheless, they are stiff and, like nylon, possess "memory," which results in poor knot retention. Multiple knots are required to ensure knot security. The first throw of a knot with polypropylene tends to slip unless tension is maintained. Polypropylene and polyethylene are among the least reactive suture materials and lose little strength in situ over a 2-year period. Both these suture materials are more suitable for use in infected wounds than the braided synthetic materials.

POLYMERIZED CAPROLACTAM

Polymerized caprolactam (Supramid, Vetafil) is a synthetic suture material used extensively in large and small animal practice. It is available for veterinary use only. The twisted fibers are made from a material related to nylon and coated to minimize capillarity.[14] Compared to catgut or silk, the material has a high tensile strength and causes little cellular reaction in tissues. Polymerized caprolactam is packaged in plastic dispenser bottles in which it is chemically sterilized; in this form, it is suitable for use in skin closure. Because of its smoothness, some knot slippage occurs with this material, and at least three knots are required for a safe tie.[16] In general, the material behaves like the other braided synthetics. The suture should not be used in the presence of infection, nor should the suture material be buried without its having been autoclaved. Either of these events can lead to the formation of a chronic draining tract that will not resolve until the suture is removed. For this reason, this material has been used primarily for skin suture. From the standpoint of economics, polymerized caprolactam has a useful place in large animal practice. Surprisingly, little has been written about its behavior in the tissues of domestic animals.

POLYESTERS

The polyesters consist of Dacron that has been coated or impregnated with various finishes. Tevdek and Ethiflex are Teflon-impregnated Dacron, whereas Polydek is Teflon-coated Dacron. Ethibond is Dacron coated with polybutylate, and Ticron is silicone-impregnated Dacron. The suture is also available in uncoated forms (Mersilene and Dacron), but these sutures naturally have more tissue drag than the coated forms.[14] Coating or impregnating the suture decreases capillary action and tissue drag, but also reduces knot-holding ability. These materials need four throws all squared, or five throws (two slip and three squared).[10] The knot-holding ability varies within the group. These suture materials are unreactive when implanted in tissues, but the shedding of the Teflon coat increases the inflammatory response.[12] It is not known whether the shedding of the Teflon coat in the tissues of large animal species has any clinical significance; if it does, it is probably minor.

The polyesters are strong sutures and are used when prolonged strength is required. Because of the multifilament nature of this material, bacteria and tissue fluids can penetrate the interstices of the polyester sutures. This can produce a nidus of infection, converting contamination to infection. Immobile bacteria have been transported inside the suture material; this is more significant than the spread of infection on the surface of the suture material.[2] Consequently, these suture materials must be used under aseptic circumstances, circumstances that unfortunately may not always exist in large animal practice.

STAINLESS STEEL

Stainless steel is an alloy of iron (iron-nickel-chromium) and is available in multi- or monofilament forms. It is difficult to handle because it is easily kinked; yet it is the strongest of all suture materials. Stainless steel holds knots well, but the knots tend to be bulky. It is one of the most unreactive suture materials and can be repeatedly sterilized, but it has a tendency to cut tissues as well as surgeons' gloves. Unlike the braided synthetics, stainless steel does not harbor bacteria and can be used in the presence of infection. Its use in large animal practice is infrequent.

MICHEL CLIPS

Michel clips are short, malleable clips with points on the ends that are used to appose wound edges. A special pair of forceps is used to bend them, and they do tend to pucker the skin once they are applied. These clips are used infrequently in large animal practice, but have been used for Caslick's operation in mares.

SKIN STAPLING DEVICES

A disposable skin stapling device (Proximate) has become available for use in man. We have used it for the past 8 years for suturing the skin of horses following laparotomy for the surgical correction of colic. One advantage of the device is its speed: the instrument closes skin incisions that are up to 2-feet long in a minute or so. This factor is important when the survival of animals could be adversely affected by a longer anesthetic time. One study showed that the use of staples saved an average of 15.5 minutes of closing time per incision.[13] The staples are well tolerated by horses and can remain in the skin almost indefinitely.

Skin staples have been shown experimentally to be more resistant to abscess formation than percutaneous sutures. Because they are metallic, they do not provide an environment conducive to bacterial growth and they do not penetrate as deeply into the relatively avascular subcutaneous tissue plane. We have noticed excellent wound healing in uninfected wounds. In abdominal surgery in which the intestinal tract has been opened, the skin incision may have received an inoculum of bacteria prior to closure, and therefore skin staples would be of benefit.[15] A small pair of forceps is available for removal of the staples once the wound has healed. We have used staples in a variety of other skin incisions in horses and found them equally acceptable. The only limitation of the device is cost, although we have used it in situations such as colic surgery, in which the cost of the staples is a small part of the total bill. We have also used skin staples in calves, other small ruminants, and llamas, although economy is a limiting factor in these species.

References

1. Artandi, C.: A revolution in sutures. Surg. Gynecol. Obstet., *150*:235, 1980.

2. Blomstedt, B., Osterberg, B., and Gergstrand, A.: Suture material and bacterial transport. Acta Chir. Scand., *143*:71, 1977.

3. Chusak, R. B., and Dibbell, D. G.: Clinical experience with polydioxanone monofilament absorbable sutures in plastic surgery. Plast. Reconstr. Surg., *72*:217, 1983.

4. Conn, J., and Beal, J. M.: Coated Vicryl synthetic absorbable sutures. Surg. Gynecol. Obstet., *150*:843, 1980.

5. Craig, P. H., et al.: A biological comparison of polyglactin 910 and polyglycolic acid synthetic absorbable sutures. Surg. Gynecol. Obstet., *141*:1, 1975.

6. Kaminski, J. M., Katz, A. R., and Woodward, S. C.: Urinary bladder calculus formation on sutures in rabbits, cats and dogs. Surg. Gynecol. Obstet., *146*:353, 1978.

7. Larsen, R. F.: Polyglycolic acid sutures in general practice. N. Z. Vet. J., *26*:258, 1978.

8. Lerwick, E.: Studies on the efficacy and safety of polydioxanone monofilament absorbable suture. Surg. Gynecol. Obstet., *156*:51, 1983.

9. Mackinnon, A. E., and Brown, S.: Skin closure with polyglycolic acid (Dexon). Postgrad. Med. J., *54*:384, 1978.

10. Magilligan, D. J., and DeWeese, J. A.: Knot security and synthetic suture materials. Am. J. Surg., *127*:355, 1974.

11. Price, P. B.: Stress, strain and sutures. Ann. Surg., *128*:408, 1948.

12. Postlethwait, R. W.: Five-year study of tissue reaction to synthetic sutures. Ann. Surg., *190*:53, 1979.

13. Ramey, D. W., and Rooks, R. L.: Consider the use of skin stapling equipment to expedite equine surgery. Vet. Med., *80*:66, 1985.

14. Stashak, T. S., and Yturraspe, D. J.: Considerations for selection of suture materials. Vet. Surg., *7*:48, 1978.

15. Stillman, R. M., Marino, C. A., and Seligman, S. J.: Skin staples in potentially contaminated wounds. Arch. Surg., *119*:138, 1984.

16. Swaim, S.: Surgery of Traumatized Skin: Management and Reconstruction in the Dog and Cat. Philadelphia, W. B. Saunders, 1980.

17. Tera, H., and Aberg, C.: Strength of knots in surgery in relation to type of knot, type of suture material, and dimensions of suture thread. Acta Chir. Scand., *143*:75, 1977.

Needles

Surgical needles are essential for the placement of sutures in tissues. They must be designed to place the suture in the tissue with a minimum of trauma; they should be rigid enough to prevent bending, yet flexible enough to prevent breaking; and they must be sharp enough to penetrate tissues with the minimum of resistance. Naturally, they must be clean and resistant to corrosion. Of the many different types of needles available, the selection of the needle is determined by the type of tissue to be sutured, its location and accessibility, and the size of the suture material.

Surgical needles have three basic components: the eye, the body (or shaft), and the point. The eye is usually of two types, closed eye or swaged (eyeless). The closed eye is similar to a household sewing needle, and the eye itself is available in a variety of shapes. Swaged-on needles are permanently attached to the suture (Fig. 4-1). The suture and needle are of approximately the same diameter. The outstanding advantage of a swaged-on needle is that tissues are subjected to less trauma, because only a single strand, rather than a double strand, of suture is pulled through the tissue. In addition, handling of the suture and needle is minimal, and it is ready for immediate use. At the end of surgery, the needle and the remaining piece of suture are discarded, and dull needles are continually culled. Tying the suture to the eye of the needle lessens the possibility of separation, but further increases the trauma as the suture material is drawn through the tissue. With a suture needle named Control Release, the suture material can be rapidly separated from the needle.

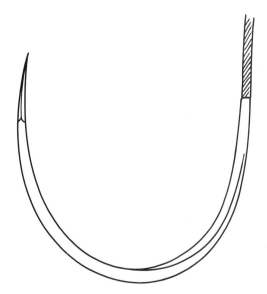

FIG. 4-1. *A swaged-on needle. The suture and needle have approximately the same diameters.*

Needles are usually curved, although some surgeons prefer to use straight needles, especially when suturing skin or bowel. Needles have a variable curvature, and they may be 1/4, 3/8, 1/2, 5/8 circle and half-curved (Fig. 4-2). Selection of a needle depends on the depth of the region to be sutured. When suturing deep in a wound, for example, the needle will have to "turn a sharp corner." In this case, a 1/2-circle or 5/8-circle needle would be most suitable. Curved needles must be used with needle holders.

The body of the needle is available in a number of different shapes: round, oval, flat, or triangular. Flat and triangular bodies have cutting edges; round or oval-bodied needles usually taper from the small diameter at the point to a larger diameter at the eye.

Needles are also available with varying types of points (Fig. 4-3). Cutting needles are designed to cut through dense, thick, connective tissue, such as bovine skin. Cutting needles can be reverse cutting, where the cutting edge is provided along the convex side of the needle, rather than on the concave surface. The purpose of a reverse-cutting needle is to minimize the excessive cutting of transfixed tissue. Another modification of the cutting needle combines the cutting point with a round needle shaft, so the needle will readily penetrate the dense tissue but not cut through it; this has been termed a Taper cut needle. One company manufactures a needle of similar concept that is useful in tough, dense tissues such as cartilage (Special K Needle). This needle readily penetrates the cartilage of the equine larynx.

Noncutting needles, or round needles, have no edges and are less likely to cut through tissues (Fig. 4-3). They are used for abdominal viscera, connective tissue, vessels, and other fragile tissues. Round (atraumatic) needles are actually round behind the tip, but the remaining portion of the shaft is oval. This design prevents angular or rotational displacement of the needle within the jaws of the needle holder.

Long-stemmed needles are also used in food animal practice. They are useful for placing heavy suture materials into the tissues, such as in vaginal prolapse in cattle.

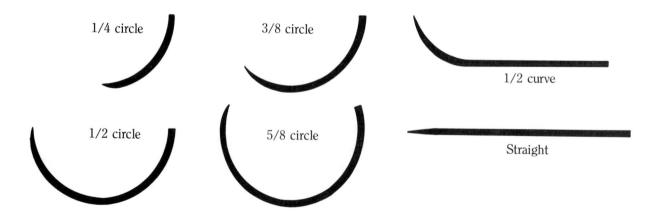

1/4 circle   3/8 circle

1/2 curve

1/2 circle   5/8 circle

Straight

FIG. 4-2. *Various needle shapes.*

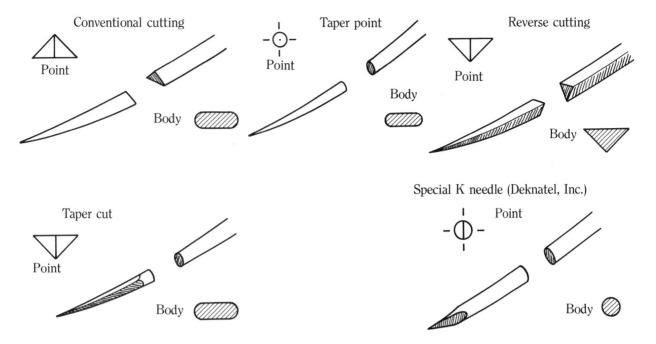

FIG. 4-3. *Various points and shaft designs of suture needles.*

5

KNOTS
AND
LIGATURES

Knots

Rapid and efficient knot tying is an essential part of any surgery. The student of surgery must continually strive to produce correct and secure knots with the desired amount of tension. The simplest knot that will perform the task should be used. This also means using the smallest size suture (without jeopardizing the strength of closure) and producing the smallest knot. This procedure reduces the amount of foreign material that the animal has to digest, extrude, or encapsulate.

Tying a secure knot is an important part of any surgical procedure. Knot failure may result in hemorrhage of major vessels, herniation, even evisceration and death. Suture ends should be cut short; however, the ends of catgut sutures should be left a little longer than other types of suture materials because they swell and untie. Generally speaking, the more secure the knot, the shorter the suture ends may be. "Sawing" (friction between the strands) frays the suture. If instruments such as clamps are to be applied to the suture, as in herniorrhaphy in foals and calves, they should not be applied to those parts of the suture material that will remain in situ.

Knotting Techniques

The square knot is the knot used most in surgery (Fig. 5-1). The knot is usually tied with needle holders, which should remain parallel to the wound, while all movements are made perpendicular to the wound. Uniform tension to the ends of the suture ensure that the knot ends up as a square and not as two half-hitches. Two half-hitches result from unequal tension on the two ends during tying (Fig. 5-1).

The granny knot is a slip knot that will not hold, especially if the strain on the ends is unequal, and its use is not recommended (Fig. 5-1).[3] Knots that tighten when the second throw is pressed home, as well as knots that end a continuous suture in which two strands are tied to one, are also prone to slippage.[1]

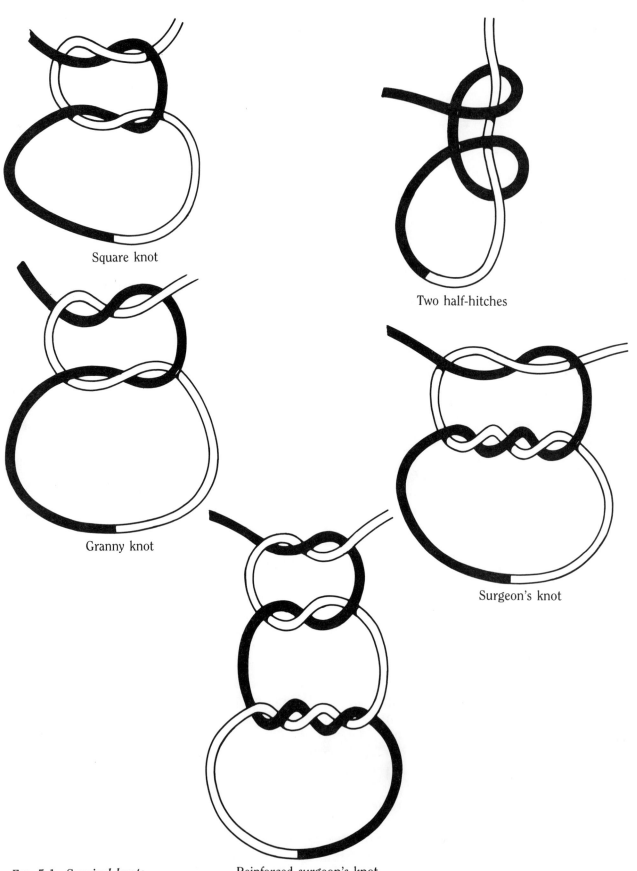

Square knot

Two half-hitches

Granny knot

Surgeon's knot

Reinforced surgeon's knot

Fig. 5-1. *Surgical knots.*

Knots stay tied because of the friction of one component against another. At least three separate throws are required to achieve the minimum amount of friction with the square knot. Monofilament suture materials, such as nylon, polypropylene, and braided synthetics, especially those that are Teflon coated, have poor knot security. With these materials, the first throw may loosen before the next throw is applied. Knotting technique warrants careful attention when using such suture materials. The surgeon can ensure knot security with braided synthetics with four throws, all squared (a double square knot) or with a knot with five throws, two slip and three squared.[1] Care must also be taken with steel because it also is prone to slippage if the knots are poorly placed. The reader is referred to Chapter 4, "Suture Materials."

A surgeon's knot is used when the first throw of a square knot cannot be held in position because of excessive tension on the wound edge (Fig. 5-1). The surgeon's knot is basically the same as a square knot, except the first suture consists of two throws. The surgeon's knot can be further reinforced by additional knots (Fig. 5-1).

Tying with the Needle Holder

In most instances, knots are tied with the aid of a needle holder (Fig. 5-2A to F). The instrument tie is recommended for most surgery because of its adaptability and because it is economical, when compared with the one-hand or two-hand tie. It is possible to use short pieces of suture material and still grasp the suture firmly.

The technique for instrument tie is as follows: a loop of the long end of the suture is made around the end of the instrument with the instrument in front of the suture (Fig. 5-2A). The short end of the suture is grasped by the needle holder, which is then pulled through the loop, setting the knot down securely (Fig. 5-2B and 5-2C). Traction must be applied in the same plane as the knot (Fig. 5-2D). The second half-hitch is begun by wrapping the long end of the suture around the instrument, but in the opposite direction (Fig. 5-2E). The short end of the suture is grasped and pulled through the loop (Fig. 5-2F). The surgeon's knot is made using essentially the same procedure, except the first loop is doubled by placing a double loop around the needle holder.

Knots should be tied with the correct tension. Excessive tension results in strangulation of the tissues, which leads to necrosis and delayed wound healing. Similarly, the wound should not be allowed to gape, either because of too few sutures or lack of tension. To relieve the tension on individual sutures, the number of sutures used to close the incision should be increased; the underlying principle is that when sutures are uniformly spaced, the tension is distributed equally among the sutures.

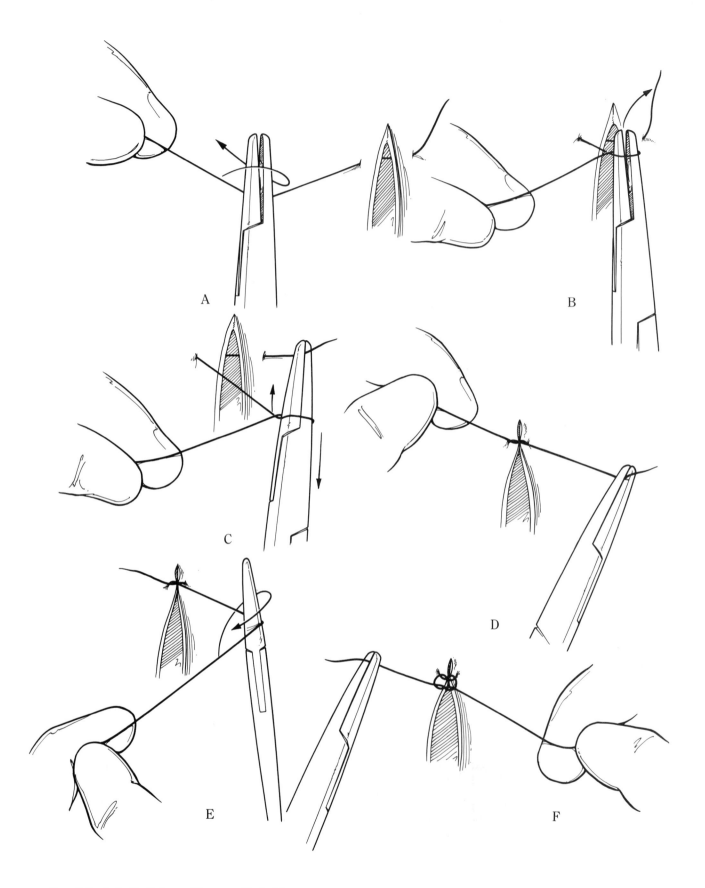

FIG. 5-2. A to F, *Tying with a needle holder.*

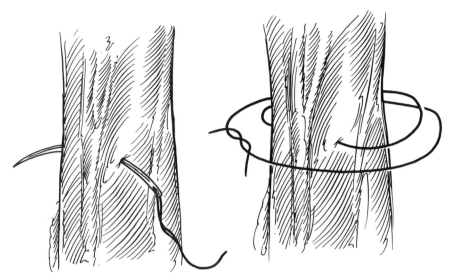

Fig. 5-3. *Transfixation ligature.*

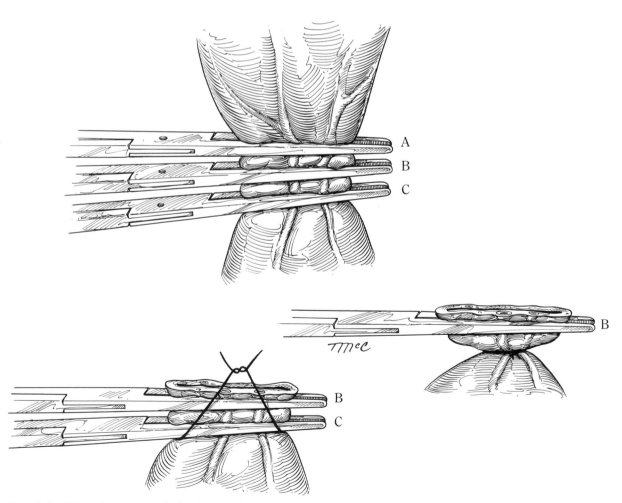

Fig. 5-4. *Three-forceps method of tissue ligation.*

Ligatures

A ligature is a loop of suture used for occluding a blood vessel either before or after it is severed. To prevent slipping, the ligature can be converted to a transfixation ligature by passing it through the middle of the vessel. It is tied around half the vessel, then around the entire vessel. Transfixation ligatures can be used to ligate several blood vessels within tissues (Fig. 5-3). As little tissue as possible should be left distal to the ligature because the stump so created will become necrotic and will have to be absorbed by the animal. Care must be taken not to cut the stump too short or the ligature may slip over the end and result in the loss of fixation. Double loops are stronger than single loops because of the distribution of friction and tensile forces. In addition, the bursting strength of a loop is inversely proportional to the volume that it encloses. In other words, the tension on the suture is proportional to the volume. Practically speaking, mass ligation of tissue is more apt to break than are ligatures around small bleeding points or isolated vessels.[2] Furthermore, vessels can recanalize within a large mass of ligated tissue.

When large amounts of tissues must be ligated, the three-forceps method can be used. The forceps are placed on the pedicle, as shown in Figure 5-4. Forceps A are distal and forceps C are proximal. The pedicle is divided between forceps A and B, and the ligature is placed proximal to forceps C. The first throw on the ligature is made, and, as forceps C are removed, the ligature is tied into the crease left by forceps C. Further throws are then placed on the ligature, and forceps B are loosened to check for hemorrhage.

References

1. Magilligan, D. J., and DeWeese, J. A.: Knot security and synthetic suture materials. Am. J. Surg., *127*:355, 1974.

2. Price, P. B.: Stress, strain and sutures. Ann. Surg., *128*:408, 1948.

3. Swaim, S.: Surgery of Traumatized Skin: Management and Reconstruction in the Dog and Cat. Philadelphia, W. B. Saunders, 1980, p. 269.

6

SUTURE

PATTERNS

Basic Suture Patterns

A wide variety of suture patterns for use under different circumstances is available to the surgeon. The student of surgery will be eager to "try out" different patterns, but will soon learn that many achieve the same purpose. The skilled, experienced surgeon uses only a few patterns, just as he selects only a few suture materials. The neophyte should learn the functions, advantages, and limitations of the various suture patterns. If one pattern does not produce optimum results, then a new technique must be mastered. Suture patterns are divided into interrupted or continuous patterns, and the following patterns are important to the student of large animal surgery.

Simple Interrupted Suture

The simple interrupted suture is the oldest and most widely used suture pattern. It is easy and relatively rapid to perform. The technique of insertion depends on the thickness of the tissue apposed. The needle and suture are inserted a variable distance from one side of the incision, cross the incision at right angles, and are inserted through the tissue on the other side. For a right-handed surgeon, this would be accomplished from right to left, and the reverse would apply for a left-handed surgeon (Fig. 6-1). The knot should be offset, so as not to rest against the incision. If this suture is used for skin closure, the point of insertion will vary, depending on the thickness of the skin. This may be 1 cm in bovine skin or 2 to 3 mm for the thin skin on the inguinal area of a foal. The simple interrupted suture should appose the wound margins, but it may invert them if it is pulled too tightly. The spacing between the sutures depends on the tension on the wound edges. Gaping of the wound edges should naturally be avoided.

Simple Continuous Suture

This continuous suture is made up of a variable number of simple bites and is tied only at the ends (Figs. 6-2 and 6-3). It is used in tissues that

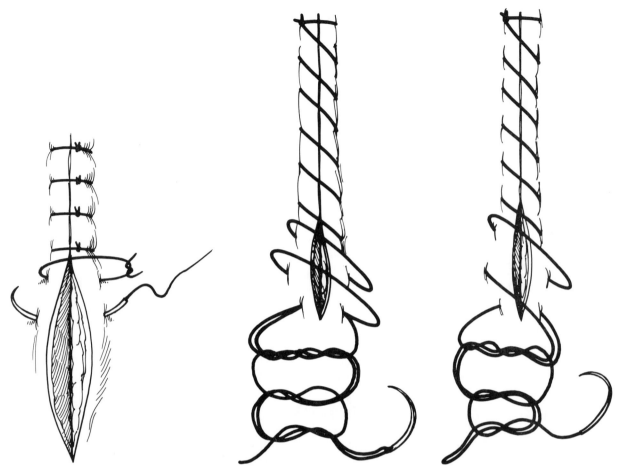

FIG. 6-1. *Simple interrupted suture.*

FIG. 6-2. *Simple continuous suture (eyed needle).*

FIG. 6-3. *Simple continuous suture (swaged-on needle).*

are elastic and will not be subjected to a lot of tension. The bites in the edges of the wound are made at right angles to the edges of the wound, but the exposed part of the suture passes diagonally across the incision. This suture pattern can be applied rapidly. Ending the suture depends on whether a swaged-on needle or a needle with an eye is used. To end the suture with an eyed needle, the needle is advanced through the tissues, and the short end of the suture is held on the proximal end of the needle passage. A loop of suture is pulled through with the needle, and the loop is tied to the single end on the opposite side (Fig. 6-2). When a swaged-on needle is used, the needle end of the suture is tied to the last available loop of suture material that is exterior to the tissues (Fig. 6-3). If any one of the sutures in a continuous suture pattern fails, the strength of the suture line will be lost. If one suture fails in an interrupted suture pattern, the remaining sutures have a better chance of maintaining the strength of the suture line.

Interrupted Horizontal Mattress Suture

This suture is illustrated in Figure 6-4*A*. The external parts of the suture lie parallel to the wound edges. To prevent eversion, the needle should be

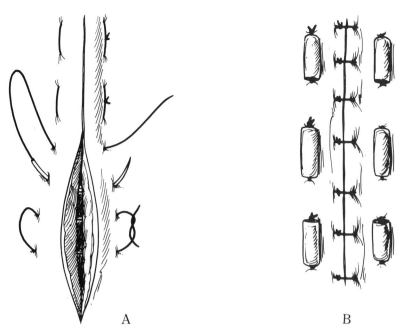

FIG. 6-4. A, *Interrupted horizontal mattress suture*. B, *Interrupted horizontal mattress sutures as tension-relieving sutures, using pieces of rubber.*

angled through the skin, and the wound edges should oppose each other gently. The horizontal mattress suture is useful in large skin wounds. It can be used in conjunction with pieces of rubber tubing or with buttons, to act as a tension suture (Fig. 6-4B). In this situation, the suture is placed some distance from the skin edges. Another pattern of sutures, such as the simple interrupted suture, is used to coapt the incision line more precisely. Because of the geometry of the horizontal mattress suture, the sutures have a tendency to reduce the blood supply to the wound edges. In such a case, a vertical mattress suture would be a better choice as a tension suture (Fig. 6-4C).

Continuous Horizontal Mattress Suture

The continuous horizontal mattress suture, illustrated in Figure 6-5, is similar to the horizontal mattress pattern, except it is continuous. Its main advantage is speed, and it is not often used in large animal surgery.

Vertical Mattress Suture

Initially, the suture and needle make a superficial bite close to the wound edge, then pass across the incision to take a small bite on the opposite side (Fig. 6-6A). The needle is then reversed in the jaws of the needle holder and is returned to the opposite side, where it takes a larger bite. If this suture is used as the sole method of skin closure, the superficial bite of the suture pattern will ensure adequate approximation of the wound edges; if used as tension-relieving sutures some distance from the wound, then simple interrupted sutures can accurately coapt the wound edges (Fig. 6-6B). Compared with the horizontal mattress pattern, the geometry of this suture allows better circulation to the wound edges and thereby decreases

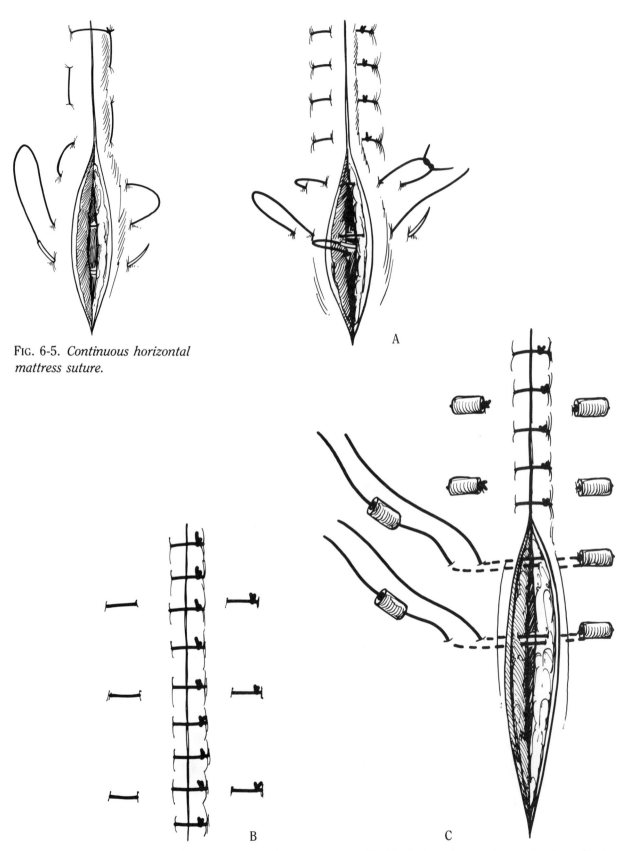

FIG. 6-5. *Continuous horizontal mattress suture.*

FIG. 6-6. A, *Vertical mattress suture.* B, *Vertical mattress suture as tension-relieving sutures.* C, *Vertical mattress suture using pieces of rubber.*

the chances of necrosis of the margins of the wound. The only disadvantages of this suture are that it uses slightly more suture material and may take longer to insert.

The vertical mattress suture is popular in repairing traumatic lacerations of the skin of equine limbs, where the blood supply may already be compromised. Like the horizontal mattress suture, it can also be used as a tension suture in conjunction with pieces of rubber tubing or with buttons. Pieces of rubber or buttons minimize tissue cutting by the suture material (Fig. 6-6C).

Near-Far-Far-Near Suture

This suture, illustrated in Figure 6-7, is a tension suture occasionally used in large animal surgery. The first bite is made close to the wound and then passes under the wound across its edges at right angles to emerge at a greater distance from the wound edge. The next part of the suture consists of crossing over the wound to the original side and inserting the needle and suture at a distance farther from the edge than the original entry point. The suture is then directed into the wound perpendicular to the edges of the wound, crosses the wound, and emerges close to the wound edge. Then the suture ends are tied. The suture is time consuming to insert, but, in our opinion, is an excellent tension suture. We have used this suture to close the linea alba of horses whenever tension on the wound edges is excessive.

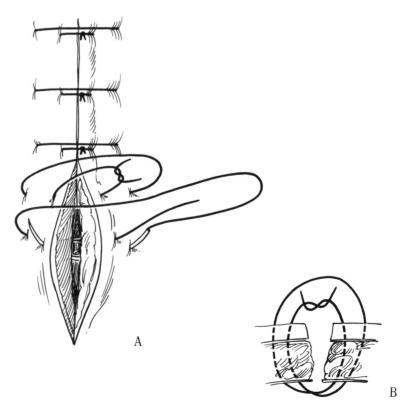

FIG. 6-7. A *and* B, *Near-far-far-near suture.*

Subcuticular Suture

This suture is used to eliminate the small scars produced around the suture holes of the more common patterns. The first part of the suture is placed by directing the needle up into the apex of the incision in the opposite direction of the incision (Fig. 6-8). The needle is then reversed and is directed down the incision. The knot is tied and, in this way, will be subcutaneous. The remainder of the suture pattern is placed like a horizontal mattress suture, with the needle crossing the incision at right angles, but advancing underneath the dermis parallel to the incision. A knot similar to the one used in the simple continuous pattern finishes the suture. The needle is then reversed and is directed back along the incision; the knot at this end should also be subcutaneous. The suture material used for this pattern can be absorbable or nonabsorbable and should be relatively unreactive and sterile.

Cruciate (Cross Mattress) Suture

The cruciate suture, illustrated in Figure 6-9, is commenced by inserting the needle from one side to the next, as one would place a simple interrupted suture. The needle is then advanced without penetrating the tissue, and a second passage is made parallel to the first. The suture ends are then on opposite sides of the wound and form an "x" on the surface of the wound.

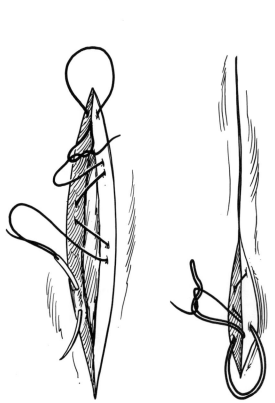

FIG. 6-8. A *and* B, *Subcuticular suture.*

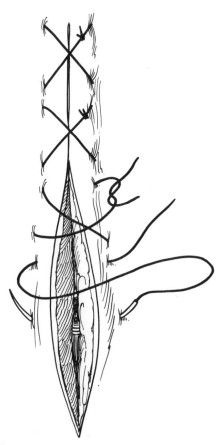

FIG. 6-9. *Cruciate (cross mattress) suture.*

This suture pattern is used by some surgeons if the skin edges are under tension.

The cruciate suture is used to close the small hole made by a hypodermic needle that is used for deflating a gas-distended bowel. The suture is used as a skin-closure technique by some surgeons.

Continuous Lock Stitch (Ford Interlocking Suture)

The continuous lock stitch is a modification of the simple continuous suture (Fig. 6-10). In this continuous pattern, the needle is passed perpendicularly through the tissues in the same direction. Once the needle is passed through the tissues, it is drawn through the preformed loop and is tightened. Each subsequent stitch is locked until the end of the incision is reached. To end the lock stitch, the needle should be introduced from a direction opposite the insertion of the previous sutures, and the end should be held on that side. The loop of suture is formed, and the single ends are tied. The interlocking suture is commonly used in the skin of cattle following a laparotomy. Good approximation of the skin edges can be obtained, especially with the thick skin on the flanks of cattle.

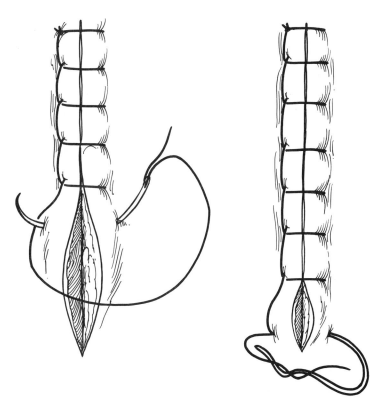

FIG. 6-10. A *and* B, *Continuous lock stitch (Ford interlocking suture).*

Suture Patterns Used for Closure of Hollow Organs

A suture pattern used for a hollow organ must be placed meticulously because of the disastrous consequences possible if infectious material should leak. In the intestinal tract, for example, gas and solid and liquid feces propelled by peristalsis place strain on the suture line. Fortunately, the walls of the healthy gastrointestinal tract are tough, pliable, and easy to manipulate. On the other hand, the friable uterus of a cesarean patient with a decomposing fetus may be difficult to suture. Another advantage of surgery of hollow organs is that the organs generally heal quickly and are remarkably secure in as short a time as a week to 10 days after surgery.

A watertight closure was once thought to be mandatory when suturing a hollow organ; however, any technique that merely opposes the wound edges is satisfactory because a fibrin clot provides an almost immediate seal. Eversion of the mucous membrane, however, is detrimental and can lead to the leakage of septic contents, resulting in peritonitis.

Classically, suture patterns used on hollow organs have been inverting sutures or opposing sutures. This section presents the inverting patterns, followed by some of the opposing patterns. When suturing the intestinal tract, the strength of a suture depends on its grasp of the tunica submucosa or fibromuscular layer. Absorbable or nonabsorbable sutures may be used to close the gastrointestinal tract. Needles used for hollow-organ surgery should be round-bodied (noncutting), with the suture material swaged on to reduce the size of the hole made on the organ wall. Noncutting needles are less likely to lacerate suture material that may have been placed in a deeper layer.

Interrupted or continuous sutures can be used in hollow-organ surgery. Interrupted sutures are safer because, if one knot becomes untied, the integrity of the entire suture line will not be jeopardized. By using interrupted sutures, the tension on each suture can be adjusted, thereby ensuring an optimum blood supply to the wound edges. Continuous sutures are rapid to place, but unlike the interrupted patterns, they compromise the wound edges.

Interrupted Lembert Suture

The Lembert suture is regarded as the classic suture of gastrointestinal surgery (Fig. 6-11). The suture is directed through the tissue from the outside, toward the cut edge of the incision. It penetrates the tunica serosa, muscularis, and submucosa, but not the mucous membrane. The suture exits on the same side and emerges close to the edge of the incision. It is reinserted close to the incision edge, passes laterad through the tunica serosa, muscularis, and submucosa and is brought up again through the tunica muscularis and serosa. The wall of the viscus automatically inverts as the knot is tied. The knot should not be so tight as to strangulate the

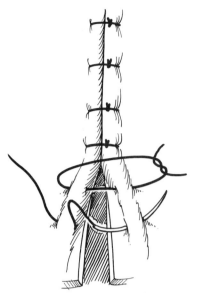

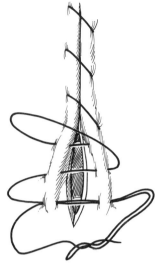

FIG. 6-11. *Interrupted Lembert suture.* FIG. 6-12. *Continuous Lembert suture.*

tissues. At no stage does the suture penetrate the lumen of the viscus; it is considered one of the safest and most useful stitches in gastrointestinal surgery and can be used as a one-layer closure. It is also suitable for use in the uterus and the rumen of large animals.

Continuous Lembert Suture

The classic Lembert suture can be performed in a continuous pattern (Fig. 6-12). The same spacing is used as in the interrupted suture, and the continuous suture is tied to itself at its proximal end and again at its distal end. The suture is commonly used in both intestinal and uterine closures and requires less time than the interrupted suture.

Interrupted Inverting Mattress Suture

The interrupted inverting mattress suture, illustrated in Figure 6-13, resembles the interrupted horizontal mattress suture (see Fig. 6-4). In this suture, the bite parallel to the incision runs through the muscle layer, and the suture material crosses externally to the left of the incision. This suture may be used to oversew the small holes left by a needle that deflated a gas-distended intestine. This suture is not often used for other purposes.

Halsted (Interrupted Quilt) Suture

The Halsted suture is a modification of the Lembert suture (Fig. 6-14). It is essentially two Lembert sutures parallel to each other and tied so the knot is on one side of the wound. When each knot is tightened, the fold on the side of the wound held by the loop and the fold in the side of the wound held by the knot are brought into contact. The suture pattern is strong, approximates well, and compresses the tissues minimally, but it probably strangulates the blood supply more than an interrupted Lembert

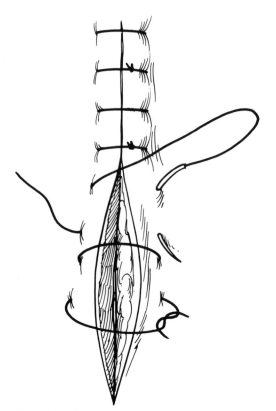

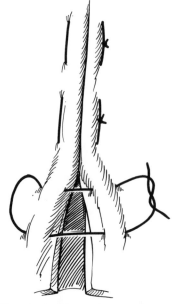

FIG. 6-13. *Interrupted inverting mattress suture.*

FIG. 6-14. *Halsted (interrupted quilt) suture.*

suture pattern. It is reportedly the suture pattern of choice for friable tissues; otherwise, it is not commonly used in large animal practice.

Cushing Suture

This is a method of continuous suturing in which the bites are made parallel to the edges of the wound (Fig. 6-15). As the suture is placed, it penetrates the tunica serosa, muscularis, and submucosa, but does not pass through the mucous membrane; hence, it does not enter the lumen of the viscus. The suture crosses the incision at right angles and is tied to itself at the proximal end and at the distal end. The Cushing suture inverts the tunica mucosa and approximates the serosa. It is generally used as the outer tier on a double-layer closure and can be executed rapidly.

Connell Suture

The Connell suture resembles the Cushing suture, but the suture material penetrates all layers of the gut wall (Fig. 6-16). The suture is tied when the first stitch has been taken and is tied again at the far end of the incision. Once outside the serosal surface, the needle and suture cross the incision and are reinserted in the tunica serosa of the opposite side at a point that corresponds to the preceding exit site. The directions of the Connell and Cushing suture are the same, and both sutures invert tissue.

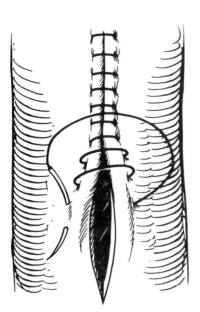

FIG. 6-15. *Cushing suture.*

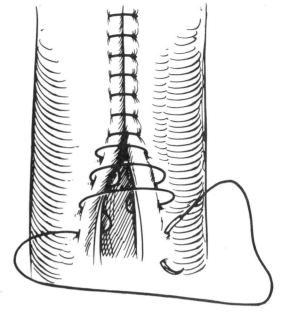

FIG. 6-16. *Connell suture.*

Parker-Kerr Oversew

This suture is a modification of the Lembert and Cushing patterns, and it is used to close the stump of a hollow viscus (Fig. 6-17). It is essentially a Cushing pattern oversewn by a Lembert pattern. The first layer of the suture pattern, which is a Cushing pattern, is performed over a pair of forceps placed on the end of the stump (Fig. 6-17A and B). The forceps are withdrawn slowly as the suture is pulled in both directions; this inverts the wound edges without opening the lumen, which would result in contamination (Fig. 6-17C). A continuous Lembert suture is then used as an oversew using the same suture (Fig. 6-17D). The needle end of the suture is brought back as the second layer to be tied at the origin of the first layer (Fig. 6-17E). The suture patterns can be reversed in this technique, using a Lembert for the pattern directly over the forceps and oversewing this with the Cushing, when the forceps have been withdrawn. The most common application of this suture pattern in large animal surgery is in the jejunocecal anastomosis in the horse.[2,7] This pattern is used in the stump of the terminal ileum. We have sometimes found it necessary to place another layer of inverting sutures over the finished Parker-Kerr oversew.

Purse-String Suture

This pattern comprises a continuous suture placed in a circle around an opening; however, the suture is tied when the entire circumference of the circle has been followed (Fig. 6-18). To aid inversion of the suture, an assistant should grasp that part of the purse string that is exactly opposite the knot and should exert upward traction. The purse string is then tightened following the release of the tissue forceps. Like the classic Cushing suture, the suture does not penetrate the lumen. Another layer of sutures may be used over the purse string, either in the form of another purse string or

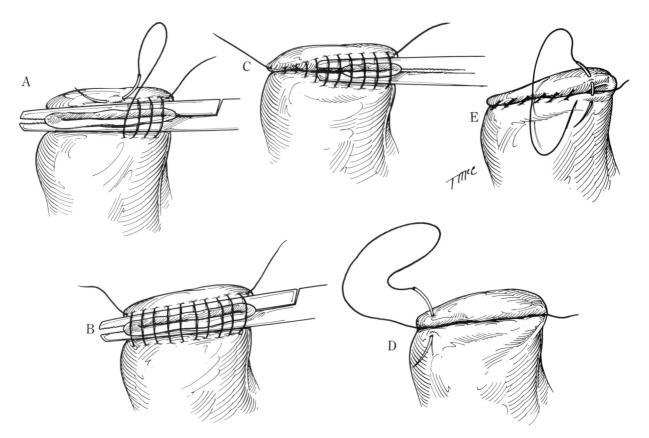

FIG. 6-17. A *to* E, *Parker-Kerr oversew.*

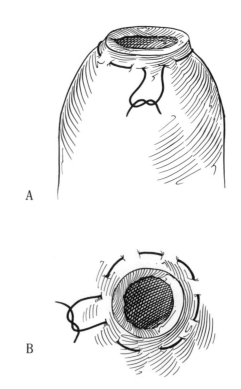

FIG. 6-18. *Purse-string suture.*

in a series of Lembert sutures. The purse-string suture is used to oversew an opening that evacuates gas in the gastrointestinal tract that is made by a needle or trocar puncture. It can also be used to stabilize permanent indwelling fistulae or cannulae.

Simple Interrupted Suture

The simple interrupted suture can be used successfully to close the intestinal tract in one or two ways. It can be used to gently oppose the wound edges, thereby causing minimal interference to the blood supply; it can also be used as a crushing suture, in which the suture is pulled tight enough, so the material tightens onto the tunica submucosa and the knot is buried. The collagenous fibers in the submucosal layer resist crushing and provide the strength for the closure.[4] In Figure 6-19A, the suture is placed through all the layers approximately 3 to 4 mm from the wound edges. The suture is then tightened, crushing all the soft tissue elements, except the collagenous fibers of the submucosal layer. The suture is cut short after at least three throws (Fig. 6-19B). An assistant can then use the end of a mosquito forceps to push the tunica mucosa back into the lumen.

Gambee Suture

The Gambee suture pattern is used for intestinal anastomosis as a single-layer closure (Fig. 6-20). The suture and needle are introduced like a simple interrupted suture and pass from the tunica serosa, through all layers, and into the lumen. The needle is then directed from the lumen through the tunica mucosa and submucosa, it crosses the incision, passes through the submucosa and mucosa, and enters the lumen of the intestine. The suture

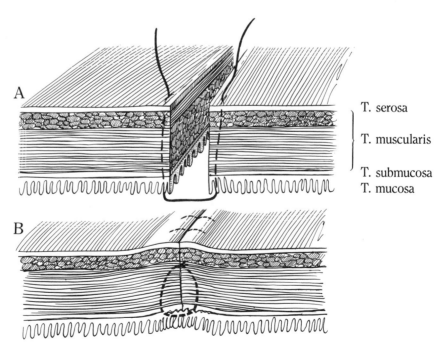

FIG. 6-19. A *and* B, *Simple interrupted suture used in bowel.*

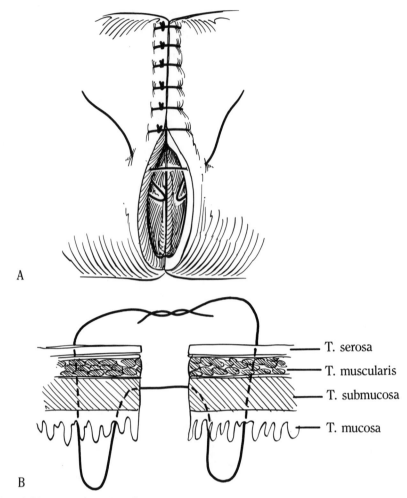

T. serosa

T. muscularis

T. submucosa

T. mucosa

Fig. 6-20. A *and* B, *Gambee suture.*

is then reintroduced through the entire thickness of the intestinal wall to emerge on the serosal surface of the bowel. The suture is tied firmly, so that the tissue compresses on itself. Although it takes longer than a simple interrupted pattern, the Gambee pattern is useful in equine gastrointestinal surgery. When this technique was evaluated experimentally in horses, it caused minimal adhesion formation and stenosis.[9,10]

Double-Layer Inverting Patterns

A two-layer inverting pattern (using Cushing, Connell, Lembert, or Halsted patterns) produces an anastomosis with higher initial tensile and bursting strength.[5] The incidence of adhesions is lower, but internal cuff formation may potentially produce intraluminal obstruction.

For end-to-end anastomosis of the small intestine a double-layer inverting anastomosis composed of a simple continuous mucosal layer and a continuous Lembert seromuscular layer has been advocated.[1] This technique inverts only one layer and results in a minimum reduction of lumen diameter. The incidence of fibrosis and suture tract inflammation is higher with this technique than with Gambee and crushing patterns; however, adhesions were not present in six horses when this technique was used, as compared to a 50% adhesion incidence with the other two techniques.[1]

Further details of intestinal resection, anastomosis, and gastrointestinal stapling are available in our advanced text.[5]

Stent Bandages (Tie-Over Dressings)

These dressings are used over areas that are difficult to apply pressure bandages to such as the proximal regions of the limbs and the torso. As well as applying some localized pressure and minimizing postoperative swelling, this bandage helps to keep dirt and bedding away from the skin incision. They also can assist in the elimination of dead space, such as the throatlatch region following modified Forssell's operation for cribbing. We have used these dressings to cover skin incisions following the closure of the linea alba for celiotomy.

For smaller incisions, a sterile gauze bandage is used. For larger incisions, we use a rolled hand towel. The bandage material should be long enough that the ends slightly overlap the ends of the incision. Following closure of the skin incision, an assistant holds the towel firmly in position. Using synthetic monofilament suture material, we insert a continuous horizontal mattress suture or interrupted horizontal mattress sutures (Fig. 6-21). As

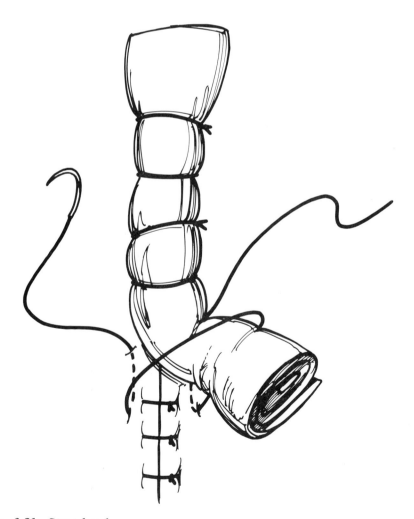

FIG. 6-21. *Stent bandage.*

the sutures are tied, slight tenting of the skin may occur. This will disappear when these sutures are removed. The stent is usually removed 4 to 7 days after surgery, depending on the procedure. The bandage helps to keep the incision dry because of its wicking effect, but it should not become moist enough to allow excessive fluid to adhere to the incision. The stent should be removed if excessive moisture persists.

Suture Patterns for Severed Tendons

Frequently, the large animal surgeon is presented with a traumatic wound involving severed tendons. If the tendon ends are not in approximate alignment, suturing may be indicated. In most situations, however, tendon lacerations are treated by external coaptation alone, such as with casts, braces, or bandages, rather than repaired with suture materials.

One has to weigh the advantages and disadvantages of suturing tendons. To appose the tendon ends properly with suture material, the tendon must be subjected to additional trauma. Nonabsorbable materials are generally used, because of their ability to maintain strength during the protracted course of tendon healing. In the face of infection or contamination, these materials may potentiate infection, or a chronic draining tract may form. Nevertheless, tendon repair is sometimes indicated to approximate the ends and to facilitate healing. If a tendon is sutured, some form of external support will be necessary to minimize extreme forces placed on the repair.

Locking-Loop Tendon Suture

Based on tendon surgery in man, the traditional suture pattern for repair of severed tendons in the horse was the Bunnell pattern or variations on this pattern. Because of the extreme loads placed on equine tendons, this pattern was prone to failure. The suture would tear out of the fiber bundles by cutting or pulling through the weak interfibrous connections. It also was believed to compromise fragile vascularity within the tendon. Improved suture patterns have since been developed. We currently use the locking-loop tendon suture (modified Kessler pattern) shown in Figure 6-22. This suture is strong, causes minimal interference with tendon blood supply, and exposes little of the suture material.[8]

The needle is inserted into the severed end of the tendon and emerges from the surface of the tendon (Fig. 6-22A). The needle is then passed transversely through the tendon just superficial to the longitudinal part of the suture (Fig. 6-22B). This results in a loop of suture locking around a small bundle of tendon fibers. When more tension is applied to the repair site, the grip of the suture loop on these fiber bundles becomes tighter. The needle is then reinserted in a longitudinal direction and passes under the transverse portion of suture material (Fig. 6-22C); this process is repeated on the other piece of tendon (Fig. 6-22D). After placement of the suture, all the loops should be tightened in turn and the suture tied snugly, so slight "bunching" occurs at the junction (Fig. 6-22E).

Monofilament nylon or polypropylene is the recommended suture material for this suture. Rough-surfaced sutures (braided or twisted) do not have sufficient glide or elasticity to permit longitudinal strain to be transmitted into locking tension. Wire is not flexible enough for this suture pattern and is not recommended.[8] The largest-diameter monofilament nonabsorbable

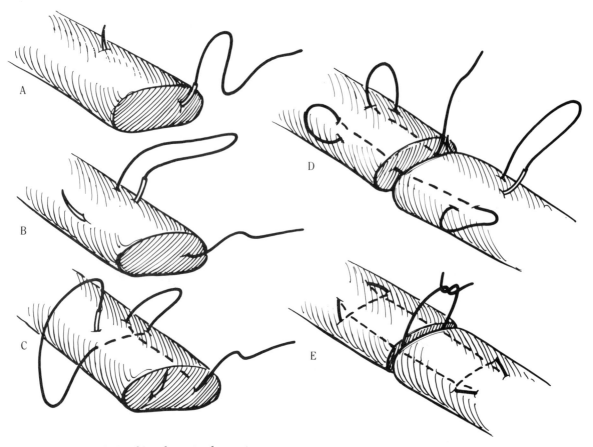

FIG. 6-22. A *to* E, *Locking-loop tendon suture.*

suture should be used. At this time, the largest commercially available suture material of this type is no. 2 nylon. A single locking-loop suture pattern with this material in equine tendon is insufficient to prevent gap formation during weightbearing, even when the area is immobilized with a cast. In vitro biomechanical studies have shown that a double locking-loop pattern should be used because it is twice as resistant to gap formation and failure than a single locking-loop pattern. Three locking-loop patterns can be used, but they may be technically difficult and time consuming to apply.[3]

Carbon fiber is not recommended for use in this pattern. Despite some earlier enthusiasm for carbon fiber for tendon repair in horses, research has shown that nylon suture is superior to carbon in the re-establishment of tension-resisting capacity.[6]

References

1. Dean, P. W., and Robertson, J. T.: Comparison of three suture techniques for anastomosis of the small intestine in the horse. Am. J. Vet. Res., *46*:1282, 1985.

2. Donawick, W. J., Christie, B. A., and Stewart, J. V.: Resection of diseased ileum in the horse. J. Am. Vet. Med. Assoc., *159*:1146, 1971.

3. Easley, K. J., et al.: In vitro comparison of the mechanical properties of four suture patterns for transected equine tendon. Vet. Surg. In press, 1989.

4. Herthel, D. J.: Technique of intestinal anastomosis utilizing the crushing-type suture. *In* Proceedings of the 18th Annual Convention of the American Association of Equine Practitioners in 1972:1973, p. 303.

5. McIlwraith, C. W., and Turner, A. S.: Equine Surgery: Advanced Techniques. Philadelphia, Lea & Febiger, 1987.

6. Nixon, A. J., et al.: Comparison of carbon fiber and nylon suture for repair of transected flexor tendons in the horse. Equine Vet. J., *16*:93, 1984.

7. Owen, R. ap R., et al.: Jejuno or ileocecal anastomosis performed in seven horses exhibiting colic. Can. Vet. J., *16*:164, 1975.

8. Pennington, D. G.: The locking-loop tendon suture. Plast. Reconstr. Surg., *63*:648, 1979.

9. Reinertson, E. L.: Comparison of three techniques for intestinal anastomosis in equidae. J. Am. Vet. Med. Assoc., *169*:208, 1976.

10. Vaughan, J. T.: Surgical management of abdominal crisis in the horse. J. Am. Vet. Med. Assoc., *161*:1199, 1972.

7

PRINCIPLES
OF WOUND
MANAGEMENT
AND THE USE
OF DRAINS

Wound Management

The aim of this chapter is to present some fundamental principles of the management of traumatic wounds in large animals. Because these problems occur frequently in the horse, the discussion is directed at this species, but the basic principles can be adapted to ruminants and swine as well. Emphasis is placed on wounds of the distal limbs, where wound management can be difficult and frustrating. Wounds can be handled in many ways. Wounds sometimes heal despite what we do, rather than because of what we do.

Large animal surgeons are often faced with wounds that owners vigorously attempted to treat with various remedies in an attempt to save money. These remedies usually retard wound healing to varying degrees and, ultimately, do not help the owner to economize. Clients should be educated in these areas and instructed to refrain from the natural instinct "to do something." Owners should be familiarized with first aid in the form of clean—or better still, sterile—dressings with pressure bandaging. These dressings will also assist in controlling hemorrhage if properly applied.

Systemic antibiotics are usually indicated for the treatment of traumatic wounds of large animals, especially the often heavily contaminated wounds. To be effective, antibiotic administration needs to be initiated as soon as possible, and adequate dosage levels need to be maintained. If an infection is already established, such as in cellulitis or phlegmon, attempts should be made to obtain a specific culture. Tetanus prophylaxis is always indicated in wounds of horses.

The use of local antibiotics or antibacterial agents is controversial. Exudate on the wound often prevents effective contact of the agent with the microorganisms. In many instances, local medications retard wound healing. If confronted with an infected wound, however, particularly when Pseudomonas species is involved, we believe that the use of povidone-iodine ointment (Betadine Ointment) is appropriate.

Initial assessment of the injured animal should include an overall, "whole-body" assessment of the patient. Vital signs should be examined, and any signs of shock or exhaustion should be noted. At the same time, a history should be taken because it may have an important bearing on the management of the injury, an example being a puncture wound or stake wound into which foreign material may have been introduced. The location of the wound is then assessed. A mental note is made of the regional anatomy because it may have a profound effect on the future usefulness of the animal. One should assess which vital structures (muscles, tendons, bones, blood vessels) have been injured and the extent of their injury. Although it is difficult to determine in some instances, one should assess the local blood supply to the region and, especially, the blood supply to the wound edges.

Primary-Intention Healing

The decision to close a wound to achieve primary-intention healing or to let it heal by secondary intention must be based on experience. Some basic premises can be used, however. Reference is continually made to the so-called "golden period;" this is the time soon after wounding during which the wound is contaminated, but not to a point where the contamination cannot be overcome by the body's natural defenses. The golden period is usually a number of hours, but its length varies, depending on the blood supply to the region, the extent of injury, the degree of contamination, and the injury's anatomic location. The classic example is the difference between a wound on the distal limb of a horse and a wound on the head. A wound on the head may heal with first intention even after a 24-hour delay, whereas a wound on the distal limb may not respond to primary closure after several hours.

Any wound that shows signs of infection, as evidenced by heat, pain, and swelling, should not be closed; it should be left open to heal by secondary intention. It may also be healed by the process of tertiary intention, whereby a secondary-intention wound is excised and closed.

ANESTHESIA AND RESTRAINT

These subjects are important if one decides to perform immediate wound closure or primary repair. Most wounds in large animals can be managed with the aid of chemical restraint (tranquilization) and local or regional anesthesia. Direct infiltration of the wound with a local anesthetic along its edges should be avoided if possible. This method of desensitizing the wound drives contamination deeper into the wound and may even open up new tissue planes; therefore, the use of regional analgesia is preferable. General anesthesia is indicated if the injury is so extensive that a local anesthetic is impractical or if the animal is too fractious. It is also indicated if extensive debridement and cast application are to be performed. The reader is referred to Chapter 2 for details on anesthesia and restraint.

EXCISION AND DEBRIDEMENT OF THE WOUND

The aim of excision and debridement is to convert a contaminated wound into a surgically clean one. These maneuvers also remove foreign material, which potentiate infection by providing a medium for bacterial proliferation.

The technique of excision and debridement involves the selective removal of dead tissue (fascia, adipose tissue, muscle) from the wound. Small, detached fragments of bone, contaminated skin edges, and edematous tissue are excised from the wound by a sharp scalpel or high-quality tissue scissors, such as Metzenbaum scissors. If possible, nerves, blood vessels, and tendons that appear viable should be left. If the wound is heavily contaminated, an initial preparation and debridement may be followed by a second preparation and debridement, with a change of gloves and instruments.

Exploration of the wound must be performed in a judicious manner. Overzealous exploration of the wound may open up new tissue planes, which will allow the spread of infection. If the possibility of a foreign body exists, however, such as in a stake wound in the inguinal region of a horse, then a thorough search for such material will be indicated.

PREPARATION OF THE WOUND

Because of the environment in which large animals reside, contamination may be so extensive that some trauma patients will require a complete hosing down, especially in the winter and spring, when barnyards are muddy. In these cases, tap water is the only practical answer, although its application directly onto the wound should be minimized. Tap water, although relatively sterile, is hypotonic and causes edema of the tissues.

To prepare the wound itself, the edges of the wound should be clipped and, in most instances, shaved. To prevent the introduction of hair into the wound, sterile, moist gauze can be placed into the wound to protect it; sterile, water-soluble lubricating jelly (KY Jelly) is also convenient for this purpose. When the edges of the wound have been clipped, the gauze is simply lifted out of the wound, or the jelly is washed out. An ample area around the wound should be clipped, in case additional exposure to deeper parts of the wound is required.

The wound should be scrubbed gently in combination with an isotonic solution (if available) and a germicidal agent. Strong disinfectants are cytotoxic and produce further cellular damage, which will prolong the inflammatory stages of wound healing. Soap solutions should also be avoided, because they, too, are irritating to the tissues. If contamination of the wound is massive, however, the advantages gained by the action of the soap may outweigh the disadvantage of irritated tissues. Povidone-iodine (Betadine) solution is widely used, but it should be diluted because strong concentrations are irritating.[2]

The cleansing agent should be administered in large volumes of the isotonic solution. This can be delivered by gravity or by low pressure with the aid of a bulb syringe. High-pressure lavage units are more effective in removing bacteria than conventional techniques; they do not, as it was once believed, force bacteria deeper into the wound or cause significant tissue injury.[1]

SUTURING TRAUMATIC WOUNDS

Certain principles are important in the suturing of traumatic wounds. The wound needs to be closed without undue tension. It is preferable to leave some of the wound edges apart, rather than to apply sutures under tension, because these sutures will produce ischemia of the wound edges and a larger defect than before. Tension-relieving suture patterns may be used to help overcome this problem, but they, too, can cause a localized ischemia. Such tension sutures include the vertical and horizontal mattress patterns that are used in combination with pieces of rubber, buttons, or gauze. In the skin edges themselves, we prefer to use the vertical mattress pattern. The reader is referred to Chapter 6, "Suture Patterns."

Dead space should be closed whenever possible; this can be accomplished by deep closure with absorbable suture material or by using a pattern that will pull the skin down onto the defect. Braided synthetic materials should be avoided in the deeper layers. If used in the face of contamination, they become readily infected and harbor this infection until they are removed by the surgeon or extruded by the animal. The newer synthetic absorbables, such as polyglycolic acid, polyglactin 910, and polydioxanone (see Chap. 4), are useful for this purpose; if infection does result, they will maintain tensile strength longer than a material such as catgut. Noncapillary, nonreactive synthetic material, such as nylon or polypropylene, should be used for tension-relieving sutures that can be applied to the wound edges.

Drains are indicated in the treatment of traumatic wounds in which unobliterated dead space or the likelihood of fluid accumulation exists. The use of drains is detailed later in this chapter.

OTHER CONSIDERATIONS

Other than antibiotics and tetanus prophylaxis, the judicious use of nonsteroidal, anti-inflammatory drugs should be considered. Drugs such as phenylbutazone are often indicated, especially for horses. Unlike high dosages of corticosteroids, these drugs have little to no effect on the course of wound healing. They diminish pain from inflammation, improve the overall "well being" of the horse, encourage ambulation, and thereby stimulate circulation, especially in the limbs. Corticosteroids are not usually used in the treatment of traumatic wounds, unless the surgeon is treating a separate problem.

Postoperative bandages help to obliterate dead space and to prevent postoperative edema. Their use is recommended, especially in injuries to the limbs of the horse. In this region, edema can become such a problem that the suture line can be disrupted. A nonadhering, sterile dressing should always be applied to the wound to prevent disruption of the skin edges when the bandages are changed. Cast application is commonly indicated for wounds of the distal limbs. Without the support of the cast, certain distal limb injuries of the horse break down, and when allowed to heal by second intention, these wounds produce exuberant granulation tissue. In this category of injuries are wounds to the bulbs of the heels and the pastern.

Secondary-Intention Healing

When the surgeon is presented with a wound that has gone beyond the golden period, or if tissue loss is so extensive that primary closure is impossible, the wound is left to heal by secondary intention. In this process, the wound fills with granulation tissue, and the skin re-establishes continuity by epithelialization or wound contraction. Wound contraction is an active process characterized by the centripetal movement of the whole thickness of the surrounding skin, which results in diminished wound size. It is the major process for re-establishment of skin continuity in wound healing by secondary intention, with the exception of the distal limbs. In the distal limbs, epithelialization plays the major role in skin closure. The resulting fragile epithelium is devoid of hair follicles and sweat glands.

Wound healing by this process needs constant attention if one wishes to obtain the best functional and cosmetic results. While the wound is "granulating in," it should receive daily cleansing. The intact skin that is ventral to the wound should be protected from serum scald with a bland ointment, such as petrolatum jelly. Once the granulation bed has become established, topical antibiotics are unwarranted because of the innate resistance to infection of this tissue. Parenteral antibiotics are only used in the initial stages of healing, unless signs of diffuse infection develop.

In the distal limbs of horses, where wounds heal by secondary intention, excessive granulation tissue can become a major problem, especially in regions where there is no muscle but only tendons, ligaments, and skin covering the bone. Exuberant granulation tissue ("proud flesh") is generally not a problem above the carpus or tarsus and on the remainder of the body. A severe cosmetic deformity will invariably result if the granulation tissue is allowed to become excessive. Prevention consists of avoiding irritating and oil-based ointments, minimizing movement, and maintaining the wound under a pressure bandage or cast. If excess granulation tissue exists, it must be removed until it approximates the level of the surrounding skin; otherwise, the migration of epithelium will be severely retarded. Excision of granulation tissue with a sharp scalpel, while being careful not to disrupt the advancing epithelium at the wound edge, is the treatment of choice. Caustics and astringents are still popular, but their action is not selective, and they remove the delicate epithelium along with the granulation tissue.

If bone or tendon is exposed, as it often is in traumatic wounds of large animals, it must be covered by granulation tissue before epithelium covers the defect. Sequestration of bone usually results if the periosteum has become dried or if the initial injury has chipped off a piece of bone. As soon as it is identified, the sequestrum should be removed; this may mean incising through the already-formed bed of granulation tissue. Skin grafting is indicated in wounds in which a large defect exists or slow skin healing is anticipated. This is discussed in detail in Chapter 8, "Reconstructive Surgery of Wounds."

Tertiary-Intention Healing

Delayed primary closure, or tertiary-intention healing, is occasionally performed in the distal limbs of the horse. In this method, the wound is allowed to heal to a certain point by secondary intention. The animal may have been presented to the surgeon after considerable attempts by the owner to heal the wound by secondary intention. The wound is then prepared for surgery. The excessive granulation tissue is excised along its borders, and the skin edges are sutured closed to heal by primary intention. Bandaging or fiberglass cast application is usually necessary to minimize movement and to prevent undue tension on the suture line.

References

1. Brown, L. L., et al.: Evaluation of wound irrigation by pulsatile jet and conventional methods. Am. J. Surg., *187*:170, 1978.

2. Viljanto, J.: Disinfection of surgical wounds without inhibition of normal wound healing. Arch. Surg., *115*:253, 1980.

Use of Drains

The basic purpose of drainage is to facilitate healing by obliterating dead space or by removing unwanted material from a particular location. Indications for the use of drains include the following: when postoperative seroma formation is a potential problem; after the internal fixation of fractures when complete obliteration of dead space is not possible; for contaminated wounds; and for thoracic and peritoneal cavity drainage whenever contamination or infection is considered to be a problem. The indications for drainage cannot be sharply defined, however, and indeed are controversial. The general philosophy of "when in doubt put a drain in" has yielded to a more cautious approach, with careful analysis of the indications.

The widespread use of drains has given rise to complications in both human and veterinary patients. Potentiation of parietal abdominal wound infections has been demonstrated in both clinical cases and experimental situations.[5,7] Both latex (Penrose) and Silastic drains potentiate infection. The problems caused by using Penrose drains for peritoneal drainage following abdominal surgery have also been emphasized.[10] Many valid indications for the use of drains still exist, but one should be more critical of the type of drain used, the number of times it is used, and how it is used. With regard to any drain, one should pay careful attention to aseptic technique at the time of placement and the postoperative management of the drains. Drainage should not be used as a substitute for meticulous debridement or careful closure of a wound.

The simplest method of wound drainage is the open technique, in which the skin is left unsutured. This technique is commonly used in large animal surgery when a primary closure cannot be performed. When a primary closure is performed and drainage away from the incision is desired, some form of artificial drainage is necessary.

At present, the latex Penrose drains and the perforated tube drains of plastic or Silastic (Redi-Vacette Perforated Tubing) are the most commonly used drains in large animal surgery. The Penrose drain is a thin, latex tube usually 7 to 12 mm in diameter (2.5-cm diameter drains are also available); it functions by capillary action and gravity flow, with drainage occurring around the drain, rather than through the lumen. Fenestration of these drains is contraindicated, because it decreases the surface area of the drain. In many cases, the use of a Penrose drain in a wound is sufficient to minimize the postoperative accumulation of blood or fluid. Penrose drains become walled off from the wound rapidly, however, with a decrease in their efficacy, and they also predispose the depths of the wound to retrograde infection from airborne and skin contamination.

In a typical wound closure, the drain is inserted with the ends exiting remote from the incision, and the incision is sutured. The external ends of the drain are sutured to the skin. The stab incisions through which the drains exit should be of sufficient size to allow drainage to occur around them. The drain may also be inserted so that only one end emerges from the wound, and the deep end of the drain is retained within the wound by a suture that can be removed later (Fig. 7-1). A dependent region for the emergence of at least one end of the drain should be selected. The drain should not be brought out through the primary incision because it encourages drainage through the incision. Daily cleansing of the drain, and bandage covering if possible, should be performed to minimize the occurrence of retrograde infection. In addition, retrograde infection is time related, and the drain should be removed as soon as it is considered nonfunctional. In addition, the drain itself acts as a foreign body, and a daily drainage of less than 50 ml/day may be purely drain induced.[3]

Penrose drains are easy to insert and do not need the continuous management that suction drains do. Their use should be restricted to wounds and the obliteration of subcutaneous dead space, however. That Penrose drains may potentiate infection if used in the peritoneal cavity is well documented, and they should not be used for this purpose. Penrose drains may also be used effectively in the treatment of hygromas. In these cases, fluid removal by drains can facilitate obliteration of the cavity by granulation tissue. It is also believed that the "foreign-body" effect of the drains may be advantageous in stimulating a granulation response in these cases. Stab incisions are made dorsally and ventrally into the hygroma, using aseptic technique. Fibrin and debris within the cavity are removed, and the drains are inserted (Fig. 7-2). The drains may be left in place 10 days to 2 weeks.

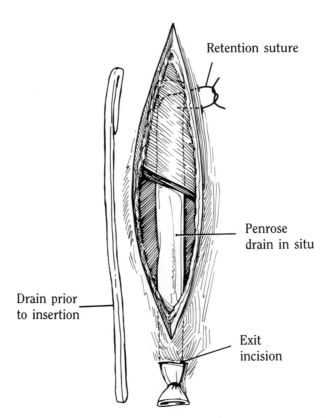

Retention suture

Penrose
drain in situ

Drain prior
to insertion

Exit
incision

FIG. 7-1. *Penrose drain with one and emerging from wound. Retention can be removed later and the drain extracted from the exit incision.*

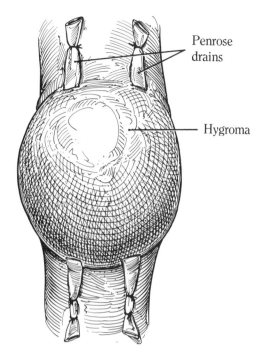

Penrose drains

Hygroma

FIG. 7-2. *Penrose drain used for treatment of hygroma.*

When more than overflow drainage is necessary, suction is applied through an implanted drain. A fenestrated tube drain is laid in the wound and exited through the skin by using a trocar (Fig. 7-3*A*), to form a tight seal around the drain (Fig. 7-3*B*). Constant suction can then be applied externally, and fluid can be evacuated from a deep tissue space. It is important that wound closure be airtight. Various evacuators are available commercially, but a simple and economical technique is the use of a syringe, as illustrated in Figure 7-3. The three-way stopcock is used to reduce further the possibility of retrograde infection when the syringe is emptied and suction is reapplied. The drains are heparinized prior to insertion; however, the suction pulls tissue into the holes in the drain, and clogging eventually results. The drains are generally effective long enough to eliminate the acute accumulation of serum following orthopedic surgery and for other procedures in which the dead space cannot be completely obliterated. Patency of tube suction drains can be prolonged by inserting a soft rubber section into the drainage system and regularly stripping the catheter.[6]

Whenever these drains can be managed appropriately and it is possible to maintain the negative pressure apparatus on the animal, the use of sealed, continuous suction drainage is definitely superior to the use of Penrose drains.[2] These drains should not be used as a substitute for hemostatic control and atraumatic technique during surgery, however.

Peritoneal drainage following laparotomy in large animals is indicated in only a few instances. We perform drainage for a few hours after equine abdominal surgery if any amount of lavage fluid has been left in the abdomen at closure. In this case, a centrally fenestrated tube drain is placed with the nonfenestrated ends and exits cranially and caudally. The drain is removed within 12 hours. With peritoneal drainage of longer duration, the fenestrations

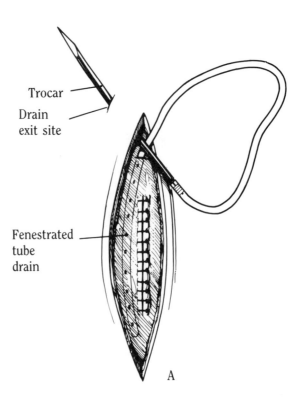

Trocar

Drain
exit site

Fenestrated
tube
drain

A

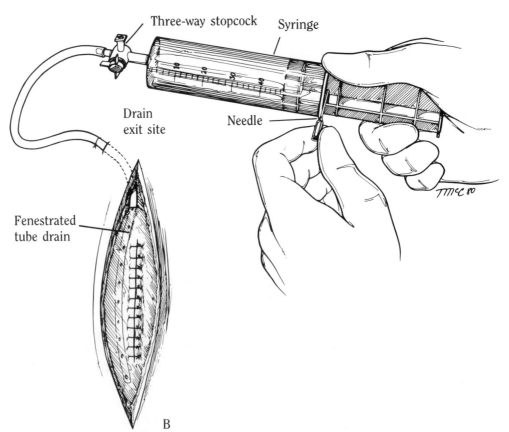

Three-way stopcock   Syringe

Drain
exit site

Needle

Fenestrated
tube drain

B

FIG. 7-3. A, *Using a trocar to exit a fenestrated drain.* B, *Syringe technique for suction drainage.*

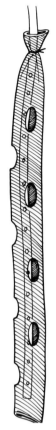

FIG. 7-4. *Sump-Penrose drain combination.*

of a tube drain will become clogged by fibrin, adhering omentum, or viscera. The ideal method for peritoneal drainage is the use of a sump-Penrose combination. A sump drain is a double-lumen, fenestrated tube drain that incorporates a smaller air vent. The air vent allows air to enter the drained region with the object of displacing fluid into the drain (an example of this is the Shirley wound drain).[8] By placing such a drain within a Penrose drain (Fig. 7-4), occlusion of the fenestrations of the central tube drain is delayed, and drainage efficiency is increased. The placement of gauze around the sump drain prior to insertion within the Penrose drain is another modification claimed to increase efficiency.[9]

Sophisticated, intra-abdominal sump drains, which also allow sterile irrigation, have been developed for man.[1,4] Whenever air or fluid ingress systems are used, careful technique is mandatory to prevent the introduction of infection. Bacterial filters should be used with the air channel of sump drains. If any ingress flushing system is to be combined with drainage, it is recommended that the flushing or irrigation be performed through a separate tube positioned through a separate entry site.

References

1. Formeister, J. F., and Elias, E. G.: Safe intra-abdominal and efficient wound drainage. Surg. Gynecol. Obstet., *142*:415, 1976.

2. Fox, J. W., and Golden, G. T.: The use of drains in subcutaneous surgical procedures. Am. J. Surg., *132*:673, 1976.

3. Golovsky, D., and Connolly, W. B.: Observations on wound drainage with a review of the literature. Med. J. Aust., *1*:289, 1976.

4. Hanna, E. A.: Efficiency of peritoneal drainage. Surg. Gynecol. Obstet., *131*:983, 1970.

5. Higson, R. H., and Kettlewell, M. G. W.: Parietal wound drainage in abdominal surgery. Br. J. Surg., *65*:326, 1978.

6. Jochimsen, P. R.: Method to prevent suction catheter drainage obstruction. Surg. Gynecol. Obstet., *142*:748, 1976.

7. Magee, C., et al.: Wound infection by surgical drains. Am. J. Surg., *131*:547, 1976.

8. Parks, J.: Peritoneal drainage. J. Am. Anim. Hosp., *10*:289, 1974.

9. Ranson, J. H. C.: Safer intraperitoneal sump drainage. Surg. Gynecol. Obstet., *137*:841, 1973.

10. Stone, H. H., Hooper, C. A., and Millikan, W. J.: Abdominal drainage following appendectomy and cholecystectomy. Ann. Surg., *187*:606, 1978.

11. Zacarski, L. R., et al.: Mechanism of obstruction of closed-wound suction tubing. Arch. Surg., *114*:614, 1979.

8

RECONSTRUCTIVE
SURGERY OF
WOUNDS

Some wounds cannot be closed by simply suturing them together. In some of these situations, the problem can be remedied by the use of full-thickness sliding flaps.[6] This technique involves local undermining of adjacent tissue along a subcutaneous plane in such a way that the dermal blood supply is maintained. In some instances, removal of excessive scar tissue beneath the surface may facilitate primary closure of the wound. Five simple reconstructive procedures to allow primary closure are described in this chapter: four utilize various methods of sliding-flap formation, and the fifth involves the removal of excessive tissue to facilitate skin closure.

Larger defects are not amenable to sliding skin flaps, and some form of free skin graft may be appropriate. The techniques of pinch-skin grafting and punch-skin grafting are also described in this chapter. Pedicle skin-grafting techniques are not practical in the horse.

Elliptical Excision Undermining for Repair of an Elongated Defect

In this situation, an elongated defect is too wide for its edges to be sutured. Using scissors or scalpel, the surgeon undermines the adjacent skin in an elliptical fashion (Fig. 8-1A). The mobilized skin flaps can then be moved toward each other, to allow a primary closure (Fig. 8-1B). The use of tension sutures in addition to the row of simple interrupted sutures may be indicated.

Wound Closure Using Tension-Relieving Incisions

In this technique, small, tension-relieving skin incisions are made adjacent to the wound, to facilitate wound closure or, at least, to decrease the healing time for the primary defect.[1] It has been described as the "mesh-expansion technique."

The skin adjacent to the defect is undermined, and a series of stab incisions is made parallel to and approximately 1 cm from the skin edge (Fig. 8-2A). Three rows of stab incisions are made on each side of the wound in a staggered fashion, with the adjacent rows approximately 1 cm apart

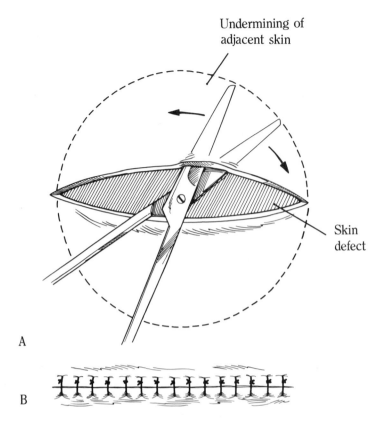

FIG. 8-1. A *and* B, *Elliptical excision undermining for repair of an elongated defect.*

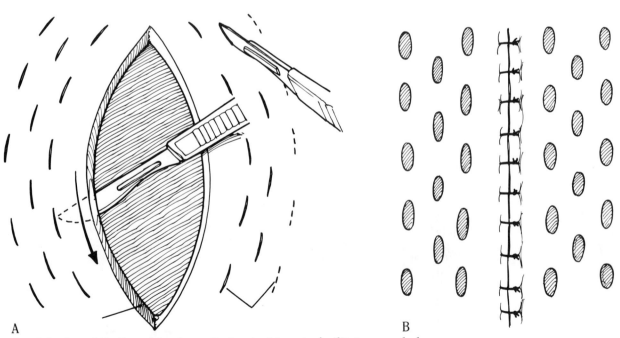

FIG. 8-2. A *and* B, *Use of tension-relieving incisions to facilitate wound closure.*

(Fig. 8-2A). The size of the stab incisions varies. In the initial description of the technique, the use of 10-mm stab incisions allowed sufficient expansion in fresh wounds and resulted in more rapid healing than when 7-mm tension-relieving incisions were used. In older wounds, however, with fibrosis and thickening of the surrounding skin, longer incisions (approximately 15 mm) are recommended. When the stab incisions have been made, the original wound edges are drawn into apposition and are sutured (Fig. 8-2B).

Wounds are managed postoperatively with bandaging or casting, depending on the individual case. The need for adequate postoperative support of the suture line needs to be recognized. Based on previous work, undermining can be performed for at least 4 cm on either side of the wound, without detrimental effects.[1] The release of blood and exudate through the stab incisions may facilitate the success of the technique by aiding revascularization and preventing hematoma and seroma formation.

Sliding H-Flap

This technique is used for the repair of rectangular or square defects. As illustrated in Fig. 8-3A, two flaps are generally created; however, if skin is not available on both sides, half of the H-plasty may be used.[6] The actual defect serves as the crossbridge of the letter H, and two arms are created (Fig. 8-3A). Triangles are cut at either end of each arm to prevent puckering of the skin when the flaps within the "H" are undermined and are slid together (Fig. 8-3A). Vertical mattress sutures are preplaced in the undermined flaps to act as tension sutures. The two flaps are then brought together and are sutured in a simple interrupted pattern (Fig. 8-3B). When performed correctly, sliding of the flaps together closes the triangular defects. These incision lines are also sutured in a simple interrupted pattern (Fig. 8-3B).

Z-Plasty

Z-plasty has two major indications. It may be used as a relaxation procedure for elliptical defects, and it can be used for scar revision of the palpebra when scar formation has produced acquired ectropion.

The use of Z-plasty as a relaxation procedure for elliptical incisions is illustrated in Figure 8-4. A Z-incision is made adjacent to the elliptical defect (Fig. 8-4A). The central incision of the "Z" (AB) should be perpendicular to the elliptical defect and centered over the area of greatest tension. The two triangles created by the incision should be equilateral; that is, having angles of 60°. The triangles are undermined to create two skin flaps. These skin flaps are then interchanged (Fig. 8-4B), and they are sutured in place (Fig. 8-4C). The principle behind this technique is that the interchange of the two flaps lengthens the original line (AB) by 50%.

In the second situation, illustrated in Figure 8-5, a linear scar (AB) has excessive tension along its longitudinal axis that results in an acquired ectropion of the upper eyelid (Fig. 8-5A). If a Z-plasty is performed in the

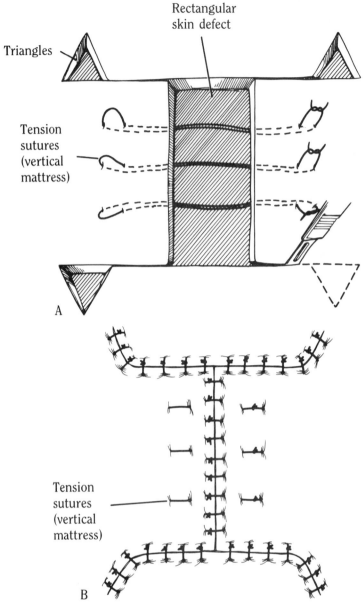

Rectangular
skin defect

Triangles

Tension
sutures
(vertical
mattress)

A

Tension
sutures
(vertical
mattress)

B

Fig. 8-3. A *and* B, *Sliding H-flap.*

previous manner, with AB as the central arm of the "Z," then tension will
be relieved, and the upper eyelid will be relaxed (Fig. 8-5*B*).

Removal of Excessive Scar Tissue (Debulking)

A cross section of a typical situation in which exuberant granulation
tissue or scar tissue coexists with incomplete skin closure is illustrated in
Figure 8-6*A*. A dotted line indicates the incision for removal of the excess
tissue, which is removed with sharp dissection (Fig. 8-6*B*); this allows the
primary closure of the skin over the dead space (Fig. 8-6*C*). Placement of
a subcutaneous drain is appropriate in this situation.

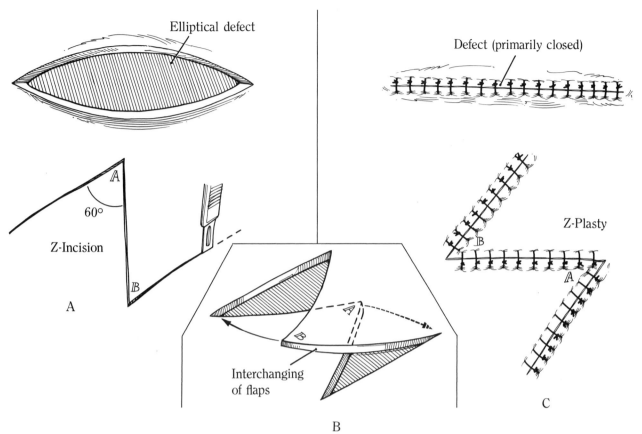

FIG. 8-4. A *to* C, *Z-plasty as relaxation procedure.*

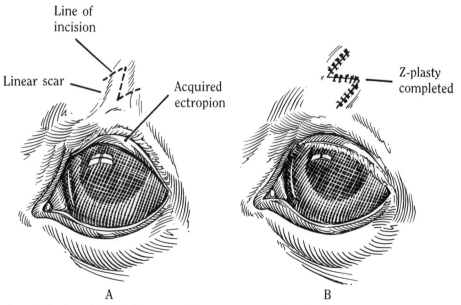

FIG. 8-5. A *and* B, *Z-plasty to relieve ectropion of eyelid.*

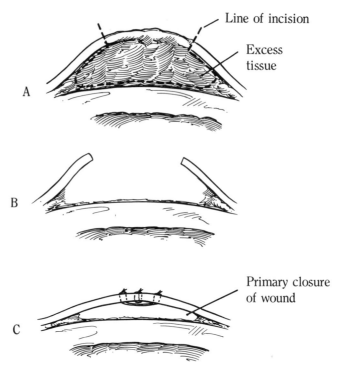

Line of incision

Excess tissue

A

B

Primary closure of wound

C

Fig. 8-6. A *to* C, *Removal of excessive scar tissue (debulking) to allow primary closure of a wound.*

Pinch-Skin Grafting

Several methods of free-skin grafting are available, including full- and split-thickness and mesh grafts.[2,3,5] If these grafts "take," the results are usually cosmetically superior to those of pinch-skin grafts or punch-skin grafts. The typical indication for a free-skin graft in large animals is for the large, slowly healing region of granulation resulting from a laceration to the distal equine limb, however. In these situations, results with full-thickness grafts have not been satisfactory. Results with split-thickness grafts have been better, but it is a complex and costly procedure. The grafting technique described here may be successful in the presence of a hostile grafting bed and when prevention of limb motion is not as critical.[4] Even if the graft does not take, its presence seems to stimulate epithelialization from the periphery. This grafting technique may be performed in the standing patient, and it is a useful, simple technique for the veterinarian in the field.

Ideally, the granulation bed should be healthy, free of infection, and level with edges of the skin prior to the skin graft. These requirements cannot be met in all situations. In many instances, however, regular trimming, topical medication, and bandaging improve the chances of a successful outcome.

The graft donor site is near the fold of the flank and is prepared for aseptic surgery. The area is anesthetized by the subcutaneous administration of local analgesic solution in the shape of an inverted "U." Because granulation tissue is devoid of nerves, analgesic infiltration of the recipient site is unnecessary. This site is prepared with dilute povidone-iodine solution (Betadine Solution) in sterile saline solution using sterile sponges.

When both the wound and the donor site have been prepared, a series of small, shallow "pockets" are made in the granulation tissue bed. The openings of the pockets should point upward, and each pocket should be parallel and 1 to 2 mm below the surface of the wound (Fig. 8-7A). The pockets are best produced with a no. 15 scalpel blade. Each pocket is about 0.5 cm square and the pockets are approximately 1 cm apart (Fig. 8-7B). Enough pockets are placed in the granulation bed to cover the wound completely. When all the pockets have been made, it is beneficial to apply pressure to the wound for 3 to 4 minutes to reduce the hemorrhage from the newly created pockets in the granulation bed.

Using fine tissue forceps, such as Brown-Adson forceps, the surgeon elevates the smallest possible pinch of skin (2 to 3 mm in diameter) at the donor site and excises it using a new, sharp scalpel blade (Fig. 8-7C). Several such pinches are transferred to a damp gauze moistened with saline solution or blood, and the grafts are then implanted in the wound. The pinches of skin are flattened as necessary and are inserted in each pocket of the granulation bed, just as one would insert a coin into a watch pocket (Fig. 8-7D).[4] Naturally, the graft is inserted with the epithelial side facing out. This procedure is repeated until all the pockets have been filled. The wound is carefully dried, ensuring that the grafts are not extruded from their pockets. The wound is then covered with one or more sterile, nonadherent dressings and is bandaged.

The horse is confined to a box stall to ensure minimal movement at the surgical site. The first 2 weeks of bandaging are critical for graft survival, and it is important that the position of the bandage be maintained. Unless otherwise indicated, the bandage is first changed 5 days following surgery. At this time, considerable exudate will have accumulated over the wound bed; this should be carefully wiped off, using sterile, saline-soaked sponges. The wound should not be scrubbed vigorously. At this stage, it is too early to assess the degree of "take," and the wound should be rebandaged in a similar manner. Bandages are then changed every 4 to 7 days or as necessary. The grafts can usually be identified in 2 to 3 weeks; failure to identify grafts at this time does not necessarily imply an unsuccessful result. As noted before, the procedure typically enhances the rate of epithelialization at the periphery of the wound and reduces healing time.

Punch-Skin Grafting

Punch-skin grafting is similar to pinch-skin grafting, except cylindrical plugs of skin are inserted into cylindrical holes in the granulation tissue.[7] The advantages to punch grafting parallel those of pinch grafting. Punch-skin grafting is preferred by some clinicians. The technique can be applied to a thinner granulation tissue bed than pinch grafts, which require a certain depth to create tissue pockets.[7] It is also believed that a more cosmetic result may be obtained.

The general principles of recipient and donor site preparation are the same as in pinch grafting. When the recipient site has been aseptically

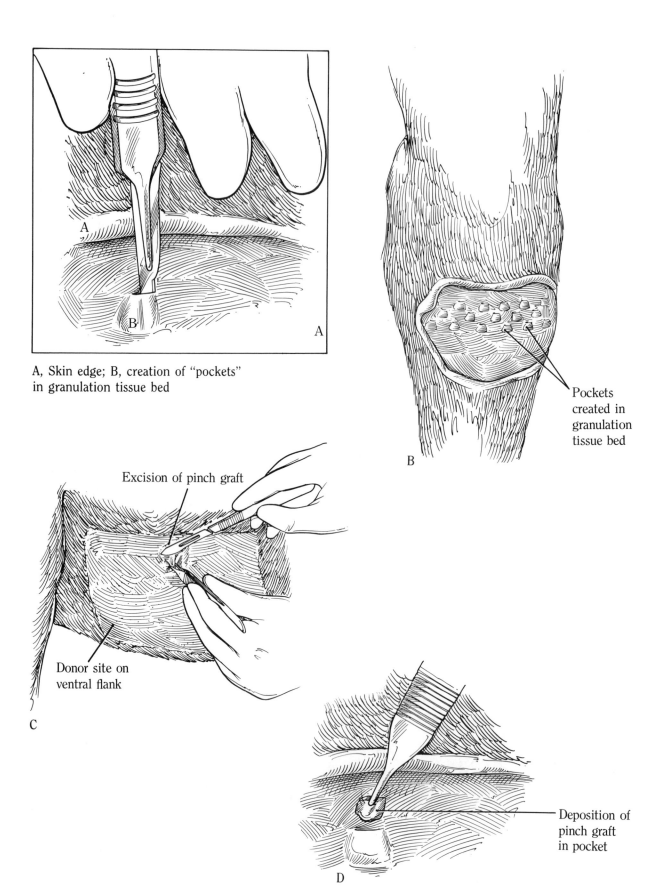

A, Skin edge; B, creation of "pockets"
in granulation tissue bed

Pockets
created in
granulation
tissue bed

B

Excision of pinch graft

Donor site on
ventral flank

C

Deposition of
pinch graft
in pocket

D

FIG. 8-7. A *to* D, *Pinch-skin grafting.*

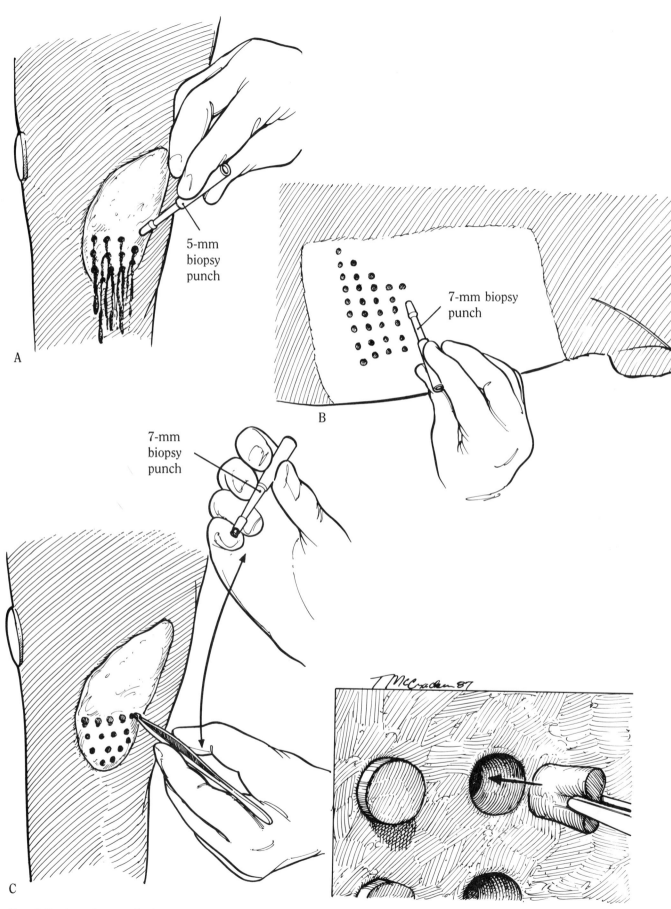

A

B

7-mm
biopsy
punch

5-mm
biopsy
punch

7-mm biopsy
punch

C

FIG. 8-8. A to C, Punch-skin grafting.

prepared, small circular holes are made in the granulating bed using a 5-mm biopsy punch* (Fig. 8-8A). These recipient holes are spaced about 7 mm apart in every direction over the entire surface of the wound. Blood clots forming in the recipient areas are removed prior to placement of the grafts or are prevented by filling the recipient holes with cotton swabs.[7]

Donor grafts are taken from the ventrolateral abdominal area using a 7-mm biopsy punch (Fig. 8-8B). The donor grafts are then placed one at a time into the recipient site (Fig. 8-8C). The 7-mm donor grafts have a tendency to contract and therefore fit snugly into the 5-mm diameter recipient holes. A sterile nonadherent dressing is placed on the wound after surgery, and a bandage is applied.

Immobilization of the area with a bandage splint or half-cast is recommended. Otherwise, aftercare is as previously described for pinch-skin grafting.

References

1. Bailey, J. V., and Jacobs, K. A.: The mesh expansion method of suturing wounds on the legs of horses. Vet. Surg., *12*:78, 1983.

2. Boyd, C. L.: Equine skin autotransplants for wound healing. J. Am. Vet. Med. Assoc., *151*:1618, 1967.

3. Hanselka, D. V.: Use of autogenous mesh grafts in equine wound management. J. Am. Vet. Med. Assoc., *164*:35, 1974.

4. Mackay-Smith, M. P., and Marks, D.: A skin-grafting technique for horses. J. Am. Vet. Med. Assoc., *152*:1633, 1968.

5. Meagher, D. M.: Split-thickness autologous skin transplantation in horses. J. Am. Vet. Med. Assoc., *159*:55, 1971.

6. Stashak, T. S.: Reconstructive surgery in the horse. J. Am. Vet. Med. Assoc., *170*:143, 1977.

7. Stashak, T. S.: Skin grafting in horses. Vet. Clin. North Am. (Large Anim. Pract.), *6*:215, 1984.

* Keyes Skin Punch, Aloe Medical Instruments, Dallas, Texas.

9

Medial Patellar Desmotomy

This procedure is performed for the treatment of upward fixation of the patella.[2] Upward fixation of the patella may be seen in horses that are debilitated or poorly conditioned. In many instances, appropriate conditioning and the development of quadriceps muscle tone with training in a young horse resolve the problem. Such conservative methods of treatment should be used first. Medial patellar desmotomy should be considered a "last resort." Upward fixation of the patella may also be seen in horses with straight conformation. We have seen cases of osteochondritis dissecans that adopt this conformation and may mimic signs of intermittent upward fixation of the patella. There may be distention of the femoropatellar joint as well. Good-quality radiographs of the stifle joint are indicated to rule out osteochondritis dissecans, especially in young horses.

Anesthesia and Surgical Preparation

This surgical procedure is performed with the animal standing. Depending on the temperament of the animal, tranquilization may be indicated. The area of the middle and medial patellar ligaments is clipped and surgically prepared. The tail is wrapped to avoid contamination of the surgical site. Two milliliters of local anesthetic are injected subcutaneously over the medial border of the middle patellar ligament. A 20-gauge, 1-in. needle is then inserted through this bleb, and the subcutaneous area around the distal part of the medial patellar ligament is infiltrated with local anesthetic.

Additional Instrumentation

This procedure requires a blunt-ended bistoury (tenotomy) knife.

Surgical Technique

A 1-cm incision is made over the medial border of the middle patellar ligament close to the attachment of the ligament to the tibial tuberosity.

(The site of the skin incision in relation to the patellar ligaments is illustrated in Figure 9-1A). Curved Kelly forceps are then forced through the heavy fascia and are passed beneath the medial patellar ligament. This creates a channel for the insertion of a bistoury knife beneath the medial patellar ligament (Fig. 9-1B). The bistoury knife is inserted so the side of the knife lies flat beneath the patellar ligament. When the knife is positioned, the cutting edge is then turned outward (Fig. 9-1C). With the left index finger palpating the end of the knife through the skin to ascertain its correct position, the surgeon cuts the ligament with a sawing movement (Fig. 9-1D). One must ensure that the blade of the bistoury knife completely encloses the medial patellar ligament before it is severed. Once the ligament has been severed, the tendon of the sartorius muscle feels like a tense band medially and may lead the inexperienced operator to believe that the medial patellar ligament has not been completely severed. One or two sutures of nonabsorbable material are placed in the skin incision.

Postoperative Management

Antibiotics are not used routinely. Hand-walking is useful to control local swelling. The horse should be rested and hand-walked for a minimum of 2 weeks and preferably 4 to 6 weeks. Even with experienced operators, instances of severe swelling and lameness of varying duration are observed occasionally.

Comments

Complications that can arise during surgery include severing of the wrong ligament or inadvertent entrance into the femoropatellar joint with the bistoury (this can potentially occur if the desmotomy is performed too proximad). A complication that can be seen postoperatively is dehiscence of the skin incision and cellulitis (phlegmon) of the limb. These complications can be avoided by careful attention to aseptic technique during the procedure.

The prognosis is generally favorable, provided surgery is performed before any secondary gonitis develops. Unfortunately, the procedure is often performed on horses with undiagnosed lameness in which upward fixation of the patella is not the problem. In these cases, the results are less satisfactory.

A condition resembling chondromalacia patellae of man and associated with medial patellar desmotomy has been observed in our clinic.[1] On radiographs, spurring or fragmentation of the distal patella is noted. When viewed arthroscopically, cartilage lesions varying from softening and fibrillation to dissection and fragmentation of the articular cartilage have been seen. It is suggested that the lesions may be caused by maltracking of the patella within the trochlear groove, more lateral positioning of the patella resulting from loss of the medial tensile pull of the medial patellar ligament. That medial patellar desmotomy is the cause of the problem has yet to be proved, however.

References

1. McIlwraith, C. W.: Unpublished data, 1984 to 1987.

2. Stashak, T. S. (Ed.): Adams' Lameness in Horses, 4th Ed. Philadelphia, Lea & Febiger, 1987, p. 737.

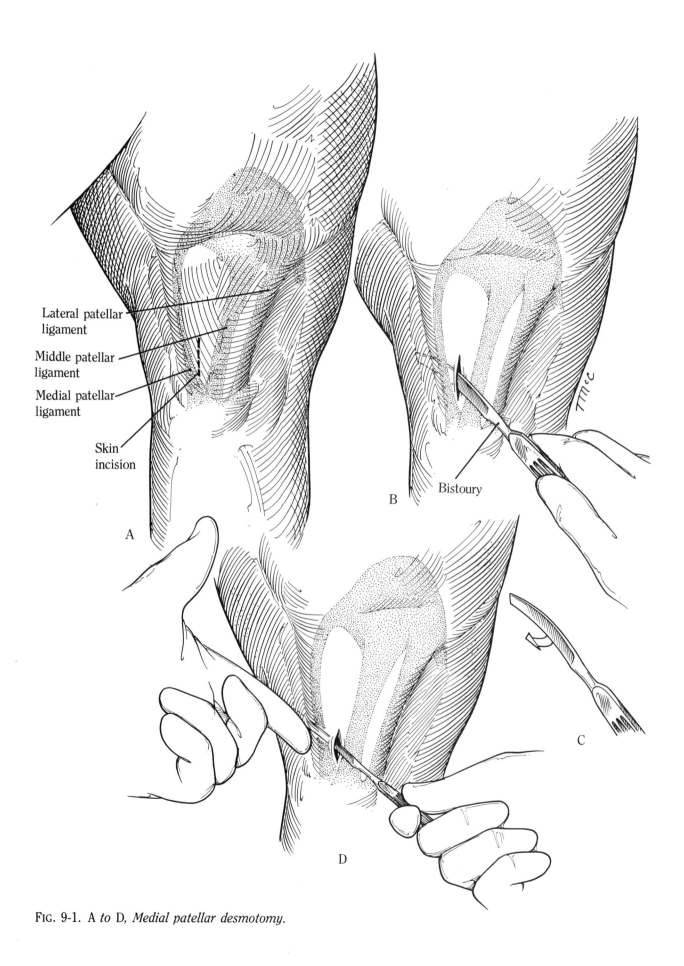

Lateral patellar
ligament

Middle patellar
ligament

Medial patellar
ligament

Skin
incision

A

B

Bistoury

C

D

FIG. 9-1. A *to* D, *Medial patellar desmotomy.*

Cunean Tenectomy

Cunean tenectomy is one of the treatments for bone spavin (degenerative joint disease of the distal intertarsal and tarsometatarsal joints).[3] The cunean tendon is the medial branch of the insertion of the tibialis cranialis muscle; it passes obliquely over the distal intertarsal and tarsometatarsal joints where a small bursa is interposed between the tendon and bone. The rationale for the surgery is that it may remove a source of pain caused by the tendon creating pressure on the spavin region.[3] The operation is used extensively in the Standardbred as treatment for the syndrome known as cunean bursitis. In a statistical analysis of cases treated by this surgical procedure and by other means, however, the operation had limited advantage over conservative methods.[1]

In the opinion of those who have performed many cunean tenectomies, this is essentially a "tendon-lengthening" operation. If the surgical site is examined at autopsy months after surgery, the severed ends will have re-established continuity.

Cunean tenectomy is also used as a surgical approach to the distal intertarsal and tarsal metatarsal joints as part of surgical arthrodesis of these joints. Surgical arthrodesis of these joints is used to treat bone spavin cases refractory to more conservative treatments. Surgical arthrodesis of these joints is beyond the scope of this book, but it is described in our advanced techniques textbook.[2]

Anesthesia and Surgical Preparation

This surgical procedure may be performed with the recumbent animal under general anesthesia or with the standing animal under local anesthesia. For the latter procedure, the limb is clipped, shaved, scrubbed, and prepared for the infusion of local anesthetic. Generally, local anesthetic is infused in an inverted "U" pattern dorsal to the proposed site of the incision. Alternatively, anesthetic can be infused above and below the tendon and into the cunean bursa, to distend it. A twitch or tranquilization may be required. The surgical site is prepared for aseptic surgery following infiltration of the local anesthetic.

Surgical Technique

The incision for the cunean tenectomy can be either a vertical incision almost perpendicular to the direction of the cunean tendon or an incision that parallels the direction of the fibers of the cunean tendon. If the surgeon is attempting the operation for the first time, we recommend that he make a *vertical* incision. This allows the surgeon a certain margin of error if the incision is too distal or too proximal.

If the second method is used and the incision is made in the direction of the fibers, the surgeon must be confident that it is placed directly over the middle of the tendon. To help locate the incision, firm digital palpation is made over the area of the tendon on the medial aspect of the hock; the distal limit of the chestnut is a good landmark (Fig. 9-2A). If this incision is too proximal or too distal, it cannot be modified like the vertical incision. The technique described here has the incision following the direction of the cunean tendon.

The incision is made through the skin and subcutaneous tissues and onto the cunean tendon; at this point, the tendon will be visible. A pair of

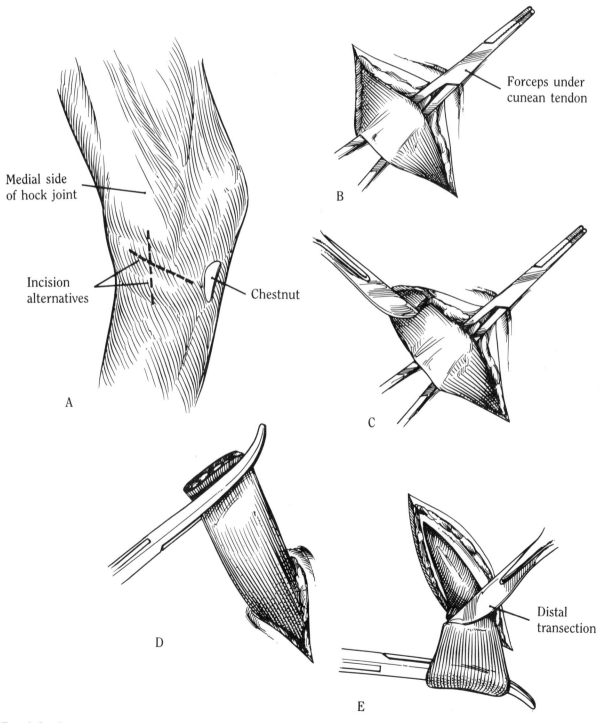

FIG. 9-2. *Cunean tenectomy.*

forceps are directed under the cunean tendon and into the cunean bursa, to emerge from the proximal edge of the tendon (Fig. 9-2B). The tendon is then incised at its proximal end (Fig. 9-2C), and the distal portion of the tendon is grasped with the forceps (Fig. 9-2D). As much of the cunean tendon is removed as possible. The tendon is incised at its distal end near the chestnut (Fig. 9-2E).

Following removal of a portion of the tendon, the skin is closed using a synthetic, monofilament, nonabsorbable suture (nylon or polypropylene) in a simple interrupted or vertical mattress pattern. If the animal is under general anesthesia, the surgeon may elect to close the subcutaneous tissues with an absorbable suture before the skin closure. The limb is bandaged using a suitable nonadherent dressing in combination with an elastic adhesive bandage that does not extend above the hock joint.

Postoperative Management

Tetanus prophylaxis is administered, but antibiotics are not used routinely. The bandage is kept in place for approximately 10 days; at the end of this time, the initial bandage and the skin sutures are removed. Exercise generally commences as soon as the skin sutures are removed.

References

1. Gabel, A. A.: Treatment and prognosis for cunean tendon bursitis-tarsitis of Standardbred horses. J. Am. Vet. Med. Assoc., *175*:1086, 1979.

2. McIlwraith, C. W., and Turner, A. S.: Equine Surgery: Advanced Techniques. Philadelphia, Lea & Febiger, 1987.

3. Stashak, T. S. (Ed.): Adams' Lameness in Horses, 4th Ed. Philadelphia, Lea & Febiger, 1987.

Lateral Digital Extensor Tenotomy

Lateral digital extensor tenotomy (myotomy) is indicated for the treatment of equine stringhalt. Although the exact cause of stringhalt is unknown, resection of the tendon and muscle belly leads to partial or even complete relief of the condition.[2] The lateral digital extensor muscle originates at the collateral ligament of the stifle, fibula, and lateral tibia; it proceeds distad, lateral to the tibia, and enters the tendon sheath just caudal to the lateral malleolus of the tibia. The tendon sheath is nonpalpable where it is covered by the fascia and extensor retinaculum of the hock. The tendon then continues distad and is palpable as it emerges from the tendon sheath at the level of the proximal third of the metatarsus (Fig. 9-3A). The following technique involves resection of the tendon plus a large portion of the muscle belly of the lateral digital extensor tendon. The original operation involved removal of the tendon plus 2 cm of muscle belly; the modified technique was designed to improve the surgical success rate.

Anesthesia and Surgical Preparation

It is preferable to perform this technique of lateral digital extensor tenotomy with the patient under general anesthesia because more attention can be paid to asepsis and hemostasis. If only a small amount of the muscle is removed, the surgery can be performed under local anesthesia with the animal standing. In this situation, the local anesthetic should be injected about 2 cm above the lateral malleolus of the tibia directly into the muscle belly of the lateral digital extensor. The second injection of local anesthetic should be made in the area below the hock and above the lateral digital extensor tendon, just before it joins the long digital extensor tendon.

The area over the surgical site is clipped and shaved. Two surgical sites are prepared: the first is a large area over the muscle belly, above the hock, and the second is a smaller area over the distal end of the tendon where it merges with the long digital extensor tendon (Fig. 9-3A).

Surgical Technique

The distal incision is made over the lateral digital extensor tendon immediately proximal to its junction with the long digital extensor tendon. An incision is made directly over the tendon; the tendon is exposed and isolated by dissecting bluntly beneath the tendon and elevating it using either curved Kelly forceps or Ochsner forceps (Fig. 9-3B). Pulling on the tendon at this stage reveals movement of the corresponding muscle belly of the lateral digital extensor tendon; this will assist the surgeon in locating the incision over the muscle belly.

The second incision is made over the muscle belly parallel to the direction of the muscle fibers. The incision should continue through the overlying fascia until the fleshy portion of the muscle belly is visible (Fig. 9-3C). The fascia overlying the muscle belly is thick, and the fibers are directed diagonally. Once the muscle belly is freed (Fig. 9-3D), the surgeon goes to the first incision over the distal aspect of the lateral digital extensor tendon and severs the tendon (Fig. 9-3E). Prior to severing the tendon, one should make sure that the tendon in the distal incision corresponds to the muscle in the proximal incision. Then a pair of Oschner forceps are placed under the musculotendinous junction; by exerting traction on it, the entire tendon is stripped from its sheath, which overlies the lateral aspect of the hock (Fig. 9-3F). The muscle belly is then elevated from the incision and is severed at an oblique angle (Fig. 9-3G).

The surgeon should attempt to oversew the muscle stump. This may be difficult because of excess tension, but we believe it reduces postoperative seroma formation. The stump of the muscle is oversewn by grasping the fascia surrounding the muscle belly on the one side and apposing it to the fascia on the opposite side of the muscle belly. Simple horizontal mattress sutures are placed using a synthetic absorbable material. The fascia is closed with simple interrupted sutures of an absorbable suture material, followed by closure of the subcutaneous tissues with a similar material in a simple interrupted or continuous pattern (Fig. 9-3H). The skin is closed with a synthetic, monofilament, nonabsorbable suture material in a simple interrupted pattern. The distal incision is closed in one layer using a similar material in the skin. The wounds are covered with nonadherent dressings, and the entire limb is bandaged.

If the condition is bilateral, the horse is rolled over (if it is under general anesthesia), and the identical procedure is performed on the other pelvic limb.

With the original technique, in which only a small amount of muscle belly is severed, postoperative bandaging is less critical. With this modified muscle-belly severing technique, however, bandaging is essential to minimize seroma formation caused by hemorrhage from the muscle stump. A bandage for this purpose consists of soft cotton and extends from the proximal tibia distad to the pastern.

Postoperative Management

Bandaging is generally required for 2 to 3 weeks, and sutures are removed 2 to 3 weeks postoperatively. Box-stall rest is indicated until the surgical sites are healed. When the sites are healed, hand-walking is commenced for about 2 weeks. After this period of hand-walking, normal training is resumed. Dehiscence of the skin sutures sometimes occurs because of the stringhalt nature of the gait, and although it has been suggested that the wounds be resutured,[2] it is preferable to allow healing by secondary intention.

Comments

The results of surgery are unpredictable probably because the underlying cause of the condition is unknown. Stringhalt probably has a neurologic basis and has been termed a distal axonopathy.[1] Axonal degeneration of certain nerves in the hindlimb has been observed. To complicate matters

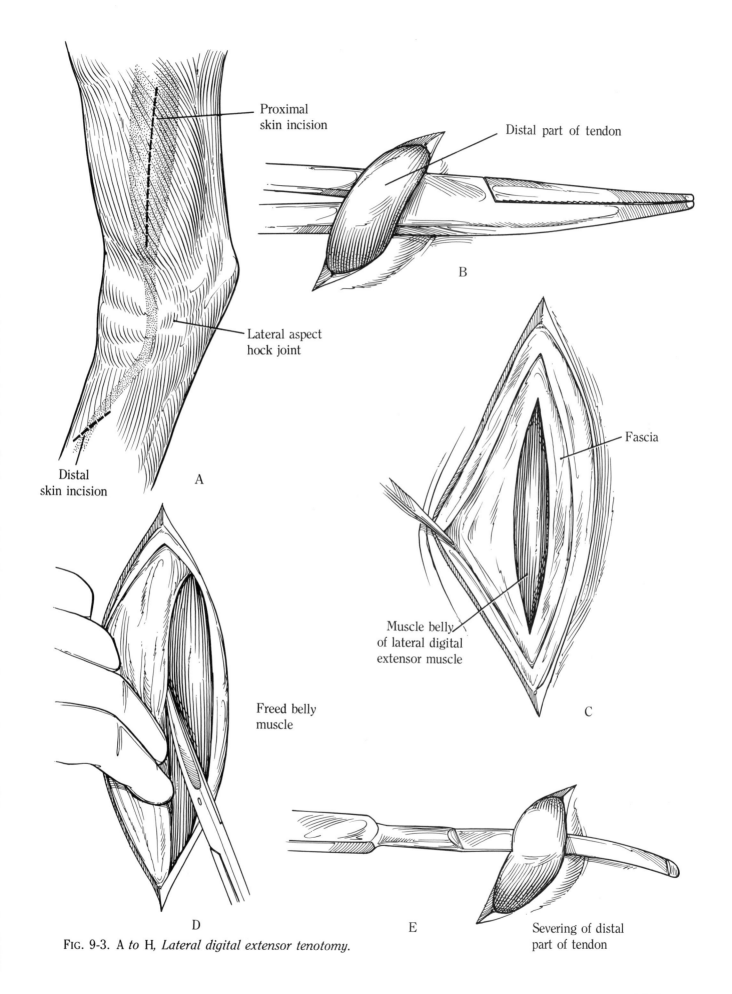

Proximal
skin incision

Lateral aspect
hock joint

Distal
skin incision

A

Distal part of tendon

B

Fascia

Muscle belly
of lateral digital
extensor muscle

C

Freed belly
muscle

D

Severing of distal
part of tendon

E

FIG. 9-3. A *to* H, *Lateral digital extensor tenotomy.*

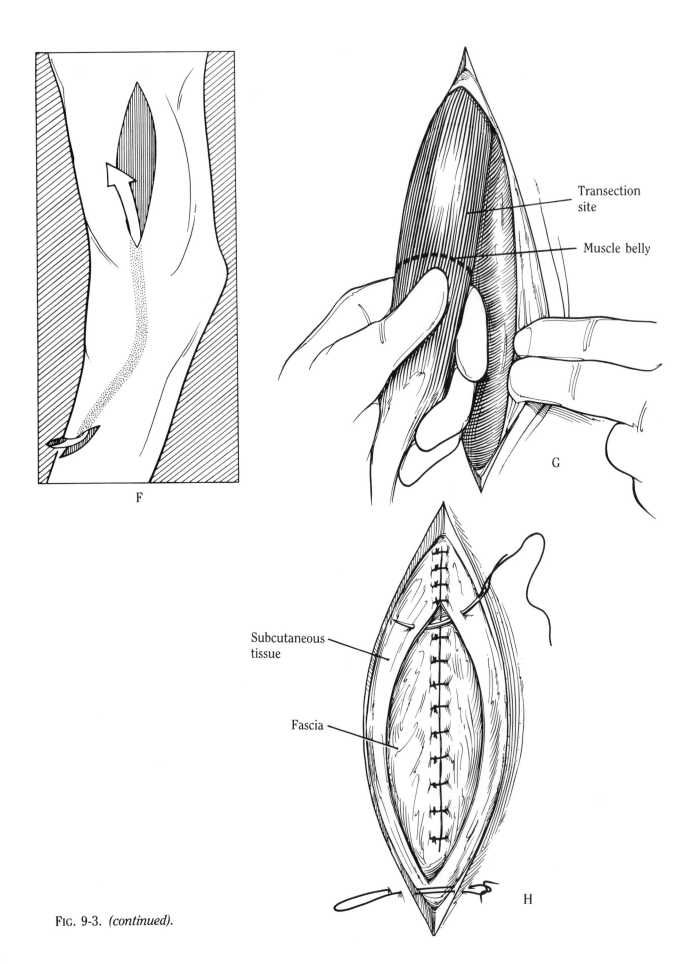

F

Transection
site

Muscle belly

G

Subcutaneous
tissue

Fascia

H

FIG. 9-3. *(continued)*.

further, pathologic changes have also been seen in the left recurrent laryngeal nerve, as well as in nerves in the forelimbs in horses with stringhalt. Possible causes of this axonopathy have been suggested, including vitamin deficiency or exposure to some toxin. The clinical signs of stringhalt vary with weather, and certain climatic conditions may facilitate production of certain mycotoxins in the soil. Outbreaks of stringhalt have occurred when horses graze on certain plants. It has been seen in association with the plant *Hypochaeris radicata,* which may contain a neurotoxic agent.[1] The predominant clinical sign of stringhalt, hyperflexion of one or both of the hindlimbs, is at variance with the pathologic findings seen in the nerves, including those in the left recurrent laryngeal nerve. It has been proposed that damage to the large, more vulnerable nerve fibers from the muscle spindles produces the exaggerated flexion of the hindlimbs early in the course of the disease.[1]

Clients are advised of these aspects when they present a horse to the clinician for surgery. We go ahead with surgery if the client still wishes it; despite the uncertain pathogenesis, the operation offers the only real treatment possibility.

References

1. Cahill, J. I., Goulden, B. E., and Jolly, R. D.: Stringhalt in horses: a distal axonopathy. Neuropathol. Appl. Neurobiol., *12*:459, 1986.

2. Stashak, T. S. (Ed.): Adams' Lameness in Horses, 4th Ed. Philadelphia, Lea & Febiger, 1987, p. 723.

Inferior Check Ligament Desmotomy

An inferior check ligament (deep digital flexor accessory ligament) desmotomy is indicated in cases of flexure deformity of the distal interphalangeal, or coffin, joint (deep digital flexor (DDF) tendon contracture) that have not responded to conservative methods of therapy. It is also indicated in cases of flexure deformity of the metacarpophalangeal, or fetlock, joint when contracture of the DDF unit is considered to be a significant factor.[1,2]

In terms of function and cosmetics, inferior check desmotomy is a better technique than deep flexor tenotomy for the treatment of distal interphalangeal flexure deformities, except when the dorsal surface of the hoof is beyond vertical.[3]

Anesthesia and Surgical Preparation

Surgery is performed with the patient under general anesthesia and in lateral recumbency. A lateral or medial approach may be used, but the lateral approach avoids the medial palmar (common digital) artery on the medial side; it is the easiest approach and is recommended for the inexperienced surgeon. A medial approach has one advantage, however, in that, if a blemish develops, it will be on the medial side of the limb and may not be as obvious. The animal is positioned so that the side of the leg to be operated on is uppermost. Then the carpometacarpal area is clipped and is surgically prepared.

Surgical Technique

A 5-cm incision is made over the cranial border of the DDF tendon and is extended from the proximal quarter of the metacarpus to halfway down the metacarpus. The position of the incision is illustrated in Figure 9-4*A*, and the relevant anatomy is illustrated in Figure 9-4*B*. Following the skin incision, the loose connective tissue over the flexor tendons is dissected bluntly, and the paratenon is incised (Fig. 9-4*C*). The superficial and deep flexor tendons must be identified, but they need not be dissected from each other. Blunt dissection is directed craniad to expose the inferior check ligament, and a cleavage plane is identified between the proximal part of the DDF tendon and the inferior check ligament. This cleavage plane is used to separate the check ligament from the DDF tendon (Fig. 9-4*D*). Forceps are inserted between the check ligament and the DDF tendon to separate the structures; then the check ligament is lifted from the incision and is incised with a scalpel (Fig. 9-4*E*). This surgical manipulation sometimes disrupts the synovial sheath of the carpal canal, the distal extremity of which extends most of the way down inside the cleavage plane. This event seems to be of little consequence, however. The foot of the patient is then extended manually. The ends of the check ligament become separated, and complete severance of all parts of the check ligament can be ascertained.

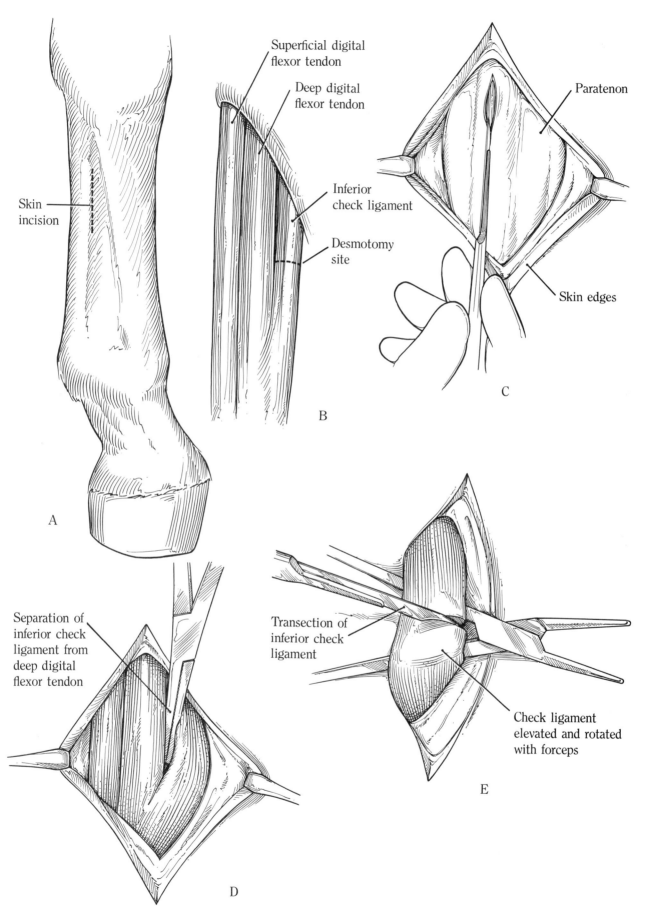

Skin incision

Superficial digital flexor tendon

Deep digital flexor tendon

Inferior check ligament

Desmotomy site

A

B

Paratenon

Skin edges

C

Separation of inferior check ligament from deep digital flexor tendon

D

Transection of inferior check ligament

Check ligament elevated and rotated with forceps

E

FIG. 9-4. A *to* E, *Inferior check ligament desmotomy.*

The paratenon and superficial fascia are closed in a single layer with simple interrupted sutures of synthetic, absorbable material. The skin is closed with nonabsorbable sutures in a suture pattern of the surgeon's choice.

Postoperative Management

A sterile dressing is placed over the incision, and the limb is bandaged from the proximal metacarpus to the coronary band. To apply more pressure over the surgical site (in an attempt to minimize swelling and reduce the potential blemish) a 4-in. roll of gauze bandage is placed over the incision and is held in position with pressure from an overlying bandage. The hoof is trimmed to normal conformation. Phenylbutazone (1 to 2 g) is administered intravenously to reduce postoperative pain and to facilitate lowering of the heel. Antibiotics are not administered routinely. Toe extensions may be indicated in more severe cases. Sutures are removed at 12 to 14 days, and bandaging may be discontinued 3 to 4 days later.

Comments

The effect of inferior check ligament desmotomy on long-term athletic function has been addressed in a retrospective study of 40 horses treated for flexure deformities of the distal interphalangeal joint.[4] Nine months to 4 years after surgery, 35 horses were not lame and were used as athletes. Of the other 7 horses, 6 had complications related to the deformity, whereas 1 had complications resulting from surgery.[4]

References

1. McIlwraith, C. W.: Diseases of joints, tendons, ligaments and related structures. *In* Adams' Lameness in Horses, 4th Ed. Edited by T. S. Stashak. Philadelphia, Lea & Febiger, 1987.

2. McIlwraith, C. W.: Tendon disorders of young horses. *In* Equine Medicine and Surgery, 3rd Ed. Edited by R. A. Mansmann and E. S. McAllister. Santa Barbara, CA, American Veterinary Publications, 1982.

3. McIlwraith, C. W., and Fessler, J. F.: Evaluation of inferior check ligament desmotomy for treatment of acquired flexor tension contracture. J. Am. Vet. Med. Assoc., *172*:293, 1978.

4. Wagner, D. C., et al.: Long-term results of desmotomy of the accessory ligament of the deep digital flexor tendon (distal check ligament) in horses. J. Am. Vet. Med. Assoc., *187*:1351, 1985.

Superior Check Ligament Desmotomy (After Bramlage)

Superior check ligament (accessory ligament of the superficial digital flexor) desmotomy was initially described as a surgical treatment for metacarpophalangeal flexural deformities in young horses.[1] Reported results vary,[4,7] however, and it is now recognized that the superficial digital flexor (SDF) tendon is not necessarily the primary unit in metacarpophalangeal flexural deformities.[6] In cases where the SDF appears to be the most involved structure, superior check ligament desmotomy may be indicated.

More recently, superior check ligament desmotomy has been reported as a treatment for superficial digital flexor tendinitis in racehorses. In a prospective study of the treatment, by superior check desmotomy of 36 horses with SDF tendonitis of 40 limbs, the operation improved the success rate in returning the horse to racing without recurrence of the injury.[2,3] The rationale for the surgery is that it interrupts the transfer of the weight-bearing load on the tendon to the distal radius, bringing the muscle and tendon proximal to the superior check ligament (and therefore enhanced elasticity to the functional unit) into use during weight-bearing.[2]

Anesthesia and Surgical Preparation

Surgery is performed with the patient under general anesthesia and either in lateral recumbency with the affected leg down or in dorsal recumbency with the leg suspended. The latter position is preferable in terms of hemostasis. The leg will have been clipped previously from midradius to midmetacarpus. The medial side of the antebrachium is surgically prepared.

Surgical Technique

A 10-cm skin incision is made cranial to the cephalic vein, over the flexor carpi radialis tendon and extending from the level of the distal chestnut proximad. The incision is continued through the subcutaneous tissue and antebrachial fascia (Fig. 9-5A). A transverse branch of the cephalic vein may or may not require ligation (the incision can often be continued under it). The fascial sheath of the flexor carpi radialis is incised (Fig. 9-5B), and Gelpi retractors are placed to expose the medial wall of the sheath, which adheres to the superior check ligament. A stab incision is made through the craniolateral wall of the sheath and superior check ligament (Fig. 9-5C). The incision is continued proximad and distad to sever the ligament completely. Complete incision through the check ligament is evidenced by visualizing the muscular portion of the radial head of the deep digital flexor tendon beneath and separation of the superficial digital flexor muscle palmad (Fig. 9-5D). An artery (nutrient artery for the superficial digital flexor tendon) may be present at the proximal border of the check ligament. After complete transection of the ligament, the membranous roof of the carpal synovial

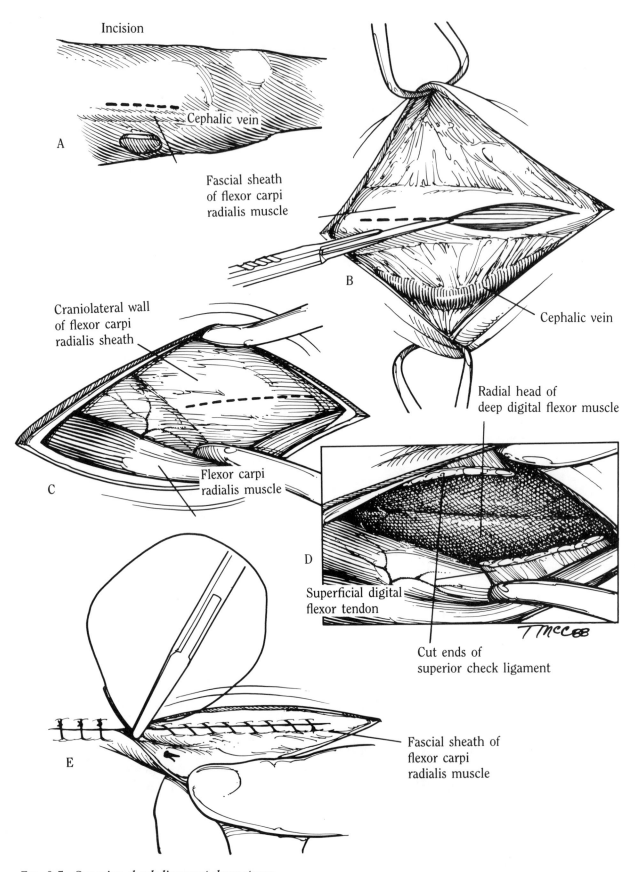

Incision

Cephalic vein

A

Fascial sheath
of flexor carpi
radialis muscle

B

Cephalic vein

Craniolateral wall
of flexor carpi
radialis sheath

C

Flexor carpi
radialis muscle

Radial head of
deep digital flexor muscle

D

Superficial digital
flexor tendon

Cut ends of
superior check ligament

E

Fascial sheath of
flexor carpi
radialis muscle

FIG. 9-5. *Superior check ligament desmotomy.*

sheath is seen distally, and the muscle belly of the radial head of the deep digital flexor tendon is seen in central and proximal areas of the incision.

The incision in the flexor carpi radialis sheath is closed with simple interrupted sutures of 2-0 synthetic absorbable material. The antebrachial fascia and subcutaneous tissue is closed with a continuous suture of 2-0 synthetic nonabsorbable material (Fig. 9-5E). The skin is closed with interrupted sutures of 2-0 nonabsorbable material.

Postoperative Management

A sterile dressing is placed over the incision, and a pressure bandage is applied. Phenylbutazone is administered postoperatively, but antibiotics are not used routinely. Sutures are removed at 12 to 14 days, and bandaging may be discontinued 3 to 4 days later.

Comments

The technique described is a modification of that previously described.[5] The approach is more caudal, and the limits of the superior check ligament are more easily defined. In addition, the closure of the medial wall of the flexor carpi radialis sheath facilitates elimination of dead space and minimizes the potential for hematoma formation and adhesions.

References

1. Bramlage, L. R.: Personal communication, 1987.

2. Bramlage, L. R.: Superior check ligament desmotomy as a treatment for superficial digital flexor tendonitis: initial report. *In* Proceedings of the 32nd Annual Convention of the American Association of Equine Practitioners in 1986:1987, p. 365.

3. Bramlage, L. R., et al.: Superior check ligament desmotomy for treatment of superficial digital flexor tendonitis. Equine Vet. J. In press.

4. Fackelman, G. E.: Flexure deformity of the metacarpophalangeal joints in growing horses. Compend. Contin. Educ., *9*:51, 1979.

5. Jann, H. W., Beroza, G. A., and Fackelman, G. E.: Surgical anatomy for desmotomy of the accessory ligament of the superficial flexor tendon (Proximal check ligament) in horses. Vet. Surg., *15*:378, 1986.

6. McIlwraith, C. W.: Diseases of joints, tendons, ligaments, and related structures. In *Lameness in Horses,* 4th Ed. Edited by T. S. Stashak. Lea & Febiger, Philadelphia, 1987, p. 339.

7. Wagner, P. C., et al.: Management of acquired flexural deformity of the metacarpophalangeal joint in Equidae. J. Am. Vet. Med. Assoc., *187*:915, 1985.

Superficial Digital Flexor Tenotomy

Superficial digital flexor tenotomy is indicated for the treatment of selected cases of flexure deformity of the metacarpophalangeal (fetlock) joint. This condition has been described previously as superficial digital flexor (SDF) tendon contracture, but it has become evident that more than the SDF tendon is involved.[3] The deep digital flexor tendon is commonly involved, and in a chronic case, the suspensory ligament may be involved as well. In an appropriate patient, however, tenotomy of the superficial flexor tendon may return the fetlock to normal alignment.

The technique of superior check (accessory ligament of the SDF) desmotomy has been advocated as an alternate treatment for flexure deformity of the metacarpophalangeal joint.[1] Effective division of the superior check ligament is more difficult than inferior desmotomy, however, and the value of the operation in treating flexure deformities of the metacarpophalangeal joint is controversial.[1,2,4] At the present time, we anticipate that SDF tenotomy will continue to be used to treat selected cases of flexure deformities of the fetlock joint.

Anesthesia and Surgical Preparation

This technique may be performed with the appropriate patient under local analgesia or in lateral recumbency under general anesthesia. The midmetacarpal area is prepared surgically.

Surgical Technique

Tenotomy may be performed blindly through a stab incision using a tenotomy knife or under direct visualization through a larger skin incision. The latter technique is illustrated here.

A 2-cm skin incision is made over the junction of the superficial and deep digital flexor tendons at the level of midmetacarpus (Fig. 9-6*A*). The paratenon is incised, and forceps are used to separate the SDF tendon from the deep digital flexor tendon. A cleavage plane is obvious (Fig. 9-6*B*). When the SDF tendon is separated, it is incised with a scalpel (Fig. 9-6*C*). Following tenotomy, the skin is sutured with nonabsorbable material.

When the surgeon has become familiar with the technique under direct visualization, it is simple to perform the surgery blindly by inserting a tenotomy knife blade through a small skin incision, manipulating it between the superficial and deep digital flexor tendons, rotating it 90°, and then severing the tendon. The stab incision is closed with a single suture.

Postoperative Management

A sterile dressing is placed over the incision, and the leg is bandaged from the proximal metacarpus distad. Phenylbutazone, 1 to 2 g, is administered

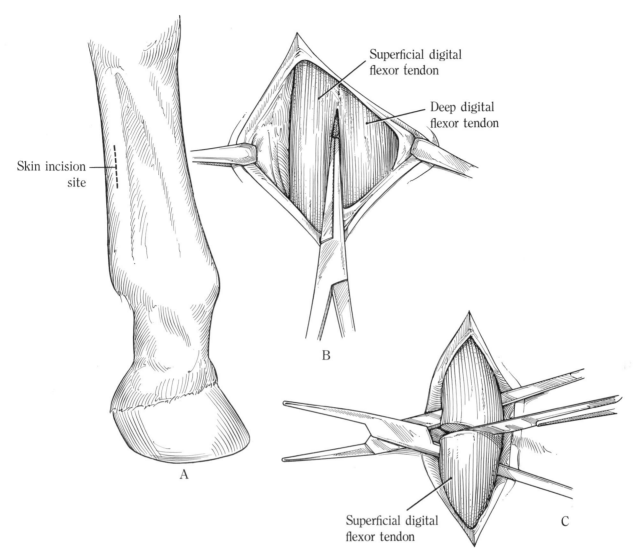

Skin incision site

Superficial digital flexor tendon

Deep digital flexor tendon

B

Superficial digital flexor tendon

C

A

FIG. 9-6. A *to* C, *Superficial digital flexor tenotomy.*

to facilitate return to function, and the animal is placed on an exercise regimen immediately. The sutures are removed 10 to 12 days after the operation, at which point bandaging is discontinued. If this technique fails to correct the deformity, additional procedures, such as inferior check desmotomy, may need to be performed. In addition, in some cases, inferior check ligament desmotomy is the initial treatment of choice in patients with flexure deformities of the metacarpophalangeal joint.[2,3]

References

1. Fackelman, G. E.: Flexure deformity of the metacarpophalangeal joints in growing horses. Compend. Contin. Educ., *1*:S1, 1979.

2. McIlwraith, C. W.: Diseases of joints, tendons, ligaments, and related structures. *In* Adams' Lameness in Horses, 4th Ed. Edited by T. S. Stashak. Philadelphia, Lea & Febiger, 1987, p. 339.

3. McIlwraith, C. W.: Tendon disorders of young horses. *In* Equine Medicine and Surgery, 3rd Ed. Edited by R. A. Mansmann and E. S. McAllister. Santa Barbara, CA, American Veterinary Publications, 1982.

4. Wagner, P. C., et al.: Management of acquired flexural deformity of the metacarpophalangeal joint in Equidae. J. Am. Vet. Med. Assoc., *187*:915, 1985.

Deep Digital Flexor Tenotomy

Deep digital flexor (DDF) tenotomy is indicated for the treatment of severe cases of flexural deformity of the distal interphalangeal joint and also as an aid in the management of chronic refractory laminitis.[3,4] If a distal interphalangeal joint flexural deformity has progressed to the extent that the dorsal surface of the distal phalanx has passed beyond vertical, secondary contraction of the joint capsule and peritendinous attachments of the distal segment of the deep flexor tendon may lock the digit in its fixed position. In such cases, a good response to inferior check ligament desmotomy cannot be anticipated, but the patient may respond to a DDF tenotomy.

Tenotomy of the DDF tendon at the midmetacarpal level has been successful,[3,4] but because of the possibility of distal peritendinous adhesions, the technique of transection at the midpastern level is logical and is described here.

The most common explanation for pedal bone rotation in horses with severe laminitis is separation of the interdigitating sensitive and insensitive laminae at the dorsal aspect of the hoof wall and the continued pull of the DDF tendon on the palmar aspect of the distal phalanx.[2] The rationale for DDF tenotomy in cases of severe laminitis is to reduce the dynamic forces favoring rotation and to reduce the pressure of the distal phalanx on the corium of the sole.[1] Results of a retrospective study support the technique's effectiveness as a salvage procedure in horses with chronic refractory laminitis.[1]

Anesthesia and Surgical Preparation

Surgery is performed with the patient under general anesthesia and in lateral recumbency. A pneumatic tourniquet and Esmarch's bandage are advantageous, to provide hemostasis. The leg is clipped from above the fetlock down to and including the coronary band. The palmar aspect of the pastern is shaved, and the area is surgically prepared.

Surgical Technique

A 3-cm skin incision is made on the midline of the palmar aspect of the pastern starting 1 cm proximal to the heel bulbs and extending proximad (Fig. 9-7A). Dissection is continued through the subcutaneous tissue to expose the digital flexor tendon sheath. The tendon sheath is incised in the same line and to the same limits of the skin incision, to expose the DDF tendon (Fig. 9-7B). Curved forceps are placed under the tendon, and it is transected with a scalpel (Fig. 9-7C). The tendon ends will retract.

The incision in the tendon sheath is closed with 2-0 absorbable suture in a simple continuous pattern (Fig. 9-7D). The subcutaneous tissue may be closed in a simple continuous pattern (optional), and the skin is closed with interrupted sutures using synthetic nonabsorbable material.

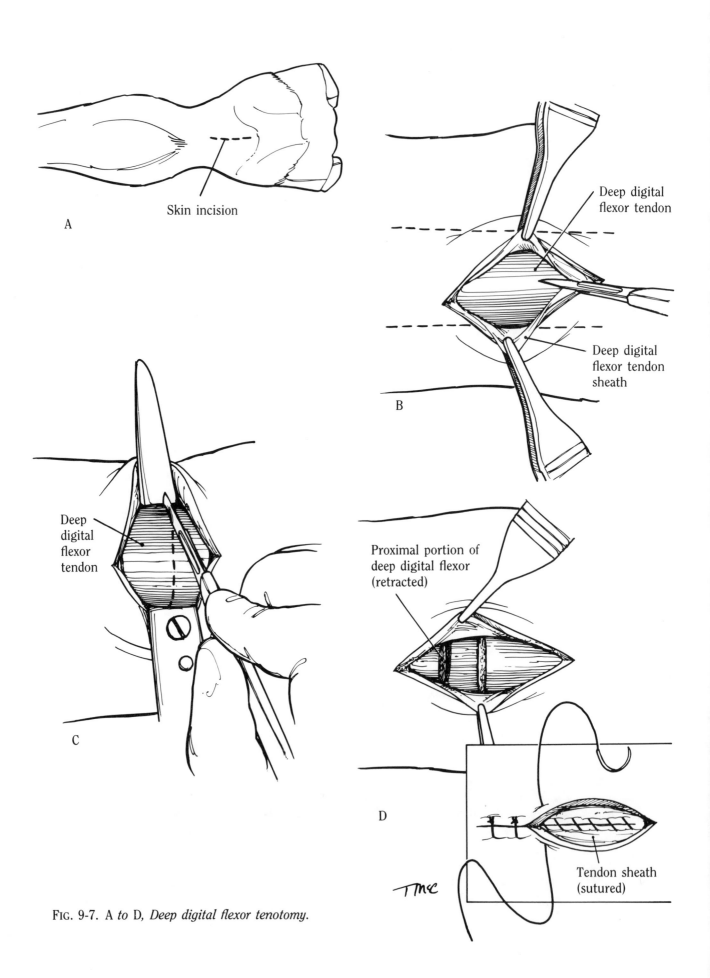

Skin incision

A

Deep digital flexor tendon

Deep digital flexor tendon sheath

B

Deep digital flexor tendon

C

Proximal portion of deep digital flexor (retracted)

D

Tendon sheath (sutured)

TMc

FIG. 9-7. A *to* D, *Deep digital flexor tenotomy.*

Postoperative Management

A sterile dressing is placed over the incision, and the limb is bandaged from the hoof to the carpus. Phenylbutazone is administered as necessary. In cases of flexural deformity, the hoof is trimmed by shortening the heels as much as possible. This may be done gradually. Hand-walking is performed. Corrective shoeing may also be necessary. If postoperative dorsiflexion develops, shoes with caudally extended branches should be applied.

In horses with laminitis, shoeing and dorsal hoof wall resection are important adjunctive therapies. Reversed, extended heel shoes have been recommended initially, with later substitution with flat shoes and pads.[1]

Comments

Both closure and resection of the synovial sheath have been recommended by different authors.[1,3] We recommend closure of the synovial sheath, based on the finding in one study that closure did not apparently impair tendon healing.[1]

References

1. Allen, D., et al.: Surgical management of chronic laminitis in horses: 13 cases (1983-1985). J. Am. Vet. Med. Assoc., *189*:1605, 1986.

2. Coffman, J. R.: Biomechanics of pedal rotation in equine laminitis. J. Am. Vet. Med. Assoc., *156*:219, 1970.

3. Fackleman, G. E., et al.: Surgical treatment of severe flexural deformity of the distal interphalangeal joint in young horses. J. Am. Vet. Med. Assoc., *182*:949, 1987.

4. McIlwraith, C. W.: Diseases of joints, tendons, ligaments, and related structures. *In* Adams' Lameness in Horses, 4th Ed. Edited by T. S. Stashak. Philadelphia, Lea & Febiger, 1987, p. 339.

Sectioning of the Palmar (or Plantar) Annular Ligament of the Fetlock

This surgical procedure is indicated for the treatment of constriction of or by the palmar or plantar annular ligament.[1,3] The problem is associated with injury or infection, and the condition may develop in several ways. Direct injury to the annular ligament with subsequent inflammation may cause fibrosis, scarring, and a primary constriction of the ligament; the constricted ligament, in turn, exerts pressure on the superficial flexor tendon. A primary injury to the superficial flexor tendon with subsequent tendinitis ("bowed tendon") can have the same result because it is associated with swelling of the superficial digital flexor (SDF) tendon against the inelastic annular ligament. In some situations, both types of injury may be involved.

The restriction of free tendon movement and tenosynovitis result in pain and persistent lameness. Prolonged permanent damage to the tendon may result. The syndrome can also arise as a primary chronic digital sheath synovitis of unknown cause, with excess production of synovial fluid and fibrous tissue deposition at the proximal reflection of the synovial sheath onto the flexor tendons.[2] Some authors have considered this pathogenesis to be the most common (the cause of the synovitis remains obscure).[2] Fluid distention of the digital flexor tendon sheath above and below the constricted annular ligament causes the characteristic "notched" appearance on the palmar (or plantar) aspect of the fetlock.[1]

Anesthesia and Surgical Preparation

The patient is placed under general anesthesia with the affected leg uppermost. The use of an Esmarch's bandage and a pneumatic tourniquet facilitates the surgery. A routine preparation for aseptic surgery is performed from the proximal metacarpus distad.

Surgical Technique

OPEN TECHNIQUE

A skin incision is made over the lateral edge of the SDF tendon behind the palmar or plantar blood vessels and nerves. The incision is about 8 cm long and extends from above to below the proximal and distal limits of the annular ligament (Fig. 9-8A). Once the skin incision is made, the lateral palmar or plantar nerve needs to be identified, and the sparse subcutaneous tissue behind this structure must be separated. The incision is continued through the annular ligament and digital tendon sheath; one must be careful not to incise the flexor tendons (Fig. 9-8B). The incision needs to pass behind the palmar or plantar border of the sesamoid bone. The incision in the annular ligament is extended to complete sectioning of the entire ligament, and the flexor tendons are examined for adhesions to the tendon sheath (Fig. 9-8C). The normal vinculum (mesotendon) should not be mistaken for an adhesion.

Neither the tendon sheath nor the annular ligament is sutured. The subcutaneous tissues are sutured closed with simple interrupted sutures of synthetic absorbable material. It is important that this closure be tight to prevent leakage of synovial fluid from the tendon sheath and the subsequent development of synovial fistulae. The skin is closed with nonabsorbable sutures.

CLOSED TECHNIQUE

This simplified version of the surgery can be performed with the patient under anesthesia (preferred) or standing. Although it does not allow complete visualization of the tendon sheath contents, it does obviate potential problems of wound dehiscence and synovial fistulation that have been experienced with the open technique.

A 2-cm skin incision is made over the proximal outpouching of the digital flexor sheath, and a subcutaneous tunnel is created distad to the distal extremity of the annular ligament using Mayo scissors (Fig. 9-8D). Mayo scissors are then positioned so that one arm is in the subcutaneous tunnel and one within the sheath and, with appropriate care to avoid the palmar or plantar vessels and nerve, the annular ligament is incised (Fig. 9-8E). Attention is also paid not to sever tendinous tissue within the sheath, and one must know the limits of the annular ligament. The subcutaneous tissue and skin of the small incision are closed with 2-0 synthetic absorbable and 2-0 synthetic nonabsorbable suture, respectively.

Postoperative Management

A sterile dressing is placed over the incision, and a pressure bandage is applied. Antibiotics are not used routinely. Hand-walking is begun in 3 days and is maintained on an increasing plane to preclude the formation of adhesions. The sutures are removed at 14 days, and bandaging is maintained for 3 weeks. With uneventful healing, the main criterion for returning the horse to work is the time necessary for healing of the tendinitis in the superficial flexor tendon. If extensive changes have not occurred in the superficial flexor tendon, the prognosis is good, but the presence of adhesions or gross pathologic changes decreases the probability for a success.

Comments

Dehiscence of the incision and the development of synovial fistulation are rare complications of the open technique. Such patients are placed on antibiotics, and careful wound management and bandaging are performed. The use of the closed technique virtually obviates this complication.

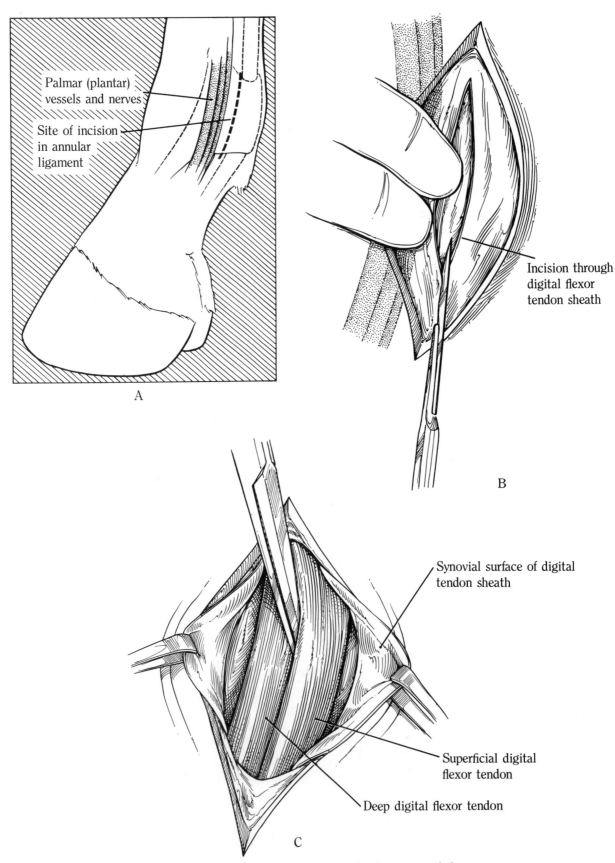

Palmar (plantar)
vessels and nerves

Site of incision
in annular
ligament

A

Incision through
digital flexor
tendon sheath

B

Synovial surface of digital
tendon sheath

Superficial digital
flexor tendon

Deep digital flexor tendon

C

FIG. 9-8. A *to* E, *Sectioning of the palmar (or plantar) annular ligament of the
fetlock; open and closed techniques.*

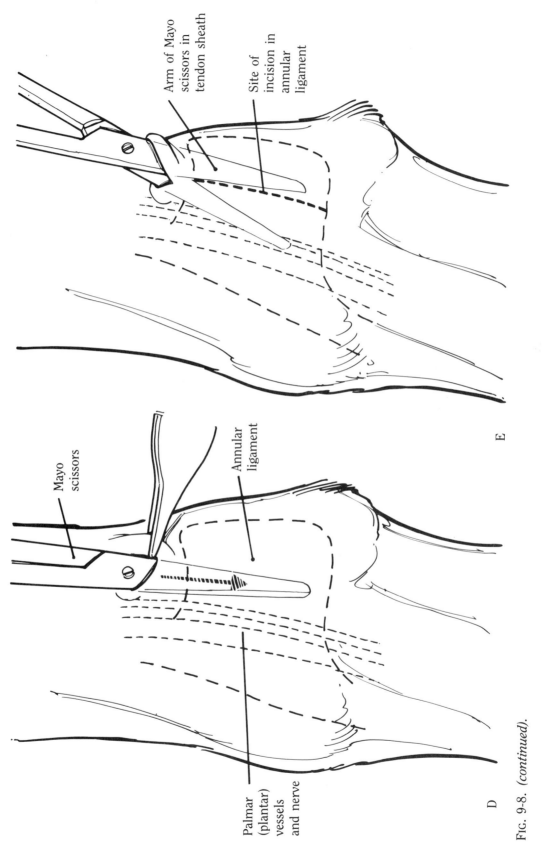

Arm of Mayo scissors in tendon sheath

Site of incision in annular ligament

E

Mayo scissors

Annular ligament

Palmar (plantar) vessels and nerve

D

Fig. 9-8. *(continued)*.

References

1. Adams, O. R.: Constriction of the palmar (volar) or plantar annular ligament in the fetlock in the horse. VM/SAC, *70*:327, 1974.

2. Gerring, E. L., and Webbon, P. M.: Fetlock annular ligament desmotomy: a report of 24 cases. Equine Vet. J., *16*:113, 1984.

3. McIlwraith, C. W.: Diseases of joints, tendons, ligaments, and related structures. *In* Adams' Lameness in Horses, 4th Ed. Edited by T. S. Stashak. Philadelphia, Lea & Febiger, 1987, p. 339.

Palmar Digital Neurectomy

Palmar, or posterior, digital neurectomy is used to relieve pain from navicular disease, fracture of the navicular bone, and selected lateral-wing fractures of the distal phalanx.[2] This surgical procedure is not benign, and it is not a panacea; a number of potential complications should be explained to the owner prior to surgery. In the hands of a good operator, however, palmar digital neurectomy is a form of long-term relief from the pain of those conditions just listed.

Anesthesia and Surgical Preparation

Neurectomy may be performed under local analgesia with the animal standing or under general anesthesia. If the surgery is performed with the animal standing, it is preferable to inject the local analgesic agent over the palmar nerves at the level of the abaxial surface of the sesamoid bones. The nerves can be palpated in this area, and the infiltration of this area avoids additional trauma and irritation at the surgery site. If neurectomy is performed in a field situation immediately following the use of a diagnostic block of the palmar digital nerve, however, this same block may be used for the surgical procedure. General anesthesia is convenient to use, and for the more involved technique of epineural capping, it is certainly indicated.

The area of the surgical incision is clipped, shaved, and prepared for surgery in a routine manner. Plastic adhesive drapes are useful to exclude the hoof as a source of contamination.

Additional Instrumentation

This procedure requires an iris spatula for the epineural capping technique.

Surgical Technique

In both the simple guillotine method and the technique of epineural capping, the approach to the nerve is the same. In the simple guillotine technique, an incision 2 cm long is made over the dorsal border of the flexor tendons (Fig. 9-9A). If epineural capping is to be performed, the incision is generally 3 to 4 cm long and is continued through the subcutaneous tissue. It is important that the tissues be subjected to minimal trauma. An incision over the dorsal border of the flexor tendons generally brings the operator close to the palmar digital nerve. Variation exists, but the relationship of vein, artery, nerve, and the ligament of the ergot assists the surgeon's orientation (Fig. 9-9B). The palmar digital nerve is identified just palmar to the digital artery approximately 1 cm below the skin surface and deep to the ligament of the ergot. At this stage of the dissection, the surgeon should look for accessory branches of the palmar digital nerve. These branches are commonly found near the ligament of the ergot. If an accessory branch is found, a 2-cm portion is removed using a scalpel.

The nerve is identified and is dissected free of the subcutaneous tissue. The structure can be identified as nerve if it puckers after it is stretched, if scraping its surface reveals the longitudinal strands of the axons, or if a small incision into the nerve body reveals cut transverse sections of bundles of nerve fibers. The nerve is severed at the distal extremity of the incision. Then a hemostat is placed on the nerve, which is stretched while being cut with a scalpel at the proximal limit of the incision (Fig. 9-9C). This sharp incision is made in such a fashion that the proximal portion of the nerve springs up into the tissue planes and out of sight. It is believed that the severance of untraumatized nerve and its retraction up into the tissue planes helps to reduce the problems of painful neuromas.

The subcutaneous tissue may be closed with sutures of synthetic absorbable material (generally, this is not performed with the animal standing). The skin is closed with interrupted sutures of nonabsorbable material.

EPINEURAL CAPPING

The technique of epineural capping has been suggested as a means of reducing the incidence of painful neuroma,[1] but controlled studies with an adequate number of cases that compare techniques are lacking. An inexperienced surgeon's use of epineural capping with undue trauma may well have more complications than the faster guillotine method performed atraumatically. Both techniques are presented for the reader's choice, however.

Surgical dissection and exposure of the nerve are accomplished as in the guillotine technique, except the incision is longer. A section of nerve 3 to 4 cm long is exposed and is freed from all fascia and connective tissue. The nerve is severed as distally as possible and is raised from the incision. The end of the nerve is then held with forceps, and the epineurium is carefully reflected (Fig. 9-9D). The epineurium is reflected for 2 to 3 cm, and two incisions are made through half the nerve on each side (Fig. 9-9E). The nerve is then severed distal to these cuts, and the epineurium is pulled back over the severed end and is ligated with 2-0 silk or nylon (Fig. 9-9F). The subcutaneous tissue and skin are sutured as described in the guillotine technique.

A modified technique of epineural capping involving cryosurgery has also been developed.[3] Following reflection of the epineurium, a sterile cryoprobe is placed on the proximal portion of the nerve, and the tissue is frozen to $-30°C$, using a double freeze-thaw cycle. The nerve tissue is then transected, leaving 5 mm of frozen tissue to retract proximally into the epineural sheath. This method is an attempt to minimize neuroma formation.

Postoperative Management

Antibiotics are not used routinely. A sterile dressing is placed on the incision, and a pressure bandage is maintained on the leg for at least 10 days. To minimize postoperative inflammation, 2 g of phenylbutazone are administered following surgery. Sutures are removed 10 days after the operation, and the horse is rested for 4 to 6 weeks. Complications of neurectomy include painful neuroma formation, rupture of the deep digital flexor tendon, reinnervation, persistence of sensation because of failure to identify and sever accessory branches of the nerve, and loss of the hoof wall.[2]

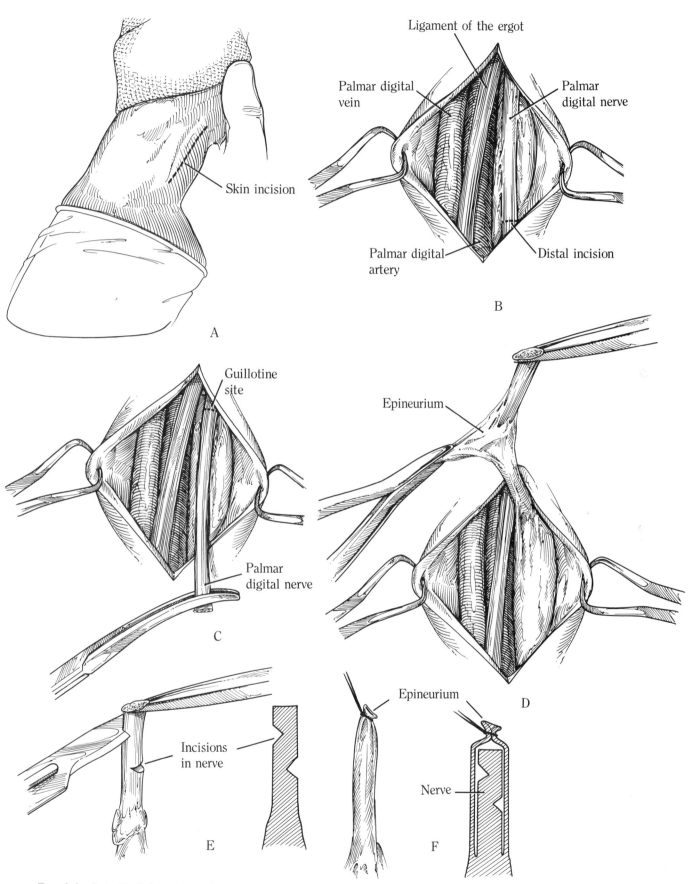

Skin incision

Ligament of the ergot

Palmar digital vein

Palmar digital nerve

Palmar digital artery

Distal incision

A

B

Guillotine site

Palmar digital nerve

Epineurium

C

D

Incisions in nerve

Epineurium

Nerve

E

F

FIG. 9-9. A *to* F, *Palmar digital neurectomy.*

References

1. Evans, L. H.: Procedures used to prevent painful neuromas. *In* Proceedings of the 16th Annual Convention of the American Association of Equine Practitioners in 1970:1971, p. 103.

2. Stashak, T. S. (Ed.): Adams' Lameness in Horses, 4th Ed. Philadelphia, Lea & Febiger, 1987.

3. Tate, L. P., and Evans, L. H.: Cryoneurectomy in the horse. J. Am. Vet. Med. Assoc., *177*:423, 1980.

Amputation of the Small Metacarpal and Metatarsal (Splint) Bones

Amputation of the small metacarpal or metatarsal (splint) bones is indicated when these bones are fractured. The distal half of the bone is usually the site of the fracture. The lameness caused by fractures of the splint bone is generally mild and may be an incidental finding in a radiographic examination. If the skin has been broken, osteitis or osteomyelitis at the fracture site may result. These cases are accompanied by more soft-tissue swelling and lameness than are closed fractures of the splint bone.[3] In horses performing fast-gaited work, particularly the Standardbred, suspensory desmitis may accompany the fracture. In this case, the suspensory desmitis, rather than the fractured splint bone, may limit the prognosis for return to athletic soundness.[2,6] Occasionally, undisplaced fractures of the splint bone heal following suitable rest, but constant movement at the fracture site generally results in nonunion with an attending callus.[3] The decision to remove the fractured distal end of a splint bone is often controversial. Dealing with the suspensory desmitis alone may be sufficient, and removal of the distal splint bone may be unnecessary.[6]

If infection and accompanying osteomyelitis are present, surgical debridement-curettage or sequestrectomy may be necessary to resolve the infectious process, regardless of the health of the suspensory ligament.

Anesthesia and Surgical Preparation

General anesthesia is recommended for this operation. The horse is either placed in lateral recumbency with the affected splint bone uppermost or in dorsal recumbency with the injured leg suspended. The latter method has advantages when more than one splint is to be operated on, and it achieves natural hemostasis during the surgical procedure.

A tourniquet facilitates the surgery if the animal is in lateral recumbency. The surgical site is shaved and prepared for aseptic surgery, unless the limb has already been prepared and wrapped in sterile bandages. Then the surgical site is draped using sterile plastic adhesive drapes, followed by routine draping methods.

Additional Instrumentation

This procedure requires a curved osteotome, chisel, and mallet.

Surgical Technique

A variable-length incision is made directly over the splint bone, extending from approximately 1 cm distal to the distal extremity of the splint bone to approximately 2 cm proximal to the proposed site of amputation (Fig. 9-10*A*). The subcutaneous fascia is incised along the same line as the incision, but not through the periosteum. The distal end of the splint bone is undermined with the aid of sharp dissection and is freed from surrounding fascia (Fig. 9-10*B*). Then the end is grasped firmly with forceps, such as Ochsner forceps. With further sharp dissection, the splint bone is separated from its attachments to the third metacarpal or metatarsal bone. Some of the attachments to the third metacarpal or metatarsal bone may need to be severed with the aid of a chisel (Fig. 9-10*C*). A curved osteotome can also be used to sever these attachments.

The splint bone should be amputated above the fracture site or the area of infection with the aid of a chisel or osteotome. The splint bone, as well as its surrounding periosteum, should be removed (a large curette is sometimes necessary to remove diseased bone adequately) as a unit.[1] The proximal end of the splint bone should be tapered to avoid leaving a sharp edge (Fig. 9-10*C*), and any loose fragments removed or flushed out of the surgical site. If infection is present, unhealthy scar tissue must be excised with sharp dissection, and all sequestra removed. Any bleeding should be controlled at this time. When infection is present, generally the region is vascular because of acute and chronic inflammation.

If the fracture or infectious process is proximal, the remaining portion of splint bone proximal to the amputation site may be short. In this case, the proximal portion of the splint bone should be fixed to the third metacarpal or metatarsal bone with a stainless steel bone screw employing the "lag" screw principle.[1,5] If this is not performed, the proximal fragment may become displaced because of the inadequate amount of interosseous ligament holding it in place.

When amputating a lateral splint bone in the pelvic limb, one must be careful to avoid incising the large, dorsal metatarsal artery III (great metatarsal artery), which lies above and between the third and fourth metatarsal bones in the interosseous space.[4] If large amounts of fibrous tissue are present because of an infectious process, the artery may be difficult to dissect from the soft tissue component. If the artery is inadvertently severed, it can be ligated without causing problems associated with loss of blood supply to the distal limb.

Following removal of the splint bone, the subcutaneous tissue should be closed with a synthetic absorbable suture. Considerable dead space may result from removal of the bone, especially if much bony and fibrous tissue reaction was present. Some patients with a severe infectious process or significant dead space may require a Penrose drain for a few days (see Chap. 7). Only in rare instances is an ingress-egress system of flushing indicated. The skin should be closed with a monofilament nonabsorbable suture using a simple interrupted pattern. The incision is covered with a nonadherent dressing and is placed under a pressure bandage.

Postoperative Management

Tetanus prophylaxis is administered. Antibiotics are used in cases of acute (active) osteitis or osteomyelitis, although with appropriate preoperative wound management and thorough wound debridement, the infection usually

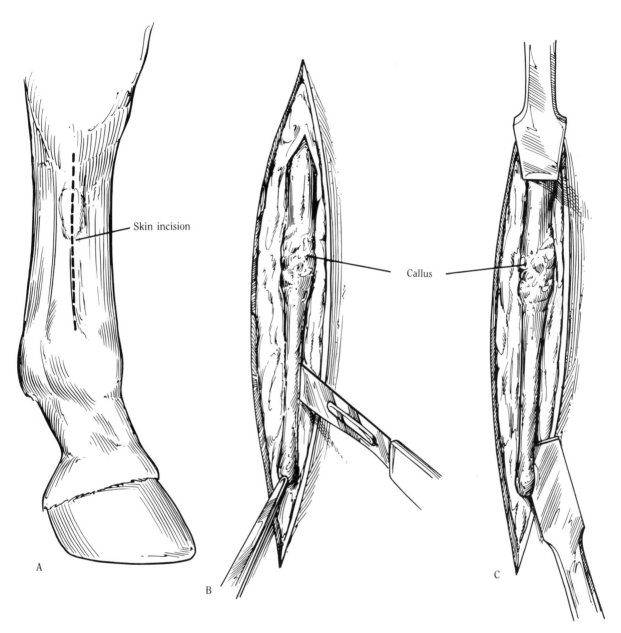

Skin incision

Callus

A

B

C

FIG. 9-10. A *to* C, *Amputation of the small metacarpal and metatarsal (splint) bones.*

resolves without the need for preoperative antimicrobial therapy.[1] The limb should be kept under a pressure bandage for 3 to 4 weeks. Despite careful hemostasis, the surgical procedure is generally accompanied by some hemorrhage. It is therefore wise to change the bandage in the first 1 to 2 days postoperatively. After that time, pressure bandages are changed every 5 to

7 days, or sooner if needed. If drains are in place, they should generally be removed second or third postoperative day. Skin sutures should be removed 10 to 14 days after surgery.

References

1. Allen, D., and White, N. A.: Management of fractures and exostosis of the metacarpals II and IV in 25 horses. Equine Vet. J., *19*:326, 1987.

2. Bowman, K. F., Evans, L. H., and Herring, M. E.: Evaluation of surgical removal of fractured distal splint bones in the horse. Vet. Surg., *11*:116, 1982.

3. Haynes, P. F.: Diseases of the metacarpophalangeal joint and the metacarpus. *In* Symposium on Equine Lameness. Vet. Clin. North Am. (Large Anim. Pract.), *2*:33, 1980.

4. Milne, D. W., and Turner, A. S.: An Atlas of Surgical Approaches to the Bones of the Horse. Philadelphia, W. B. Saunders, 1979.

5. Stashak, T. S. (Ed.): Adams' Lameness in Horses, 4th Ed. Philadelphia, Lea & Febiger, 1987.

6. Verschooten, F., Gasthuys, F., and De Moor, A.: Distal splint bone fractures in the horse: an experimental and clinical study. Equine Vet. J., *16*:532, 1984.

Arthrotomy of the Midcarpal Joint

Arthrotomy of the intercarpal joint is indicated for surgical excision of osteochondral fragments and osteophytes. Such pathologic changes can occur at other sites in those areas as well. The use of arthrotomy to remove osteochondral fragments from the carpus has generally been replaced by the technique of arthroscopic surgery, and various advantages of arthroscopy have been identified.[3] Arthroscopy requires specialized equipment and considerable learning and experience, however; we believe that arthrotomy is still a valid technique when the foregoing resources are unavailable.

The exact location of the lesion should be ascertained with preoperative radiographs of the affected limb. As with all elective surgical procedures on horses' limbs, the presence of any other problems should be ascertained prior to surgery. The technique described is only one of five approaches used to gain access to various bones of the carpal joint.[4] This approach is the most common because of the higher incidence of injuries to the distal radial and proximal third carpal bones in the fast-gaited horse. This arthrotomy approach is also used for the repair of slab fractures of the third carpal bone. This technique is considered to be advanced, however, and is presented in our book *Equine Surgery: Advanced Techniques*.[2]

Anesthesia and Surgical Preparation

The surgery is performed under general anesthesia with the horse placed in lateral recumbency and the affected limb down. Some surgeons prefer to operate with the horse in dorsal recumbency and the limb elevated, to take advantage of natural hemostasis. Prior to anesthetic induction, the patient's leg is clipped from the coronary band to midradius all the way around the leg. Following anesthetic induction, the area of surgical excision is shaved, and routine surgical preparation is performed. By preparing the limb before surgery, the anesthetic time can be reduced.

Additional Instrumentation

This procedure requires curettes, retractors, periosteal elevators, and a bulb syringe.

Surgical Technique

After draping (the use of sterile plastic adherent drapes is recommended for this procedure), the following structures should be identified: the tendinous insertion of the extensor carpi radialis muscle, the tendon of the extensor carpi obliquus muscle, the antebrachial joint, and the midcarpal joint. Identification of these structures is facilitated by flexing and extending the carpal joint. A straight 3-cm skin incision extending from the middle of the face of the radial carpal bone to the middle of the face of the third carpal bone and 5 to 8 mm medial to the extensor carpi radialis tendon is made (Fig. 9-11A).

The incision is continued through the subcutaneous fascia, carpal extensor retinaculum, and joint capsule. Synovial fluid will flow from the incision when the joint is entered (Fig. 9-11B). Any blood vessels or their visible lumens should be cauterized at this point. Using suitable retractors, the surgeon carefully retracts the edges of the incision in the carpal extensor retinaculum and joint capsule; this will expose the proximal surface of the third carpal bone and the distal surface of the radial carpal bone.

If the osteochondral chip fragments are not visible immediately, a pair of curved forceps can be used to gently probe the articular margins of the third carpal and radial carpal bones. Any movement or instability along these edges should be investigated further because they are usually the location of the offending chip fractures.

Chip fractures may be difficult to identify because they may be embedded in fibrous tissue. Rarely are they completely loose and detached. To remove the fractures from their attachments, the chip can be grasped with forceps and dissected free with a no. 15 scalpel blade. Another method is to take a small, sharp, periosteal elevator and pry the fragment loose (Fig. 9-11C). The resultant defect is then curetted down to the subchondral bone (Fig. 9-11D). This curettage has been recommended to ensure filling of the defect with granulation tissue and its subsequent metaplasic transformation to fibrocartilage and possible hyaline cartilage. How effective this healing response is, however, is controversial. Curettage has been reported to decrease the likelihood of exostosis formation postoperatively.

Closure is performed in three layers. The joint capsule and retinaculum are closed with a layer of simple interrupted sutures of absorbable synthetic material or nonabsorbable monofilament material. The sutures should not penetrate the synovial membrane. Preplacement of the sutures in the joint capsule and extensor retinaculum ensures an accurate apposition and a tight seal (Fig. 9-11E).

Following joint capsule closure, 4 to 5 ml of Ringer's solution with 1 million U of potassium penicillin are flushed into the joint using a 20-gauge needle. If any leaks are observed through the incision, additional sutures can be placed at this time (Fig. 9-11F). The subcutaneous fascia is closed with a simple continuous pattern using synthetic absorbable sutures. The skin is closed with a simple interrupted or vertical mattress pattern using synthetic monofilament sutures, and the limb is wrapped with a tight pressure bandage. Control of minute capillary ooze will be possible if the tourniquet is released when the pressure wrap has been applied.

Postoperative Management

The limb is wrapped in a firm pressure bandage for 3 weeks, during which time the bandage is changed several times. Skin sutures are removed at 10 to 12 days. Care must be taken when bandaging the carpal joint, to prevent formation of a pressure sore on the accessory carpal bone; this can be avoided by cutting a small hole over the accessory carpal bone in the back of the bandage. During convalescence, the horse is kept in a box stall. The convalescence and aftercare depend on the individual case and the

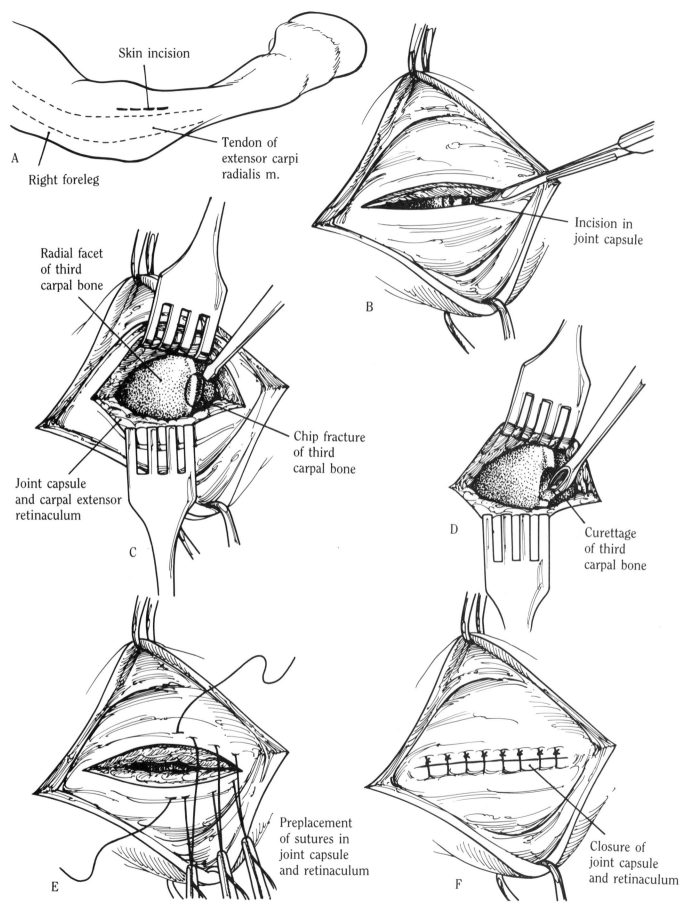

A — Skin incision

Tendon of extensor carpi radialis m.

Right foreleg

B — Incision in joint capsule

C

Radial facet of third carpal bone

Chip fracture of third carpal bone

Joint capsule and carpal extensor retinaculum

D — Curettage of third carpal bone

E — Preplacement of sutures in joint capsule and retinaculum

F — Closure of joint capsule and retinaculum

FIG. 9-11. A *to* F, *Arthrotomy of the midcarpal joint.*

severity of the injury to the carpal bone. Generally, it is 6 to 12 months before the horse should return to its athletic activities, although at 4 months, defects in the carpal bones produced by curettage have healed as well as they will.[1]

References

1. Grant, B. D.: Repair mechanisms of osteochondral defects in equidae: a comparative study of untreated and x-irradiated defects. *In* Proceedings of the 21st Annual Convention of the American Association of Equine Practitioners in 1974:1975, p. 95.

2. McIlwraith, C. W., and Turner, A. S.: Equine Surgery: Advanced Techniques. Philadelphia, Lea & Febiger, 1987.

3. McIlwraith, C. W., Yovich, J. V., and Martin, G. S.: Arthroscopic surgery for the treatment of osteochondral chip fractures in the equine carpus. J. Am. Vet. Med. Assoc., *191*:531, 1987.

4. Milne, D. W., and Turner, A. S.: An Atlas of Surgical Approaches to the Bones of the Horse. Philadelphia, W. B. Saunders, 1979.

5. Raker, C. W., Baker, R. H., and Wheat, J. D.: Pathophysiology of equine degenerative joint disease and lameness. *In* Proceedings of the 12th Annual Convention of the American Association of Equine Practitoners in 1965:1966, p. 229.

6. Riddle, W. E.: Healing of articular cartilage in the horse. J. Am. Vet. Med. Assoc., *157*: 1471, 1970.

Arthrotomy of the Fetlock Joint and Removal of an Apical Sesamoid Chip Fracture

Arthrotomy and removal of the fractured fragment comprise the treatment of choice for an apical chip fracture of the proximal sesamoid bone.[1] If left unoperated, the result will be either a fibrous union or displacement of the fragment proximad, which, in turn, can lead to exostosis formation and joint-surface irregularity.[3] In Standardbreds, conservative therapy has dramatically reduced the racing performance when preinjury values are compared to postinjury values.[3] Surgical removal carries the best prognosis for horses with proven speed, when they are operated on within 30 days of injury and have no evidence of suspensory desmitis or osteoarthritis.[3]

Anesthesia and Surgical Preparation

This surgical procedure is performed with the horse under general anesthesia, and depending on the surgeon's preference, the horse may be placed in lateral or dorsal recumbency. With dorsal recumbency and the leg suspended, natural hemostasis is achieved. If surgery is performed in lateral recumbency, Esmarch's bandage and a pneumatic tourniquet are generally used. Prior to anesthetic induction, the patient's leg is clipped from proximal cannon to coronary band all the way around the leg. Following anesthetic induction, the area of the surgical incision is shaved, and routine surgical preparation is performed. Draping may include the use of a plastic adhesive drape. The surgical preparation is performed by some surgeons prior to induction of anesthesia.

Additional Instrumentation

This procedure requires a Weitlaner retractor, bone curette, and rongeurs.

Surgical Technique

The limb is maintained in an extended position while surgical entry into the joint is made. With the leg in this position, it is easier to identify the branch of the suspensory ligament. An incision approximately 5 cm long is made over the palmar or plantar recess (volar pouch) of the metacarpo (metatarso) phalangeal joint immediately dorsal and parallel to the branch of the suspensory ligament and palmar or plantar to the distal aspect of the metacarpus or metatarsus (Fig. 9-12A). The incision extends from approximately 1 cm below the distal extremity of the splint bone to the proximal border of the collateral sesamoidean ligament. The incision is continued through the thin subcutaneous areolar connective tissue in the same line, and Weitlaner retractors are placed to facilitate exposure of the joint capsule. A 3-cm incision is made through the joint capsule (fibrous joint capsule plus synovial membrane) to enter the joint (Fig. 9-12B). Care is taken to avoid the collateral sesamoidean ligament distally and the vascular plexus on the palmar (plantar) aspect of the distal metacarpus or metatarsus proximally. Following entry into the joint, the fetlock is flexed, and the edges of the joint capsule are retracted to expose the palmar articular surface of the third metacarpus and the articular surface of the proximal sesamoid bone.[2]

The apical fragment to be removed is identified, and it is incised from the suspensory ligament using a no. 15 scalpel blade (Fig. 9-12C). Trauma to the suspensory ligament is minimized by careful, sharp dissection. As the soft tissue attachments are severed, the chip is removed using Ochsner forceps or small rongeurs (Fig. 9-12D). The fracture site is curetted smooth, and the joint is vigorously flushed with sterile Ringer's solution. The hypertrophic synovial membrane is also removed.

The fibrous joint capsule is closed with a layer of simple interrupted sutures of synthetic absorbable or monofilament, synthetic nonabsorbable material. The sutures in the fibrous joint capsule should not penetrate the synovial membrane. Preplacement of the sutures in the joint capsule facilitates accurate apposition and a tight seal. Following closure of the joint capsule, 8 to 10 ml of Ringer's solution (to which 1 million U of potassium penicillin may be added) are flushed into the joint using a 20-gauge needle (Fig. 9-12E). If any leaks are observed through the incision, additional sutures are placed. The subcutaneous fascia is closed with a simple continuous pattern using synthetic absorbable material, and the skin is closed with simple interrupted or vertical mattress sutures of monofilament nonabsorbable material. The tourniquet is removed, a sterile dressing is placed over the incision, and a firm bandage is placed on the leg.

Postoperative Management

The use of antibiotics is optional. The skin sutures are removed in 10 to 12 days, and the bandage is maintained on the leg for another 10 days. Postoperative radiographs are taken within 24 hours following surgery; these films are of value for comparative purposes if follow-up or progressive radiographs are made at a later time. Convalescent time after removal of an apical sesamoid chip should be at least 4 months, but it varies, depending on the degree of concurrent injury in the suspensory ligament and other soft tissues.

References

1. Churchill, E. A.: Surgical removal of fractured fragments of the proximal sesamoid bone. J. Am. Vet. Med. Assoc., *128*:581, 1956.

2. Milne, D. W., and Turner, A. S.: An Atlas of Surgical Approaches to the Bones of the Horse. Philadelphia, W. B. Saunders, 1979.

3. Spurlock, G. H., and Gabel, A. A.: Apical fractures of the proximal sesamoid bones in 109 Standardbred horses. J. Am. Vet. Med. Assoc., *183*:76, 1983.

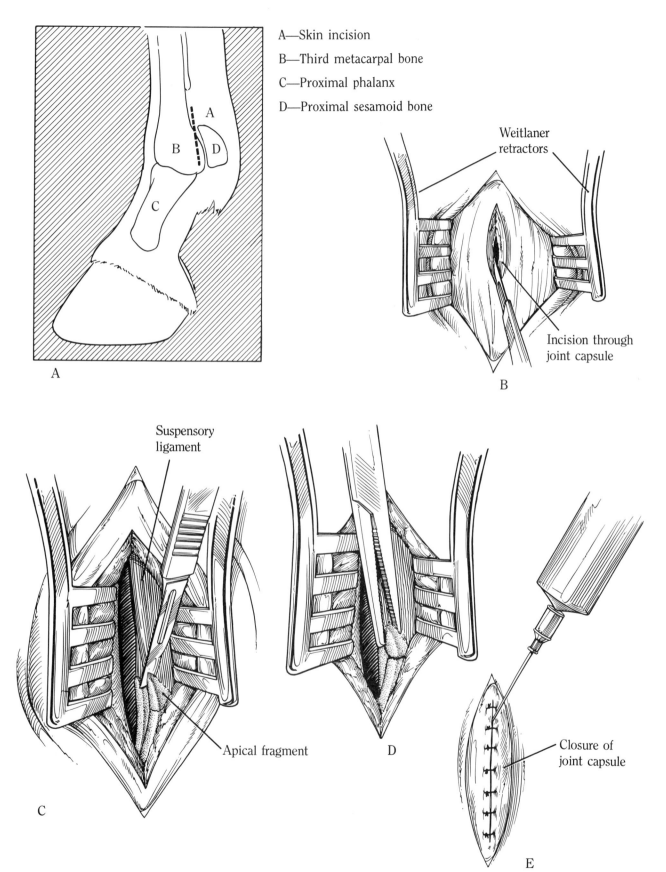

A—Skin incision

B—Third metacarpal bone

C—Proximal phalanx

D—Proximal sesamoid bone

Weitlaner retractors

Incision through joint capsule

Suspensory ligament

Apical fragment

Closure of joint capsule

FIG. 9-12. A *to* E, *Arthrotomy of fetlock joint for removal of apical sesamoid fracture.*

10

EQUINE UROGENITAL SURGERY

Castration

Castration is usually performed to facilitate the management of a particular animal when it is in the company of females or other males. Castration can be performed at any time; however, the colt is generally left entire for 12 to 18 months to allow for development of certain desirable physical characteristics. Other animals may be castrated at a later age when it is no longer desirable to maintain them as stallions. Prior to castration, it should be ascertained that the animal is healthy and that both testes are descended.

Anesthesia and Surgical Preparation

Castration may be performed on the standing animal under local analgesia or with the animal in recumbency under general anesthesia. The technique depends on the temperament of the animal, the experience of the surgeon, and in some situations, the tradition and environment in which the horse is castrated.

For castration of the standing animal, a tranquilizer or sedative may be administered to the horse, and local infiltration analgesia is performed. Following surgical preparation of the area, the skin is infiltrated on a line 1 cm from the median raphe with 10 ml of local analgesic solution; this infiltration is continued into the subcutaneous tissue. Local analgesia can be injected directly into the testis. It is also important to infiltrate the spermatic cord in the region of emasculation with a long 18- to 20-gauge needle.

For castration of the recumbent animal, several anesthetic regimens are available and suitable. Guaifenesin in combination with thiamylal sodium, xylazine followed by ketamine, or rapid induction with thiamylal sodium or thiopental sodium alone is suitable; in our opinion, the use of succinylcholine hydrochloride alone for equine castration is unacceptable practice. For a right-handed operator, the horse is cast with the left side down. The upper hind leg is tied craniad, and the surgical site is prepared; clipping or shaving is not necessary.

Additional Instrumentation

This procedure requires emasculators.

Surgical Technique

This castration technique is illustrated here in the recumbent animal. Castration is performed through separate incisions for each testis, with incisions located approximately 1 cm from the median raphe (Fig. 10-1*A*). The lower testis is grasped between thumb and forefingers, and the first skin incision is made for the length of the testis (Fig. 10-1*B*). The incision is continued through the tunica dartos and scrotal fascia, leaving the common tunic (tunica vaginalis parietalis) intact. At the same time, pressure exerted by the thumb and forefingers causes the testis, which is still contained within the common tunic, to be extruded (Fig. 10-1*C*). The testis is then grasped in the left hand (for a right-handed operator), and the subcutaneous tissue is stripped from the common vaginal tunic as far proximally as possible (Fig. 10-1*D*). The use of a gauze sponge can facilitate the stripping of the subcutaneous tissue from the common tunic. The surgeon incises the common tunic over the cranial pole of the testis (Fig. 10-1*E*) and, hooking a finger within the tunic to maintain tension, continues the incision proximad (Fig. 10-1*F*).

The testis is now released from within the common tunic. The mesorchium is penetrated digitally, to separate the vascular spermatic cord from the ductus deferens, common tunic, and external cremaster muscle (Fig. 10-1*G*). The latter structures are severed, with attention to removing as much of the common tunic as possible (Fig. 10-1*G*). The severance of this musculofibrous portion of the spermatic cord may be performed conveniently with emasculators, and the crush need only be applied for a short period of time. The testis is then grasped, and the spermatic vessels are emasculated (Fig. 10-1*H*).

Care must always be taken to apply the emasculator correctly without incorporating skin between its jaws and to prevent stretch on the spermatic cord at the time of emasculation. An optional preliminary to emasculation is to place forceps proximally on the cord as a safeguard against loss if a failure occurs during emasculation. The emasculator remains in position for 1 to 2 minutes, depending on the size of the cord, and is then released.

The skin incisions are enlarged by pulling them apart with the fingers until a 10-cm opening is obtained. The median raphe may also be removed to further facilitate drainage. Any redundant adipose tissue or fascia is also removed.

Postoperative Management

Tetanus immunization is administered, and antibiotics usually are not indicated. The horse should be kept under close observation for several hours after castration to make sure that it is not hemorrhaging; the horse should be observed periodically during the first week following surgery. Uneventful healing is the usual result with good drainage and satisfactory exercise. The animal should be forcibly exercised twice daily from the day

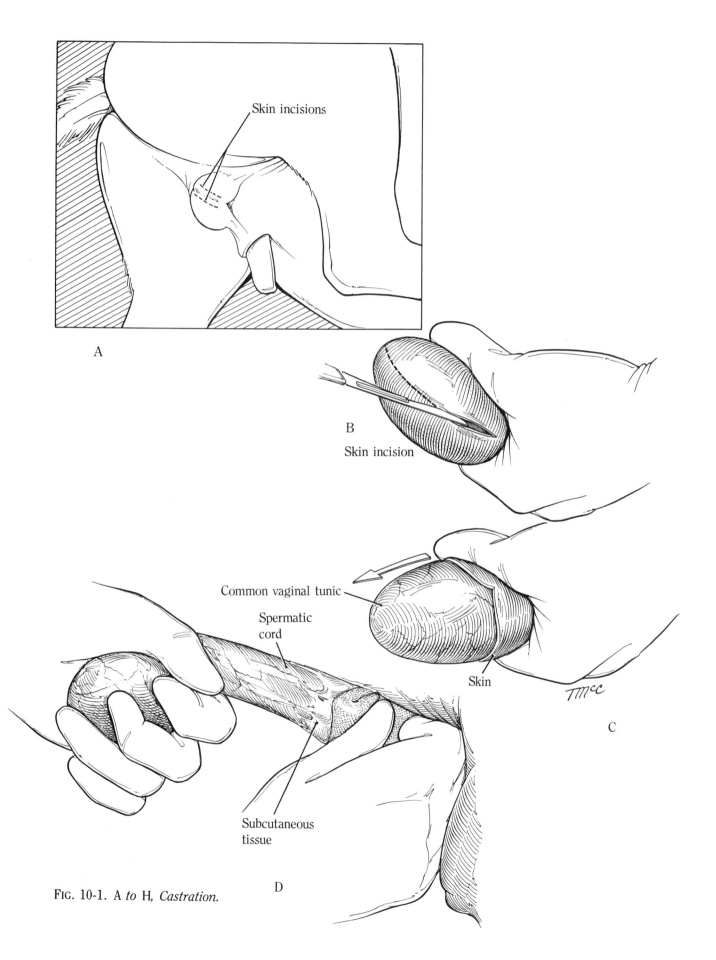

A

Skin incisions

B

Skin incision

Common vaginal tunic

Skin

Spermatic cord

Subcutaneous tissue

C

D

FIG. 10-1. A *to* H, *Castration.*

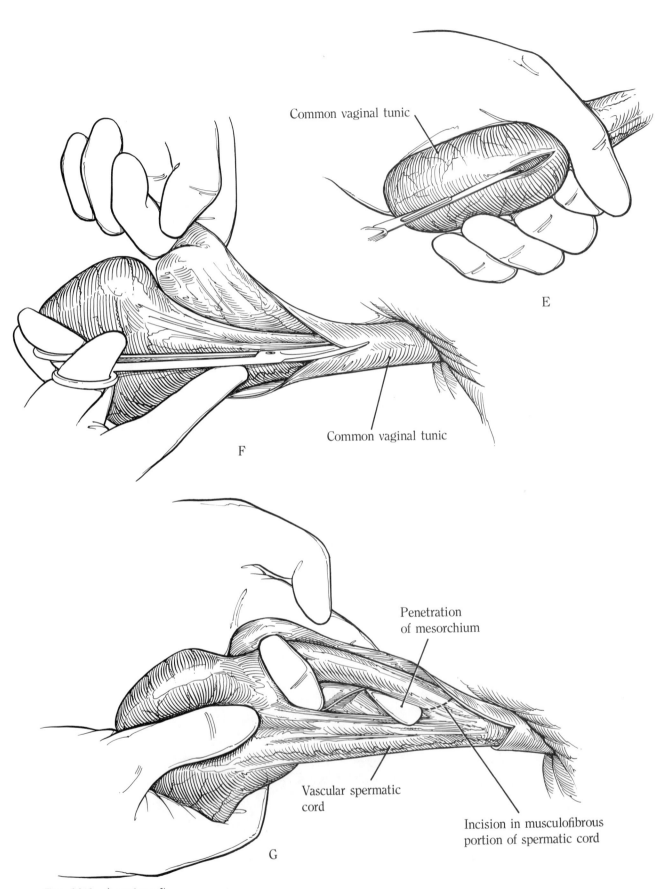

Common vaginal tunic

E

Common vaginal tunic

F

Penetration
of mesorchium

Vascular spermatic
cord

Incision in musculofibrous
portion of spermatic cord

G

FIG. 10-1. *(continued)*.

Emasculation of spermatic cord

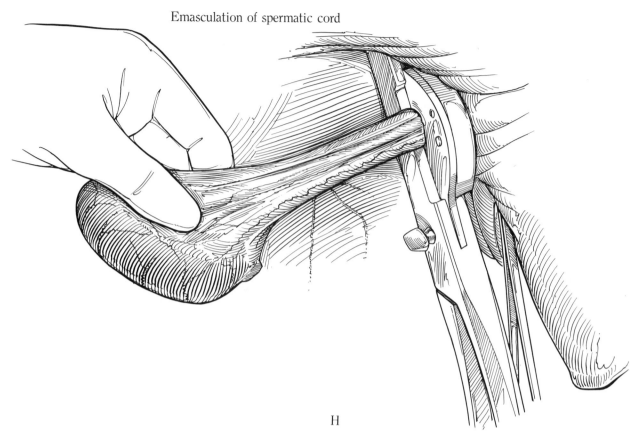

H

Fig. 10-1. *(continued).*

following surgery until healing is complete. The new gelding should be separated from mares for a week to ensure that no pregnancies will occur.[7]

A number of possible complications may arise following castration: (1) severe hemorrhage is usually associated with inadequate emasculation of the testicular artery of the spermatic cord, but considerable hemorrhage can occur from one of the branches of the external pudendal vein in the scrotal wall or septum, if accidentally ruptured,[8] or in the transected external cremaster muscle; (2) excessive swelling of the surgical site can arise because of inadequate drainage or inadequate exercise; (3) evisceration may occur through an inguinal hernia; (4) acute wound infection and septicemia may occur; (5) a hydrocele may form because of collection of fluid in a common tunic that has been inadequately resected; (6) scirrhous cord formation is due to chronic infection and generally can be related to poor technique and inadequate exercise or drainage; and (7) persistent masculine behavior can occur following removal of two normal testes. Many practitioners and horsemen believe that if a stallion is "cut-proud" (a small quantity of epididymis was not removed during surgery), he will continue to show stallion-like behavior. That removal of identifiable epididymal tissue or another piece of a long spermatic cord has resolved the problem in some instances lends some support to this idea.[8] Testicular or adrenal tissue has not been demonstrated in these removed segments, however, and the problem has been proposed to be psychologic.[4]

If one suspects that testicular tissue is still present in a "gelding," we suggest measuring testosterone levels 30 to 100 minutes after injecting 6000 to 12,000 IU of human chorionic gonadotropin (HCG).[3]

Comments

Alternate methods of castration are available. We have described two-phase emasculation preceded by separate dissection of the common tunic because we believe it is the optimal technique for the prevention of untoward sequelae. In the technique of "closed" castration, the common vaginal tunic is dissected, but not opened, and emasculation of the entire cord within the tunic is performed as a single procedure. Because several structures are enclosed within the jaws of the emasculator, there is a greater chance that a vessel will be emasculated inadequately. This technique should be restricted to patients with small testes.

In the "open" technique, the common tunic is opened with the initial skin incision, and prior dissection of the tunic from the subcutaneous tissue is not performed. This method is commonly used without any problems, but the chances of inadequate tunic removal with consequent hydrocele are increased.

A technique of primary closure in multiple layers with ablation of the scrotum has been described.[1] In this technique, the ventral scrotum is ablated. The testicles are removed by emasculation, and transfixation ligatures are considered unnecessary. Additional skin may have to be removed, so the scrotum is completely ablated when the skin edges are apposed. Closure of the subcutaneous and subcuticular tissues is performed in three or four layers. This method is certainly more time consuming than other procedures, but postoperative scrotal swelling is usually eliminated.[1]

Complications of equine castration are uncommon, but they can be life-threatening to the horse and of great concern to the surgeon. To minimize postoperative complications, good communication with the client is required. The gelding should be under observation for at least the first 24 hours because this period is when the most serious complications are likely to occur. During this time, the horse should be confined with limited exercise. This inactivity allows some swelling to occur in the region of the inguinal ring and decreases the chances of eventration. Other horses, especially mares, should be kept away because their presence may encourage the horse to rear and may thereby predispose the animal to eventration.

Minor hemorrhage may occur for several hours, but significant hemorrhage beyond about 12 hours may require surgical intervention. If the source of hemorrhage is the testicular artery, then ligation using a synthetic absorbable suture material may be required. This procedure may warrant general anesthesia if the horse is difficult to manage. Curved forceps, such as Mixter curved hemostatic forceps, are helpful.

Prolapse of abdominal contents usually involves a portion of small intestine or omentum through the internal inguinal ring. It is most likely to occur within the first few hours after castration, before swelling has closed the inguinal canal. If management of the eventration is beyond the capabilities of the surgeon, the offending viscera, unless it is extensive, can be replaced in the scrotum, the scrotum can be packed with sterile gauzes and temporarily closed with several simple interrupted sutures, and following the appropriate fluid therapy and parenteral antibiotics, the animal can be referred to an equine surgical facility.

If the eventration is to be managed where the horse was gelded because referral is out of the question, preoperative planning is essential. The appropriate instruments, drapes, and isotonic solutions for lavage must be obtained, and preoperative broad-spectrum antibiotic therapy should commence. Plans for balanced, movement-free general anesthesia must also be made.

With the animal under general anesthesia and in dorsal recumbency, the offending viscera is cleaned by lavage of balanced electrolyte solutions. The incision and scrotal area are prepared for aseptic surgery as thoroughly as possible. Debris, such as straw or blood clots, may have to be manually removed from the bowel in the earlier stages of preparation for surgery. Small segments of bowel, if viable and relatively uncontaminated, can be replaced in the abdomen. Some enlargement of the inguinal ring may be required if the bowel has become congested and edematous. Greater lengths of intestine may be sufficiently contaminated or devitalized that resection and anastomosis will be required. The internal ring may have to be enlarged, a portion of normal bowel exteriorized, and then anastomosis performed. If a portion of omentum is the only abdominal content involved, then it can be excised, and remaining healthy omentum can be replaced in the abdomen.

Closure of the internal ring is usually impossible, but closure of the external ring using preplaced simple interrupted synthetic absorbable suture material is necessary, as described in the section of this chapter on cryptorchidectomy.

Packing of the external canal, as shown in Figure 10-2J, is then performed. Fluid therapy should be instituted, as well as other adjunctive therapy for shock such as flunixin meglumine. The prognosis following eventration is always guarded. A long-term complication may be adhesion of bowel to the inguinal ring (discussed in the final paragraph of this section).

Penile paralysis (paraphimosis), a rare complication, is usually seen when phenothiazine tranquilizers have been used. If the penis is flaccid and does not retract in 4 to 8 hours, then mechanical support of the penis is indicated. Priapism is an abnormally prolonged erection of the penis, not associated with sexual desire.[5] It also has been associated with the use of phenothiazine tranquilizers, but fortunately, it is an even rarer complication of castration. Priapism has been treated medically using an anticholinergic agent, benztropine mesylate.[6] The condition has also been treated by drainage and irrigation of the corpus cavernosum penis, along with creation of a vascular shunt between that structure and the corpus spongiosum penis.[5] Description of this procedure is beyond the scope of this book, and the references should be consulted for further details.[5]

Edema of the scrotum and prepuce, a more common complication of castration, usually begins on the third or fourth postoperative day and is often associated with inadequate exercise. Simply turning the gelding out to pasture without forced exercise is often inadequate because of postoperative pain. Horses with excessive edema of the scrotum and prepuce should be checked for a temperature rise because it may indicate impending infection. To help re-establish drainage, a sterile surgical glove is donned, and the scrotal incision is opened cautiously. Parenteral antibiotics, such as procaine penicillin G, may be indicated, as well as a conscientious program of forced exercise. Phenylbutazone may be indicated to reduce soreness and to encourage pain-free movement. Longstanding chronic infections with abscess formation in the inguinal canal may need surgical exploration and abscess drainage.

Other long-term complications of castration are uncommon, but they are serious and require surgical management. Adhesions of small intestine may occur following ascending infection.[2] We have seen this condition cause a chronic low-grade colic because of incomplete obstruction of the lumen of the small intestine. Muscular hypertrophy, fibrosis, and thickening of the bowel wall aboral to the adhesion usually result. A ventral midline celiotomy, in combination with an inguinal approach, may be required to treat an adhesion in this region. Following identification of the offending bowel and the extent of the adhesion, the adhesion is broken down by carefully separating the bowel from the inguinal region. If the adhesion is of long duration, then blind transection of the adhesion with scissors may be required. With either method, the risk of tearing the intestinal wall and contaminating the abdominal cavity with intestinal contents is real and may be fatal. Peeling the bowel off the adhesion has been successful with us, but it leaves a raw, bleeding edge that itself is prone to future adhesion formation. Daily rectal examinations, if the horse's size and temperament permit, allow the surgeon carefully to "wipe away" any potentially adhering bowel from these raw surfaces.

References

1. Barber, S. M.: Castration of horses with primary closure and scrotal ablation. Vet. Surg., *14*:2, 1985.

2. Crouch, G. M., Snyder, J. R., and Harmon, B. G.: Adhesion of the ileum to the inguinal ring in a gelding. Equine Pract., *5*:32, 1983.

3. Cox, J. E.: Experiences with a diagnostic test for equine cryptorchidism. Equine Vet. J., *7*:179, 1975.

4. Pickett, B. W., et al.: Factors affecting sexual behavior of the equine male. *In* Proceedings of the 25th Annual Convention of the American Association of Equine Practitioners in 1979:1980, p. 61.

5. Schumacher, J., and Hardin, D. K.: Surgical treatment of priapism in a stallion. Vet. Surg., *16*:193, 1987.

6. Sharrock, A. G.: Reversal of drug induced priapism in a gelding by medication. Aust. Vet. J., *58*:39, 1982.

7. Shideler, R. K., Squires, E. L., and Pickett, B. W.: Disappearance of spermatozoa from the ejaculate of geldings. J. Reprod. Fertil., *27 (Suppl.)*:25, 1979.

8. Walker, D. F., and Vaughan, J. T.: Bovine and Equine Urogenital Surgery. Philadelphia, Lea & Febiger, 1980.

Cryptorchidectomy by the Noninvasive Inguinal Approach

The approach we describe can be used for both inguinal and abdominal cryptorchidism in the horse. If the testis has traversed the vaginal ring but has not reached the scrotum, the horse is considered an inguinal cryptorchid ("high flanker"). If the testis has not traversed the vaginal ring and has descended into the inguinal canal, the horse is considered an abdominal cryptorchid. In the invasive technique of abdominal cryptorchidectomy, which we use infrequently, the surgeon introduces his fingers or his entire hand into the abdominal cavity through the inguinal canal. The noninvasive technique of abdominal cryptorchidectomy is performed by traction on the gubernaculum, testis, epididymis, or ductus deferens after rupture of the vaginal process and without manual exploration within the abdominal cavity. We believe that the second technique is the most convenient and reliable method of cryptorchidectomy, and its superiority in terms of decreased hospitalization time and fewer complications has been documented.[3] We recognize little indication for a flank or paramedian approach for equine cryptorchidectomy.

A rectal examination performed on a cryptorchid patient will enable one to ascertain whether the cryptorchid testis(es) is abdominal or inguinal. Inguinal testes may be nonpalpable on external examination of the inguinal canal. The rectal palpation of the ductus deferens through the vaginal ring indicates that the testis is in the inguinal canal.[1,3] If the ductus deferens cannot be palpated passing through the vaginal ring, the testis is considered to be within the abdomen.[5] We do not routinely perform a rectal examination prior to cryptorchidectomy. Because of altered behavior frequently seen in these cases, the horses are usually fractious and are therefore at an increased risk for rectal perforation. Unlike the broodmare, these animals have not usually been subjected to routine rectal palpation, and this further increases the risk. Arabians, because of a smaller anus and rectum, may be particularly predisposed to this problem.[2]

Anesthesia and Surgical Preparation

The horse is placed under general anesthesia in dorsal recumbency with the body tilted slightly, so the side with the undescended testis is uppermost. If the horse is a bilateral cryptorchid, it should be rolled slightly to the opposite side when the second testis is operated on, to allow the bowel to gravitate away from the vaginal ring. The inguinal area is prepared for aseptic surgery in a routine manner and draped.

Additional Instrumentation

This procedure requires sponge forceps, an emasculator, and a sterile gauze bandage.

Surgical Technique

A 12- to 15-cm skin incision is made over the external inguinal ring and is continued through the superficial fascia (the site of the incision is illustrated in Fig. 10-2A). Sharp dissection is then abandoned in favor of blunt dissection with fingertips to separate the subcutaneous inguinal fascia and to expose the external inguinal ring. Large branches of the external pudendal vein are in this region, and trauma to these vessels should be avoided. Dissection is continued beyond the external inguinal ring and through the inguinal canal until the vaginal ring is located with the finger (Fig. 10-2B). With an inguinal cryptorchid, the testis contained within the common vaginal tunic would be located in the canal at this time (Fig. 10-2C). The common tunic is opened, and the testis is removed.

With an abdominal cryptorchid, however, the testis will not be located. In this situation, the vaginal ring is located, and curved sponge forceps are carefully introduced through the inguinal canal, so the jaws are placed through the vaginal ring into the vaginal process (Fig. 10-2D). The partially opened jaws of the forceps are pressed against the vaginal process and are closed (Fig. 10-2E). The forceps grasp the vaginal process and associated gubernaculum testis, and the forceps are then withdrawn (Fig. 10-2E). This is the critical part of the technique and the most difficult part for the inexperienced surgeon, because excessive force ruptures the vaginal process. The cord-like gubernaculum may then be palpated within the everted vaginal process by rolling it between the thumb and forefinger. When the gubernaculum is identified, the vaginal process is opened with Metzenbaum scissors (Fig. 10-2F), and the gubernaculum is grasped with Ochsner forceps. Traction on the gubernaculum causes the tail of the epididymis to be presented (Fig. 10-2G). Generally, gentle traction on the epididymis pulls the testis through the vaginal ring. Pushing around the vaginal ring with the fingers at the same time usually is sufficient to deliver the testis, but manual dilation of the vaginal ring is necessary in some cases.

At this point, the testis is positively identified (Fig. 10-2H) and is emasculated (Fig. 10-2I). In some instances, the testis cannot be retracted sufficiently to enable emasculation, so the cord is ligated. If the opening made in the vaginal process to deliver the testicle is considerable and if intestinal herniation is a possibility, then a sterile gauze bandage is packed over the external inguinal ring (Fig. 10-2J); this protects against herniation while normal swelling obliterates the inguinal canal. Then the skin is sutured with heavy polymerized caprolactam (Vetafil), either in a continuous pattern or with simple interrupted sutures with long ends (Fig. 10-2J). If the opening in the vaginal process is small (barely enough to squeeze the testicle through), then packing will usually be unnecessary. Surgical judgment and some experience will decide whether to pack the external ring or not.

The foregoing technique cannot be used in certain instances, such as when accidental rupture of the vaginal process, vaginal ring, or medial wall

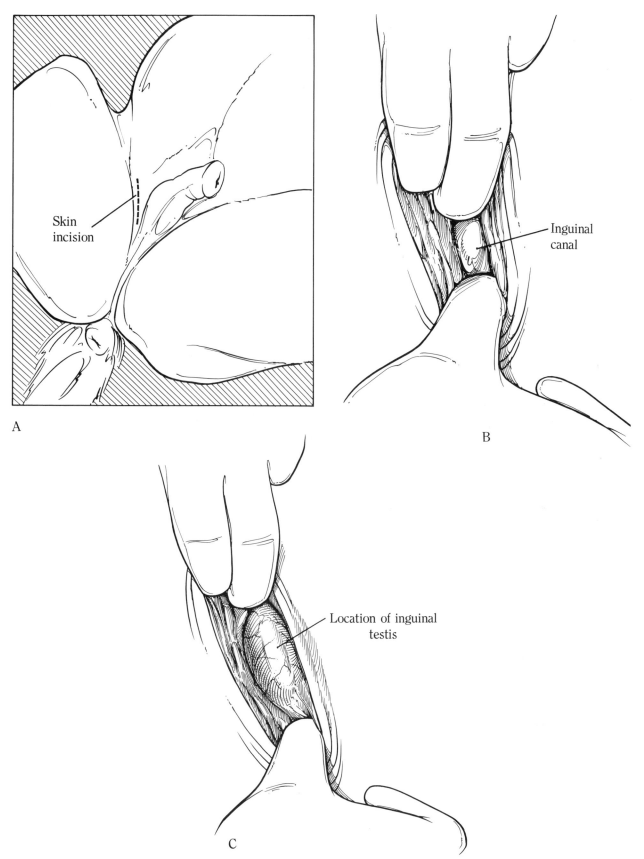

FIG. 10-2. A *to* J, *Cryptorchidectomy by the noninvasive inguinal approach.*

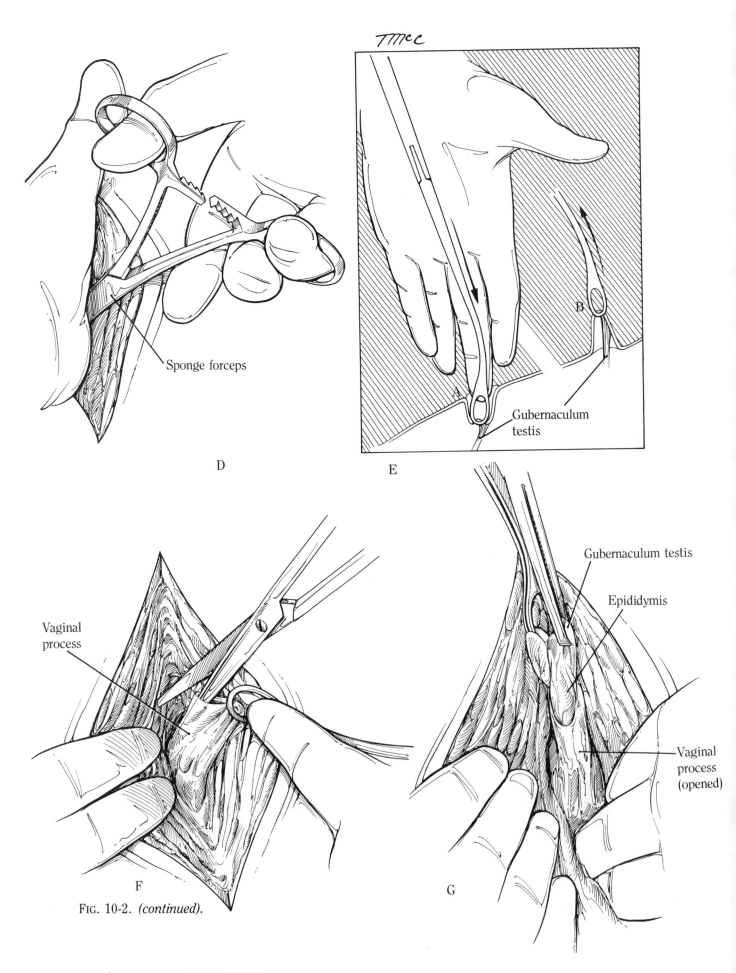

TMCC

Sponge forceps

D

Gubernaculum
testis

E

Vaginal
process

Gubernaculum testis

Epididymis

Vaginal
process
(opened)

F

FIG. 10-2. (continued).

G

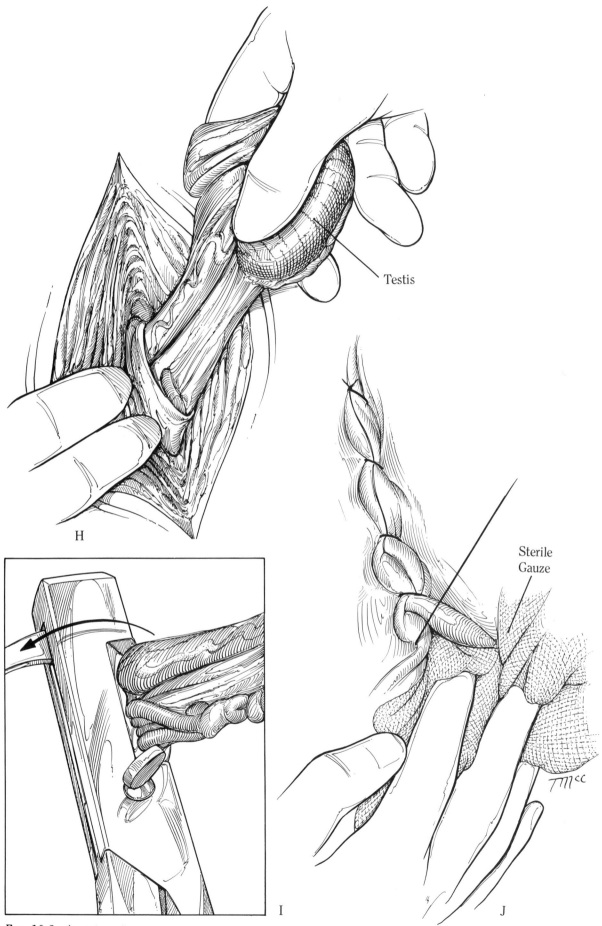

Testis

Sterile
Gauze

H

I

J

FIG. 10-2. *(continued)*.

of the inguinal canal results in the loss of vital landmarks or when the horse has been subjected to a previous, unsuccessful attempt at surgery. In these situations, the first alternative is digital exploration of the boundaries of the vaginal ring to locate the gubernaculum and the ductus deferens or epididymis. Occasionally, the testes are encountered during the digital exploration. If these methods fail to locate the testis, manual exploration of the abdomen with the entire hand may be necessary. The hand may be admitted through a dilated (ruptured) vaginal ring or through the internal abdominal oblique muscle. The internal abdominal oblique muscle forms the medial wall of the inguinal canal and is thin and easily penetrated in this location. If the testis or ductus deferens is not found immediately, the ampullae should be located at the dorsal aspect of the bladder and traced craniad to the ductus deferens and testis. Termination of the ductus deferens with no epididymis or testis suggests the absence of a testis.

Although we recommend packing the inguinal canal with a sterile gauze bandage in certain cases, suture closure of the inguinal canal is recommended when extensive rupture of the vaginal ring or considerable manual invasion of the abdominal cavity has occurred. The external inguinal ring is closed with simple interrupted sutures of no. 2 polyglycolic acid (Dexon) or polyglactin 910 (Vicryl). The strong aponeurotic condensations of the external abdominal oblique muscle support sutures well. Deeper tissues in the canal offer little support for sutures, but it is worthwhile to place a simple interrupted suture across the inguinal canal deep to the external inguinal ring to facilitate obliteration of the canal. The internal inguinal ring is inaccessible for suturing.

Postoperative Management

Tetanus immunization is administered. The internal inguinal ring area is examined rectally 24 hours after surgery. If there are no adhesions of viscera in this area, the skin sutures and gauze pack are removed, the horse is discharged, and the owner is given instructions for routine postcastration management. If suture closure of the inguinal canal is performed, we prefer to hospitalize the horse for 72 hours.

Comments

The potential postoperative complications following cryptorchid surgery are the same as described previously for routine castration. Management of the complications is the same for both procedures, and the reader is referred to the "Comments" heading of the section of this chapter on castration. Scrotal ablation and primary closure techniques have been described with apparently fewer complications, better cosmetic results (less postoperative swelling), and less postoperative discomfort. Further details of these methods are available.[3,4]

References

1. Adams, O. R.: An improved method of diagnosis and castration of cryptorchid horses. J. Am. Vet. Med. Assoc., *145*:439, 1964.

2. Arnold, J. S., Meagher, D. M., and Loshe, C. L.: Rectal tears in the horse. J. Equine Med. Surg., *2*:55, 1978.

3. Barber, S. M.: Castration of horses with primary closure and scrotal ablation. Vet. Surg., *14*:2, 1985.

4. Palmer, S. E., and Passmore, J. L.: Midline scrotal ablation for unilateral cryptorchid castration in horses. J. Am. Vet. Med. Assoc., *190*:283, 1987.

5. Stickle, R. L., and Fessler, J. F.: Retrospective study of 350 cases of equine cryptorchidism. J. Am. Vet. Med. Assoc., *172*:343, 1978.

Caslick's Operation for Pneumovagina in the Mare

The operation for pneumovagina in the mare is to prevent the involuntary aspiration of air into the vagina. Pneumovagina is caused by faulty closure of the lips of the vulva as a result of poor conformation or injury. Mares in which the lips of the vulva are tilted toward the anus are prone to vaginitis, cervicitis, metritis, and infertility due to contamination from material aspirated through the vulva. Old, thin, debilitated mares with sunken ani usually are more prone to pneumovagina. At least 80% of the vulval labia should be located ventral to the pelvic floor, and the vulval seal should be at least 2.5 cm deep and resistant to parting. In addition, the labia should be at an angle of at least 80° to the horizontal.[1] Breeding or foaling injuries may also result in pneumovagina because the skin and mucosa of the labia become misshapen, resulting in a faulty seal. Some mares, especially in racing, may aspirate air even though they have good vulvar conformation, whereas others may have overlapping vulvar lips with relatively good conformation. These mares are also candidates for Caslick's operation. This operation is also performed in combination with other surgery of the mare's perineum, such as repair of first-, second-, and third-degree perineal lacerations.[3]

Anesthesia and Surgical Preparation

Caslick's operation is performed with the animal under local anesthesia by direct infiltration of the vulvar labial margin. The surgery is best performed in a set of stocks, where dangers to the mare and operator are minimal; some mares require a twitch and, occasionally, tranquilization. Prior to the surgery, the feces should be manually removed from the rectum, and the tail should be bandaged and secured out of the surgical field. A thorough cleansing of the perineal region should be performed using a mild disinfectant solution, and all traces of the disinfectant solution should be removed by rinsing with water. Cotton or paper towels are recommended, rather than a scrub brush. Approximately 5 ml of local anesthetic are used for local infiltration into each side (Fig. 10-3A and B).

Following desensitization of the required length of mucocutaneous junction of the vulva and labia, a final preparation of the surgical site is performed using a suitable, nonirritating antiseptic applied with cotton or gauze sponges.

Surgical Technique

Using tissue scissors, the surgeon removes a ribbon of mucosa approximately 3 mm wide from each vulvar labium (Fig. 10-3C). To facilitate trimming the tissue, thumb forceps are used to grasp the ribbon of tissue and to apply downward pressure to stretch the area. A common mistake is to remove too much tissue. Most mares require that this operation be performed on successive years, and if excessive tissue is removed, subsequent repairs will be more difficult. The length of the vulva and labia to be sutured will vary, depending on the conformation of the individual mare. This length may vary from the upper half of the vulva to as much as 70% of its length. Once the ribbon of tissue is removed, the raw surface is generally much wider than one would anticipate because tissue edges under tension retract (Fig. 10-3D). This tension is due to swelling caused by the local analgesic infiltration. Bleeding from the edges usually is minimal.

When the ribbon of tissue has been removed, the raw edges are apposed using a simple interrupted suture pattern (Fig. 10-3E). A nonabsorbable, noncapillary suture material such as 2-0 nylon or 2-0 polypropylene is preferred. Vertical mattress, simple continuous, and continuous interlocking patterns, and Michel clips, have also been used successfully. The suture pattern depends on individual preference, but the raw edges should be in good apposition no matter what pattern is used (Fig. 10-3F). Skin staples have also been used successfully without prior removal of mucosa.[2]

To avoid excessive stress on the suture line at its ventral end during breeding or speculum examination, a "breeder's stitch" may be inserted ventral to Caslick's closure. The area where the stitch is placed is desensitized and is infiltrated 2 cm in all directions from where the suture is to be placed (Fig. 10-3F). Using sterile umbilical tape, the surgeon places a single interrupted suture at the most ventral part of Caslick's operation (Fig. 10-3G). The stitch should not be so ventral that it interferes with breeding, nor should it be so loose that it may lacerate the stallion's penis (Fig. 10-3H). Excessive penetration of the stallion's penis during natural cover in mares with Caslick's operation can be avoided with the use of a stallion/breeding roll.[1]

Postoperative Management

Generally, postoperative topical or systemic antibiotics are not indicated. The sutures can be removed 7 to 10 days postoperatively.

To prevent unnecessary damage at parturition, the vulvar labia should be surgically separated (episiotomy), and the operation should be performed 1 or 2 days after foaling. It may also be necessary to separate the labia during natural mating or during manipulations of the reproductive tract for examination or therapy. If the labia become separated for any reason, the surgery should be redone at the earliest opportunity to prevent pneumovagina.

Comments

Certain mares may be candidates for other procedures, such as episioplasty and urine-pooling surgery, to achieve optimal fertility.[3] A mare that still has vaginal aerophagia following Caslick's operation should be considered a candidate for additional surgery. Animals in which the perineal region is sunken beneath both tuber ischii and in which the dorsal commissure of the vulva becomes horizontal, with rostral displacement of the anus, may not respond to Caslick's operation alone. Older, multiparous mares seem to be more prone to this condition, especially if they are unthrifty.

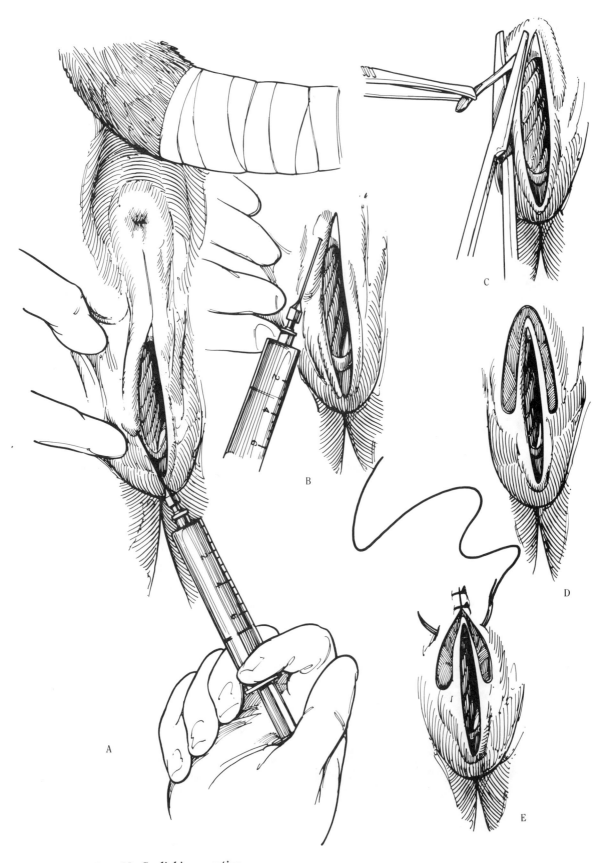

FIG. 10-3. A *to* H, *Caslick's operation.*

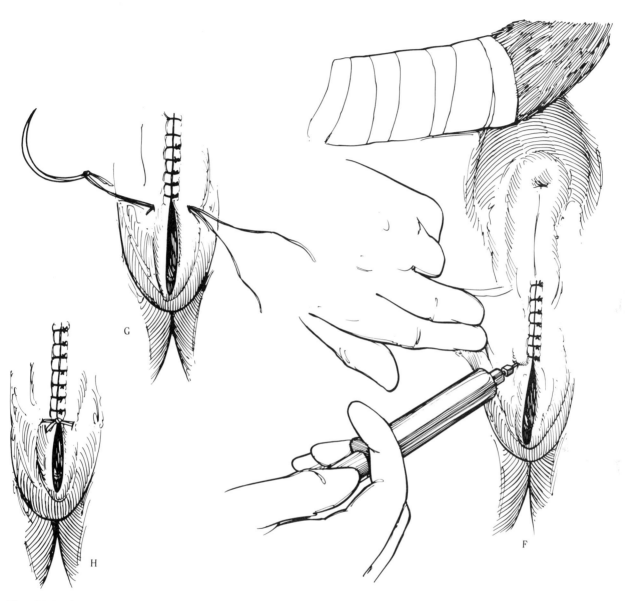

F

G

H

Fig. 10-3. *(continued).*

References

1. Ansari, M. M.: The Caslick operation in mares. Compend. Contin. Educ. Pract. Vet., *5*:107, 1983.

2. Candle, A. B., et al.: Skin staples for non-scarified Caslick procedures. Vet. Med., *78*:782, 1983.

3. McIlwraith, C. W., and Turner, A. S.: Equine Surgery: Advanced Techniques. Philadelphia, Lea & Febiger, 1987.

Urethroplasty by Caudal Relocation of the Transverse Fold

This reconstructive technique is indicated for treatment of urine pooling in the vagina. Urine pooling is more common in older, multiparous mares when sunken vaginas develop. The ventral floor of the vagina slopes cranioventrad, and uterine fluid and urine accumulate in the fornix of the vagina around the cervix. Vaginitis, cervicitis, endometritis, and temporary or permanent sterility may result. The aim of this operation is to promote caudal evacuation of urine and to prevent its pooling in the vagina.

Anesthesia and Surgical Preparation

The surgery is performed on the standing mare restrained in stocks. Tranquilization and epidural anesthesia are used. If the epidural anesthetic is ineffective, local infiltration of the surgical site can be performed. The tail is wrapped and is tied away from the surgical field. The vestibule and vagina are flushed with dilute povidone-iodine solution (not performed routinely by all surgeons), and the perineal area is prepared for aseptic surgery.

Additional Instrumentation

This procedure requires a self-retaining retractor (Glasser retractor) and long-handled surgical instruments.

Surgical Technique

A self-retaining retractor (Glasser retractor) is placed in the vulva to expose the surgical area (Fig. 10-4A). The urethral orifice opens just caudal to and underneath the transverse fold (the remnant of the hymen at the vaginovestibular junction). The transverse fold of mucosa is identified approximately 5 to 10 cm cranial to the brim of the pelvis on the floor of the vagina (Fig. 10-4B). Long-handled instruments facilitate the performance of this procedure. The transverse fold is grasped left of center with a pair of thumb forceps and is retracted caudad approximately 5 cm using moderate tension (Fig. 10-4C and D). The dotted line in the figure indicates the line of mucosal resection. Using curved scissors, the surgeon removes the lateral edge of the retracted transverse fold from the point of attachment of the thumb forceps to the junction of the fold with the vestibular wall (Fig. 10-4C and D). Then the transverse fold is positioned along the ventrolateral wall of the vestibule to ascertain the line of the proposed attachment, and a second incision is made with curved scissors in the wall of the vestibule (Fig. 10-4E and F). This incision also extends craniad to the junction of the transverse fold with the wall of the vestibule.

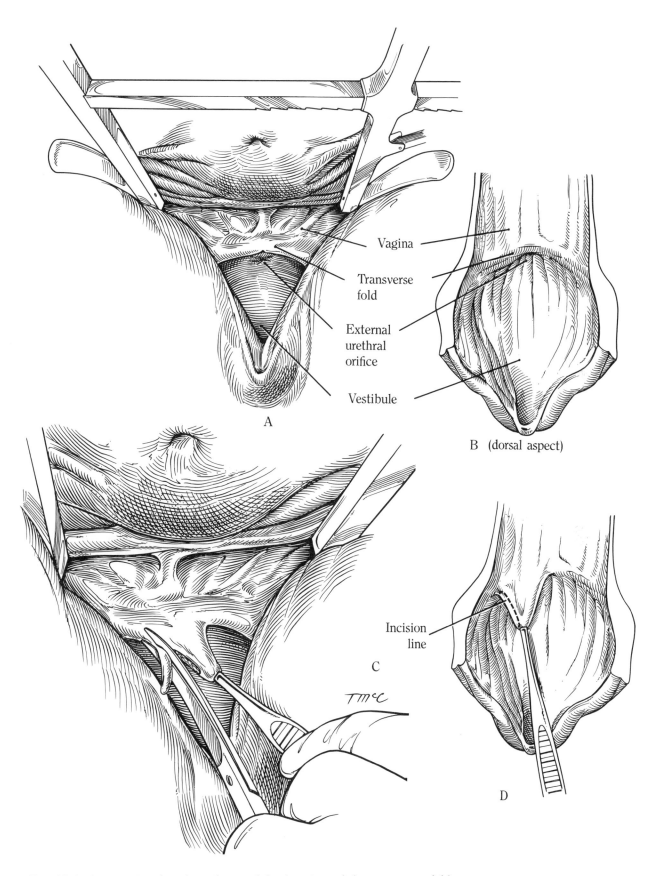

Vagina

Transverse
fold

External
urethral
orifice

Vestibule

A

B (dorsal aspect)

C

TM°C

Incision
line

D

FIG. 10-4. A *to* H, *Urethroplasty by caudal relocation of the transverse fold.*

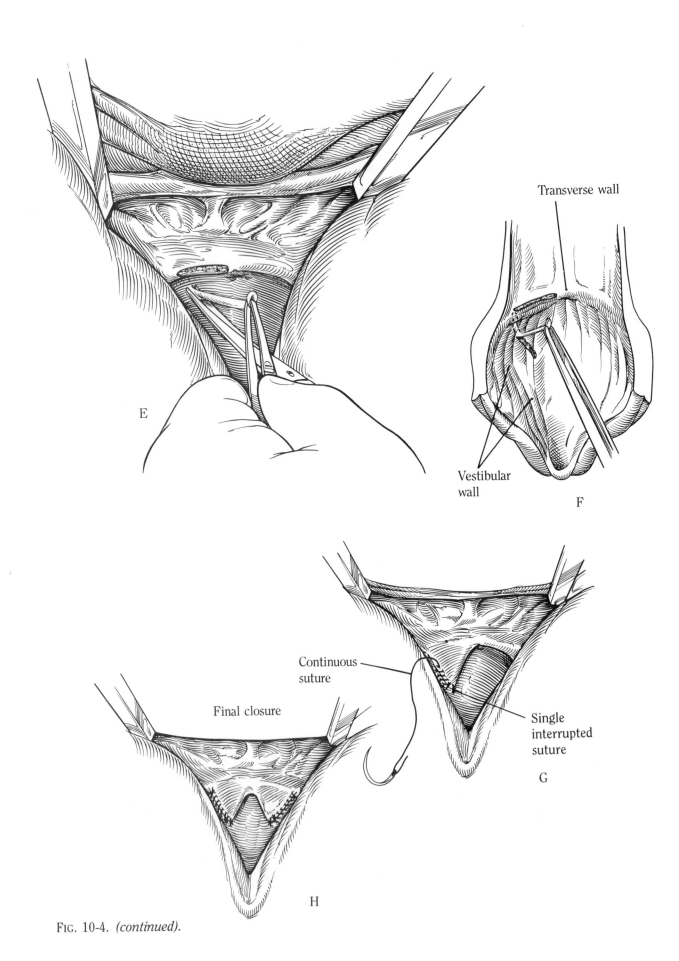

Transverse wall

Vestibular wall

F

Continuous suture

Final closure

Single interrupted suture

G

H

FIG. 10-4. *(continued)*.

The denuded line along the transverse fold is sutured to the denuded line on the ventrolateral wall of the vestibule (Fig. 10-4G). A single simple interrupted suture of nylon or polypropylene is placed at the caudal end, and the apposition is completed with a continuous suture pattern of 2-0 synthetic absorbable material; this procedure is repeated on the right side of the transverse fold (Fig. 10-4H). The transverse fold now has a "V"-shaped appearance with the apex of the "V" cranial in position. It is important to have minimal tension on the transverse fold when it is sutured into this new position; otherwise, the surgery will fail because of pressure necrosis at the sutures. In addition, the transverse fold should not be sutured more than 2 cm from the floor of the vestibule or the fold will be torn during copulation. It is also important that the new urethral aperture be of sufficient size so normal urine flow is not restricted.

Postoperative Management

Tetanus prophylaxis is provided, and a course of systemic antibiotics is instituted. The two nonabsorbable sutures are removed in 10 to 14 days. Caslick's operation is performed at the same time as the urethroplasty. The vagina is not interfered with for 2 weeks. After surgery, mares should not be sexually active for 30 to 60 days; during this time, any uterine infection should be treated. Artificial insemination should be used when possible.

Comments

This technique is usually effective in eliminating urine pooling in mares with a vaginal slope of 5 to 30°.[3] Mares with a greater slope have a less-favorable prognosis. An alternate urethroplasty technique, in which a shelf is developed to act as a tunnel, has been described and may be considered an option if the transverse-fold relocation fails to correct the problem or as the preferred procedure in many cases.[1,2] Details of this procedure are described in our advanced text.[2]

References

1. Brown, M. P., Colahan, P. T., and Hawkins, D. L.: Urethral extension for treatment of urine pooling in mares. J. Am. Vet. Med. Assoc., *173*:1005, 1978.

2. McIlwraith, C. W., and Turner, A. S.: Equine Surgery: Advanced Techniques. Philadelphia, Lea & Febiger, 1987.

3. Monin, T.: Vaginoplasty: A surgical treatment for urine pooling in the mare. *In* Proceedings of the 18th Annual Convention of the American Association of Equine Practitioners in 1972:1973, p. 99.

Cesarean Section in the Mare

This operation is indicated for treatment of various types of dystocia in the mare; the most common indications are transverse presentation,[6,7] some instances of uterine torsion,[5,7] and the production of gnotobiotic foals.[1] Although uterine torsion is best managed by a standing flank laparotomy and manual repositioning of the gravid uterus, a ventral midline celiotomy is indicated if the mare is intractable, if the uterus is ruptured, or if the torsion cannot be corrected with the animal in the standing position. In such cases, hysterotomy is performed first, making untwisting of the torsion easier.[5] Fetal manipulation with the animal under general anesthesia or fetotomy is used in many instances of dystocia. The particular method used to handle a problem commonly depends on the experience and preference of the clinician. Availability of anesthetic assistance may also be a consideration. If manipulation or fetotomy does not produce successful results in a reasonable period of time (or is not expected to do so), however, cesarean section is indicated. In general, as one achieves experience and confidence in the technique, one will undertake this operation sooner and achieve proportionately better results. Cesarean section should not be considered as a last resort in the mare. Uterine rupture, sometimes due to excessive fetal manipulation, is also an indication for cesarean section.[2]

Anesthesia and Surgical Preparation

Various anesthetic regimens have been advocated, in an effort to minimize fetal depression. Epidural anesthesia combined with chloral hydrate and guaifenesin and a low oblique flank surgical approach have been used successfully in Europe.[6,7] We prefer a ventral midline approach to the abdomen performed with the mare under general anesthesia. Although a flank incision is adequate to correct torsion of the uterus, the small paralumbar fossa makes it a poor choice for cesarean section.

Induction of anesthesia with guaifenesin, with or without thiamylal sodium, is preferred to induction with a bolus of thiobarbiturate. Methohexital sodium as an induction agent is superior to thiopental sodium for obtaining live gnotobiotic foals by cesarean section.[1] Halothane and oxygen have been used for anesthetic maintenance, and live foals have been successfully obtained.[1] The level of halothane required for maintenance of anesthesia can be minimized by performing local infiltration of the ventral midline incision line. In many situations, the foal is already dead because of the protracted dystocia and advanced involution of the uterus by the time cesarean section is performed, and whatever anesthetic regimen is considered best for the mare is appropriate.

The use of halothane as an anesthetic agent has been associated with increased bleeding of the uterine incision. This bleeding is associated with congestion of the myometrial vessels and is more significant in species that have diffuse placentation. In an experimental study of cesarean section in mares, mares anesthetized with halothane had increased bleeding from the uterine incision than mares anesthetized with methoxyflurane.[3] If an encircling suture of the incision edge is used, however, bleeding problems are avoided, and halothane remains a safe anesthetic.

If the ventral midline approach is used, the mare is placed in dorsal recumbency and is clipped and prepared for aseptic surgery in a routine manner. According to the systemic status of the patient, appropriate fluid therapy and medication are administered.

Surgical Technique

The abdomen is entered through a ventral midline incision, which is used for the ventral midline laparotomy described in Chapter 12. The uterus enclosing the fetus is located, and an incision site over a limb is chosen, just as in bovine cesarean section. This area is exteriorized as much as possible to minimize contamination of the peritoneal cavity. A more cranial limb should be chosen; otherwise, it may be difficult to close the hysterotomy incision because of caudal retraction of the uterus once the fetus is removed. The uterus is incised using a scalpel, and the foal is removed. Unless the allantochorion has already separated or will lift off easily, it should be left in the uterus.

Before closing the uterus when equine cesarean section is performed, the allantochorion is separated for a distance of 2 to 5 cm from the margin of the uterine incision, and a continuous suture of catgut is placed around the entire margin of the uterine incision for hemostasis (Fig. 10-5, inset).[7] The technique consists of a simple continuous pattern penetrating all layers of the uterus; it is necessary because the equine endometrium is only loosely attached to the myometrium, and there is little natural hemostasis for the large subendometrial veins. In addition, halothane may cause congestion of these veins. Bleeding is virtually impossible to control by clamping and ligation. If the uterus has been ruptured, a continuous suture to stop bleeding may not be necessary because hemorrhage may have ceased.[2] The uterus is closed with a double inverting layer of sutures using no. 2 polyglactin 910 (Vicryl) or polyglycolic acid (Dexon) (Fig. 10-5). The abdomen is closed as for ventral laparotomy in the horse, which is described in Chapter 12. Great care should be exercised when separating the allantochorion at the margin of the uterine incision and avoiding its inclusion in the suture lines. If rupture has occurred, copious lavage of the abdomen with warm physiologic solutions during surgery is indicated because of the increased risk of contamination from uterine contents.[2]

Postoperative Management

Tetanus prophylaxis, antibiotics, and oxytocin are administered. Appropriate fluid therapy is continued or is instituted if the patient is compromised systemically.

As soon as the mare is standing and it is safe to milk her, colostrum should be obtained and given to the foal. The foal should be introduced to the mare as soon as the mare is stable enough on her feet not to be a danger to the foal. For the next 5 to 7 days, rectal examination is indicated to assess uterine size. It is also useful to determine whether bowel is becoming adhered to the hysterotomy incision. If this complication is detected

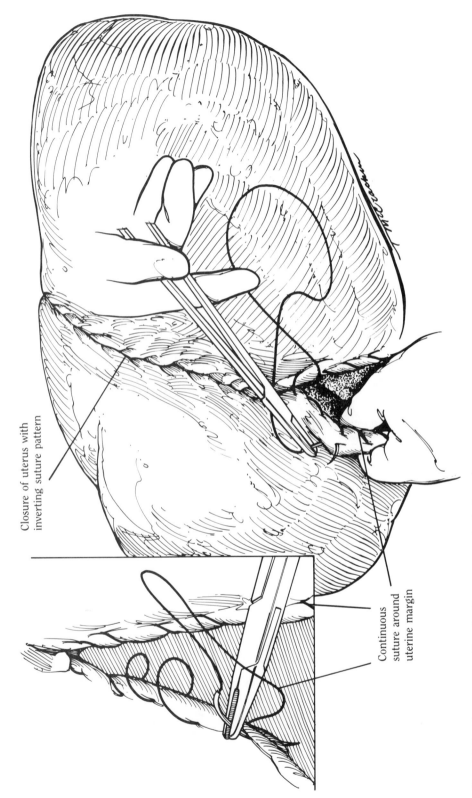

Closure of uterus with
inverting suture pattern

Continuous
suture around
uterine margin

Fig. 10-5. *Cesarean section in the mare and uterine closure.*

early enough, the adherent bowel can, using a flat hand per rectum, be "wiped off," and the fibrinous adhesions can be broken down. If left undetected, such an adhesion may mature and may become a potential source of colic at a later date. Prolonged retention of the placenta is of significant concern in the horse, and the mare should be monitored and treated for retention of fetal membranes if necessary. Immediate forced traction of the placenta should be avoided in case the uterus is torn, especially in mares that have had uterine rupture. The placenta will usually pass on its own. If not, gentle manual removal with careful separation of the placenta from the uterine wall may eventually be indicated.[2]

Comments

Although an oblique low flank laparotomy approach has been used successfully in Europe,[6,7] we believe that the ventral midline approach offers the best exposure and fewer complications during healing of the incision. As discussed in the section of Chapter 12 on ventral midline laparotomy, fears regarding dehiscence or herniation following the use of this approach are unfounded.

In women, postoperative infection can be reduced by prophylactic antibiotics, even when these drugs are administered in the immediate postoperative period, rather than preoperatively.[4] Although undesirable transfer of antibiotics is of concern in infants, we see no reason not to commence antibiotics preoperatively in mares.

References

1. Edwards, G. B., Allen, W. D., and Newcomb, J. R.: Elective caesarean section in the mare for the production of gnotobiotic foals. Equine Vet. J., *6*:122, 1974.

2. Fischer, A. T., and Phillips, T. N.: Surgical repair of a ruptured uterus in five mares. Equine Vet. J., *18*:153, 1986.

3. Heath, R. B.: Personal communication, 1980.

4. Itskovitz, J., Paldi, E., and Katz, M.: The effect of prophylactic antibiotics on febrile morbidity following cesarean section. Obstet. Gynecol., *53*:162, 1979.

5. Pascoe, J. R., Meagher, D. M., and Wheat, J. D.: Surgical management of uterine torsion in the mare: a review of 26 cases. J. Am. Vet. Med. Assoc., *179*:351, 1981.

6. Vandeplassche, M., et al.: Caesarean section in the mare. *In* Proceedings of the 23rd Annual Convention of the American Association of Equine Practitioners in 1977: 1978, p. 75.

7. Vandeplassche, M., et al.: Some aspects of equine obstetrics. Equine Vet. J., *4*:105, 1972.

Circumcision of the Penis
(Reefing)

This operation is indicated for the removal of neoplasms, granulomas (including those associated with repeated habronema infestation), and scar tissue or chronic thickening of the preputial membrane that prevents retraction of the penis.[1,2] Circumscribed lesions of the preputial ring may only require simple surgical removal and suturing of the skin edges. More extensive lesions cause deformity, and consequently, a complete ring of tissue is removed.

Anesthesia and Surgical Preparation

The horse is positioned in dorsal recumbency under general anesthesia, the penis is held in extension with towel clamps or a gauze loop around the neck of the glans, and the surgical area is prepared and draped for aseptic surgery. Catheterization of the urethra and the use of a tourniquet are optional.

Surgical Technique

Figure 10-6A shows a lesion on the internal preputial membrane with the lines of excision demarcated. If the lesion involves the cranial rim of the inner prepuce, retraction of the inner lining will be essential before the incisions are made. Two circumferential skin incisions are made cranial and caudal to the lesion (Fig. 10-6B), and the preputial membrane is tensed by the use of towel forceps. A plane of dissection superficial to the deep fascia of the penis is found, and the tissue between the two circumferential incisions is removed. A third longitudinal incision connecting the two circumferential incisions facilitates the ease of dissection. One should be careful not to cut the large subcutaneous vessels around the penis during the blunt dissection. It is necessary to ligate one subcutaneous vein on each side of the penis. We prefer not to use a tourniquet, but if a tourniquet is used, it should be released at this stage to check for bleeding vessels (minor bleeding may be controlled by electrocoagulation). Once the tissue between the two circumferential incisions is removed, two healthy skin margins are left proximally and distally, ready for reapposition (Fig. 10-6C). The edges are brought together and are closed with a layer of simple interrupted sutures of 0 polyglactin 910 (Vicryl) (Fig. 10-6D). If a subcutaneous layer is used, then no attempt is made to secure this to the underlying tunica albuginea.

Postoperative Management

Tetanus prophylaxis is administered, and the use of postoperative antibiotics is recommended. The horse is hand-walked to help minimize preputial

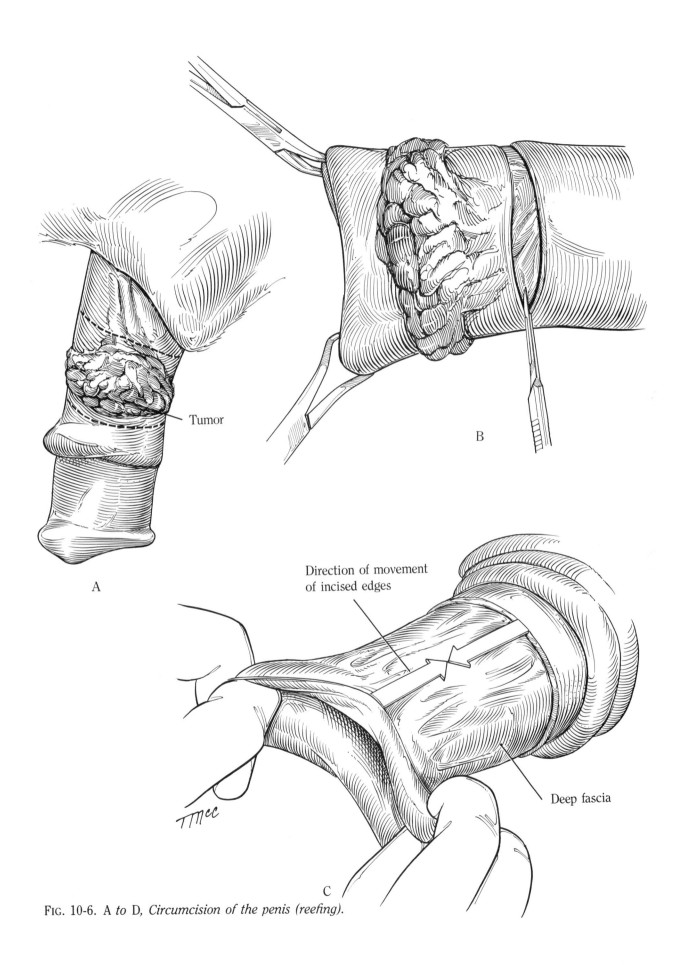

Tumor

Direction of movement
of incised edges

Deep fascia

A

B

C

Fig. 10-6. A *to* D, *Circumcision of the penis (reefing).*

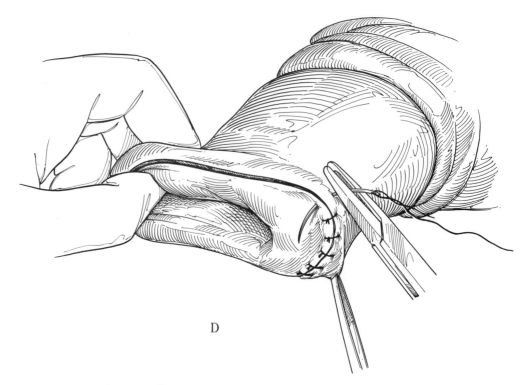

D

Fig. 10-6. *(continued).*

swelling, and sutures are removed in 14 days. If this surgery is performed on a stallion, the animal should be isolated from mares for 3 to 4 weeks.[2]

References

1. Walker, D. F., and Vaughan, J. T.: Bovine and Equine Urogenital Surgery. Philadelphia, Lea & Febiger, 1980.

2. Vaughan, J. T.: Surgery of the male equine reproductive system. *In* The Practice of Large Animal Surgery. Edited by P. Jennings. Philadelphia, W. B. Saunders, 1984, p. 1088.

Amputation of the Penis

The indications for penis amputation in the horse are invasive neoplastic lesions, granulomas associated with habronemiasis, and intractable paralysis or priapism of the penis. The procedure is illustrated as it would be performed for a squamous cell carcinoma of the glans of the penis. In this situation, the penis is amputated at a point distal to that required for penile paralysis, and the operation is therefore easier. The proximal amputations are more difficult because of the greater diameter of the penis and the reflections of the prepuce.[1]

Anesthesia and Surgical Preparation

The horse is positioned in dorsal recumbency under general anesthesia. The penis is prepared for aseptic surgery in a routine manner, and a sterile catheter is passed to identify the urethra. A tourniquet of rubber tubing is applied proximal to the site of amputation (Fig. 10-7A). The penis is also extended and stabilized using a gauze loop around the neck of the glans (not illustrated).

Surgical Technique

A triangular skin incision is made on the ventral aspect of the penis, and the incision is continued through the fascia and corpus cavernosum urethrae (Fig. 10-7B). The apex of the triangle is located on the midline in a caudal direction. The triangle has a 3-cm base with sides approximately 4 cm in length. These incisions should extend down to the urethral mucosa, and the connective tissue within the triangle is removed and discarded. With the catheter as a guide, the urethral mucosa is split longitudinally on the midline from the base to the apex of the triangular defect. Then the catheter is removed.

The edges of the urethra are sutured to the skin edges along the sides of the triangular defect using simple interrupted sutures of 2-0 polyglactin 910 (Vicryl) (Fig. 10-7C). The urethra and penis are then transected. The incision extends from the base of the triangle at a slightly oblique angle craniad towards the dorsal surface of the penis (Fig. 10-7D). The principal blood vessels encountered are the branches of the dorsal arteries and veins of the penis that lie between the deep fascia and the tunica albuginea. Other vessels lying in the loose connective tissue beneath the superficial fascia may require ligation.

The tunica albuginea is closed over the transected corpus cavernosum penis using simple interrupted sutures of 0 polyglactin 910 (Fig. 10-7E). The first suture is placed in the midline, and the next two sutures bisect these halves. Generally, seven sutures are used, and preplacement of the sutures to minimize excess tension on a single suture is preferable. The transected base of the urethral mucosa is then sutured to the skin using simple interrupted sutures of 2-0 polyglactin 910; these sutures should pass through the underlying stump (Fig. 10-7F). Alternatively, the closure can

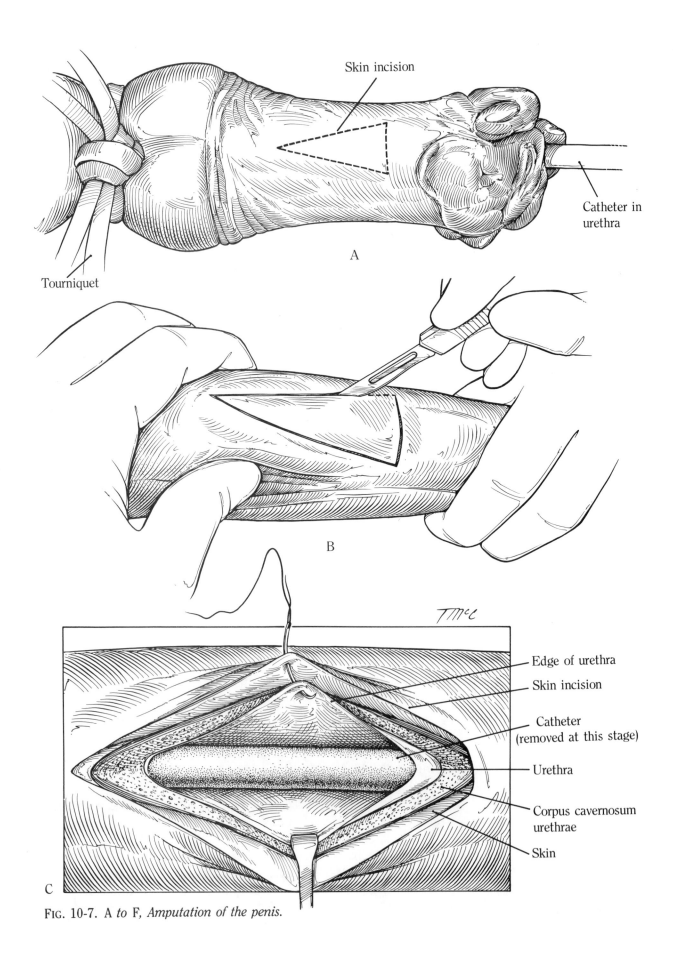

Skin incision

Catheter in
urethra

Tourniquet

A

B

Edge of urethra

Skin incision

Catheter
(removed at this stage)

Urethra

Corpus cavernosum
urethrae

Skin

C

FIG. 10-7. A *to* F, *Amputation of the penis.*

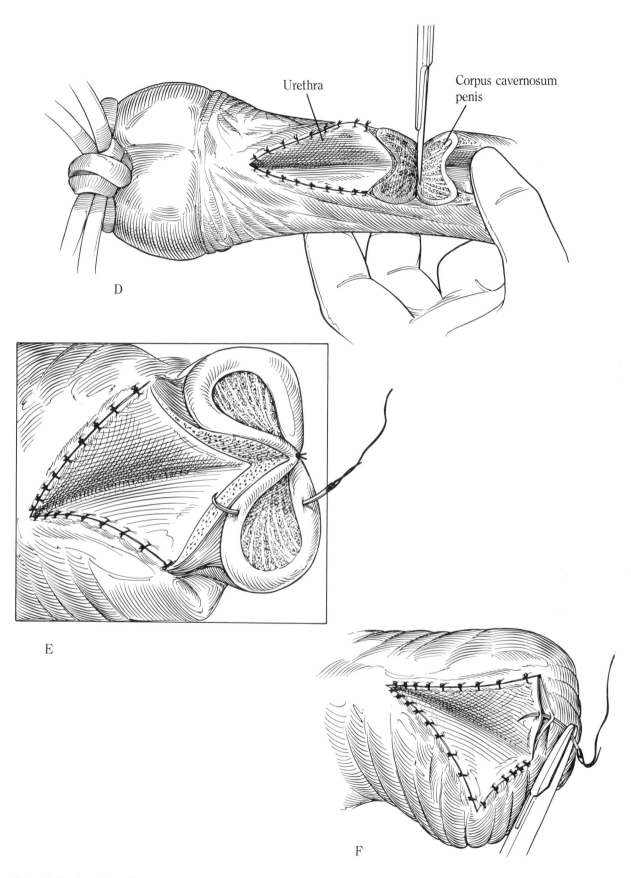

Urethra

Corpus cavernosum
penis

D

E

F

FIG. 10-7. *(continued).*

be made in one layer using simple interrupted sutures, with four bites taken through urethral mucosa, ventral and dorsal tunica albuginea, and skin. At this point, the tourniquet is removed.

Postoperative Management

Tetanus prophylaxis is administered, and systemic antibiotics may be used for 4 to 5 days. Sutures should be removed in 14 days. A stallion should not be exposed to mares for 4 weeks. Complications include hemorrhage, dehiscence, granuloma formation, and urethral stenosis. Some hemorrhage will be observed following removal of the tourniquet, but excessive hemorrhage can cause a dissecting hematoma and wound breakdown. Minor dehiscence of the suture line, if it occurs, will not cause a significant problem; granulation and epithelialization will occur. Urethral stenosis should not be a problem if the triangulation technique is used. If wound dehiscence is extensive, however, stenosis secondary to fibrosis may result.

Reference

1. Walker, D. F., and Vaughan, J. T.: Bovine and Equine Urogenital Surgery. Philadelphia, Lea & Febiger, 1980.

Aanes' Method of Repair of Third-Degree Perineal Laceration

Perineal lacerations in the mare occur during parturition when the foal's limb(s) or head are forced caudad and dorsad.

The injury is seen predominantly in primiparous mares and is usually due to violent expulsive efforts by the mare in combination with some degree of malposition of the fetus, such as dorsopubic position or footnape posture. The injury is also seen following forced extraction of a large fetus or extraction before full dilation of the birth canal.[4]

First-degree lacerations occur when only the mucosa of the vagina and vulva are involved. Second-degree lacerations occur when the submucosa and muscularis of the vulva, anal sphincter, and the perineal body are involved, but there is no damage to the rectal mucosa. Third-degree perineal lacerations occur when there is tearing through the rectovaginal septum, musculature of the rectum and vagina, and the perineal body (Fig. 10-84).[2] Reconstruction of third-degree perineal lacerations is necessary to return the mare to breeding soundness. The communication between the rectum and vagina results in the constant presence of fecal material in the vagina. Reconstruction is performed occasionally in riding horses to eliminate the unpleasant sound made by air aspirated into the vagina.

Generally, surgery is not performed on an emergency basis. The torn tissues are edematous, necrotic, and grossly contaminated, and it is advisable to wait a minimum of 4 to 6 weeks before attempting repair. Repairs attempted earlier than this are usually unsuccessful. While waiting for repair, the mare should remain under close observation. The excessive straining caused by the injury can lead to prolapse of the viscera, including eversion of the urinary bladder.[5]

The cervix should also be examined for lacerations prior to repair because lacerations of the cervix result in a poor prognosis for return to breeding soundness. Mares with lacerations of the cervix are more susceptible to endometritis and early abortion.[1] Upon discovery of the injury, tetanus immunization should be administered. Some cases may require a course of antibiotics. A preoperative diet of grass hay and alfalfa hay should be commenced to maintain proper fecal consistency.

The following technique is performed in two stages: in the first operation, a shelf is constructed between the rectum and vagina; the second operation involves reconstruction of the perineal body. The aim of two-stage repair is reduction of the incidence of straining and subsequent tearing of sutures. Delaying reconstruction of the perineal body avoids reduction in the size of the rectal lumen, minimizes the accumulation of feces, and reduces the number of muscular contractions necessary to void feces. Moreover, suturing of rectal mucous membrane is avoided in this technique, which decreases straining because of suture irritation.[3]

Anesthesia and Surgical Preparation

Feed is withheld from the mare for 24 hours. The mare is tranquilized, is placed in stocks, and an epidural anesthetic is administered (refer to Chapter 2 for details of epidural anesthesia in the horse). The tail is wrapped and tied in a cranial direction to avoid interference during surgery. Feces in the rectum and vagina are removed manually, and the perineal region is scrubbed with mild soap and water. The rectum and vagina are then cleansed with povidone-iodine solution (Betadine), and excess fluids are absorbed with moistened cotton. The perineal area is finally prepared for surgery by spraying with concentrated povidone-iodine solution.

During the first phase of the surgery, two temporary retaining sutures are placed on each side of the laceration, one at the level of the anal sphincter and one near the dorsal commissure of the vulva. These sutures are tied to the skin 8 to 10 cm lateral to the normal position of the anus and vulva. If assistants are available during surgery, they can use a pair of malleable retractors to enhance visualization of the surgical site (Fig. 10-8B).

Additional Instrumentation

The surgery is facilitated by the use of malleable retractors and long-handled needle holders, thumb forceps, and scalpel handles.

Surgical Technique

FIRST STAGE

An incision is made along the scar tissue at the junction of the rectal and vaginal mucosa, commencing at the cranial end of the shelf and moving caudad toward the operator. The completed incision should extend from the shelf formed by the intact rectum and vagina, along the scar-tissue margin, to the level of the dorsal commissure of the vulva (Fig. 10-8B).

The vaginal mucous membrane and submucosa are reflected ventrad from the line of the incision to form a flap of tissue approximately 2.5 cm wide. At the shelf, the rectum and vaginal mucosa are separated craniad for a distance of 2 to 3 cm. Hemorrhage from the incision is usually minimal and is not a problem.

At this point, the surgeon should determine whether further dissection is necessary by estimating the ease with which the vaginal mucosa can be brought into apposition. The mucosa should form the vaginal roof with minimal tension on the suture material.

Closure of the shelf is commenced by apposing the vaginal roof, using no. 1 medium chromic catgut, and tying on the midline of the vaginal roof just cranial to the defect. The knot becomes the cranial end of a continuous horizontal mattress suture pattern, inverting the vaginal mucosa and forming the first layer of the repaired roof of the vagina (Fig. 10-8C and D).

The suture pattern should penetrate the edges of the vaginal mucous membrane and should be continued caudad for one-third to half the laceration. The suture is tied and is tucked into the vagina until it is needed later in the repair (Fig. 10-8C). Catgut is used for this layer because synthetic absorbable sutures drag on the tissues, especially the vaginal mucosa.[1]

A second row of sutures of no. 2 polyglactin 910 (Vicryl) is placed between the rectum and the vaginal wall. The suture is essentially a purse-string pattern, passing through the rectal submucosa; perivaginal tissue, and vaginal submucosa on both sides of the common vault. Each suture is tied immediately after it is placed (Fig. 10-8E).

When the interrupted sutures are placed as far caudally as the newly sutured vaginal roof, the continuous horizontal mattress pattern of catgut is resumed, and the vaginal mucosa is sutured in a caudal direction to the dorsal commissure of the vulva (Fig. 10-8C). The interrupted polyglactin 910 sutures are continued caudad to the dorsal commissure of the vulva; one should keep the overall direction of this row horizontal. This method avoids narrowing of the rectal lumen. Sutures should not be placed in the rectal mucous membrane (Fig. 10-8F).

Following the first stage of the operation, the mare should receive antibiotics for about 5 days. Approximately 2 weeks of healing should be allowed before proceeding with the second stage of the operation. Any exposed polyglactin 910 sutures should be removed a few days before the second operation.

SECOND STAGE

Surgical preparation and anesthesia for the second stage of the procedure are similar to those for the first stage. The retrovestibular shelf is examined for healing, and if a small, granulating fistula remains, the second stage should be delayed until it is healed. When a large fistula remains, the shelf is converted to a third-degree perineal laceration, and the first stage is repeated. Local infiltration of lidocaine can be used, rather than epidural anesthesia.

To obtain fresh surfaces for reconstruction and healing of the perineal body, the newly formed epithelialized tissue must be removed. An incision that commences at the cranial margin of the perineal body is made; it extends peripherally along the scar tissue margin and ends at the dorsal commissure of the vulva, forming two sides of a triangle. An incision is made on the opposite side, and a superficial layer of epithelium is removed, creating two raw, triangular surfaces. The skin of the perineum is undermined and is reflected laterad to permit subsequent closure of the skin without undue tension (Fig. 10-8G).

Closure of the deep layers of the perineal body should commence cranially with simple interrupted sutures of no. 1 polyglactin 910. This closure is completed with simple interrupted sutures of 2-0 nylon placed within the epithelial edges of the rectum. The nylon and polyglactin 910 sutures are placed alternately until reconstruction of the perineal body is completed. No attempt is made to locate and to suture the ends of the anal sphincter muscle because they are usually surrounded by scar tissue. The dorsal portion of the vulvar lips are removed just as in Caslick's operation for pneumovagina. The skin of the perineum and lips of the vulva are closed with interrupted sutures of 2-0 nylon (Fig. 10-8H).

Postoperative Management

The mare is put back on feed immediately after the operation. Antibiotics are administered for 5 days, and the sutures in the perineum and lips of the vulva are removed 14 days after surgery.

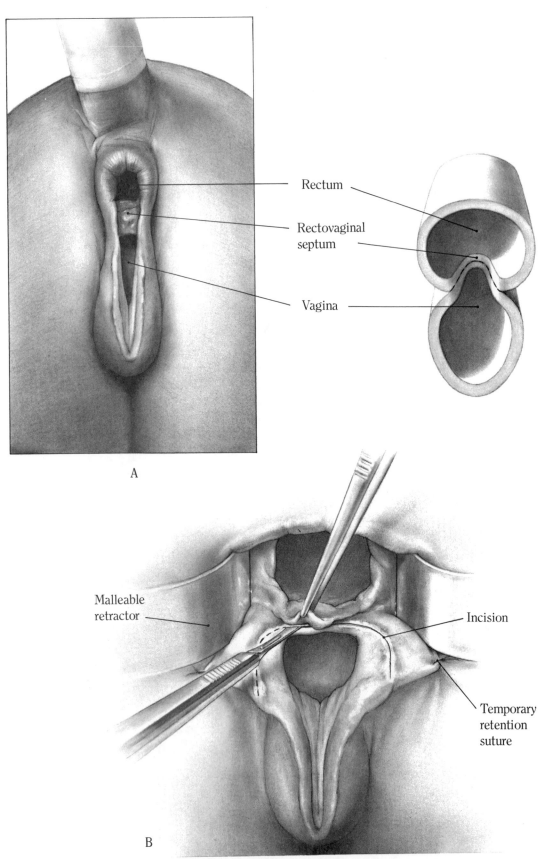

Rectum

Rectovaginal
septum

Vagina

A

Malleable
retractor

Incision

Temporary
retention
suture

B

FIG. 10-8. A *to* H, *Aanes' method of repair of third-degree perineal laceration.*

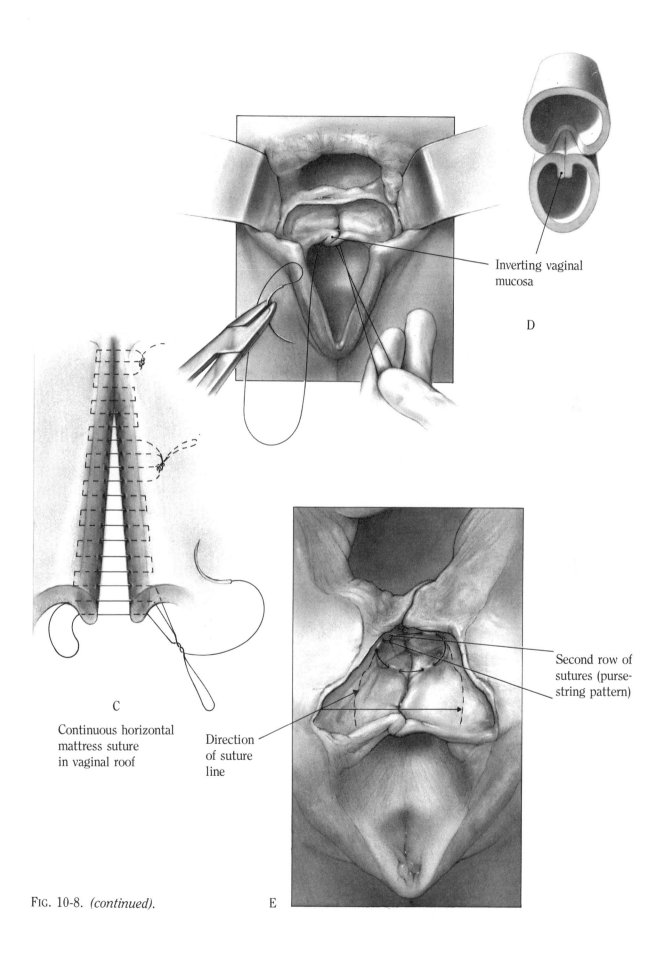

Inverting vaginal
mucosa

D

C

Continuous horizontal
mattress suture
in vaginal roof

Direction
of suture
line

Second row of
sutures (purse-
string pattern)

FIG. 10-8. *(continued)*.

E

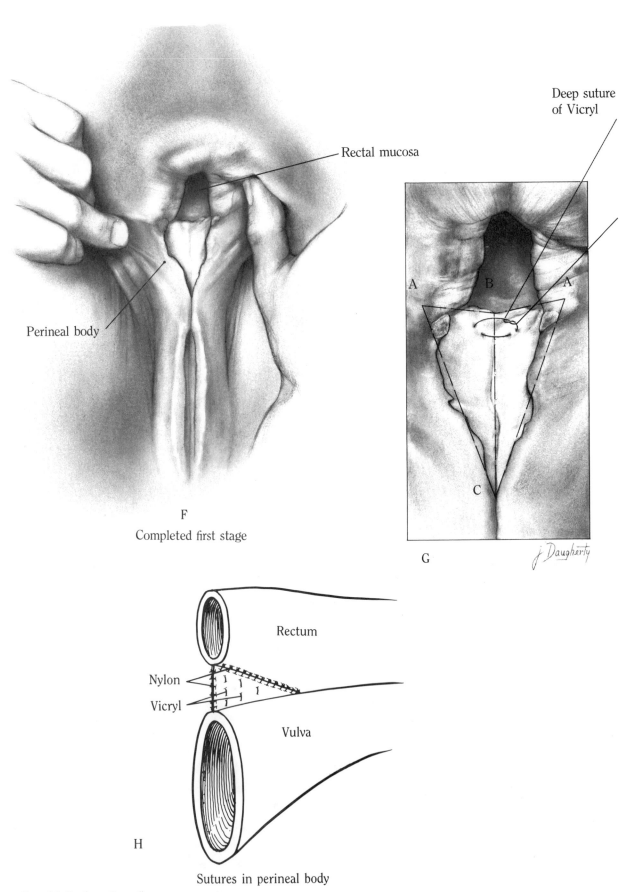

Rectal mucosa

Deep suture
of Vicryl

A   B   A

C

j Daugherty

F

Completed first stage

G

Rectum

Nylon

Vicryl

Vulva

H

Sutures in perineal body

FIG. 10-8. *(continued)*.

Following healing, the mare should be examined for endometritis and treated accordingly. A uterine biopsy may be indicated. Natural service should be postponed for 6 months to allow the region to attain some strength. Some mares require artificial insemination because of a marked reduction in the size of the vulvar opening.

In most cases, the prognosis for future pregnancies following successful repair of a third-degree perineal laceration is excellent. A fertility rate of approximately 75% can be expected.[4] Recurrence of third-degree perineal lacerations at subsequent parturitions ranges from no injury to another third-degree perineal laceration. It is advisable to have an attendant present during future foalings, to minimize the severity of damage in case dystocia occurs.[1]

The complications of this surgery include dehiscence, abscessation and cellulitis, constipation, and fistula formation. Urine pooling may occur and may require one of the urethral extension operations described elsewhere in this chapter and in our other textbook.[6]

References

1. Aanes, W. A.: Personal communication, 1981.

2. Aanes, W. A.: Surgical repair of third-degree perineal laceration and rectovaginal fistula in the mare. J. Am. Vet. Med. Assoc., *144*:485, 1964.

3. Aanes, W. A.: Progress in rectovaginal surgery. *In* Proceedings of the 19th Annual Convention of the American Association of Equine Practitioners in 1973: 1974, p. 225.

4. Colbern, G. T., Aanes, W. A., and Stashak, T. S.: Surgical management of perineal lacerations and rectovestibular fistulae in the mare: a retrospective study of 47 cases. J. Am. Vet. Med. Assoc., *186*:265, 1985.

5. Haynes, P. F., and McClure, J. R.: Eversion of the urinary bladder: a sequel to third degree perineal laceration in the mare. Vet Surg., *9*:66, 1980.

6. McIlwraith, C. W., and Turner, A. S.: Equine Surgery: Advanced Techniques. Philadelphia, Lea & Febiger, 1987.

11

SURGERY OF THE EQUINE UPPER RESPIRATORY TRACT

Tracheostomy

Tracheostomy may be performed on an emergency or an elective basis. Emergency situations include obstructions of the upper airway, such as those caused by rattlesnake bite, regional lymph node abscessation due to Streptococcus equi infection, nasopharyngeal neoplasia, excessive guttural pouch distention with inspissated pus, or postsurgical edema. Elective tracheostomy may be performed following nasal surgery such as nasal septum resection, laryngeal surgery, or whenever postoperative respiratory obstruction is anticipated. It is also indicated for retrograde pharyngoscopy and endotracheal intubation, to permit arytenoidectomy or surgery in the oral cavity,[1] as well as to provide oxygen insufflation into the trachea during any hypoxic crisis.[2]

Anesthesia and Surgical Preparation

Tracheostomy is usually performed with the horse in a standing position. The hair is clipped over the middle third of the neck, and the area is scrubbed surgically. The surgical site is anesthetized by infusing local anesthetic subcutaneously along the proposed incision line for about 10 cm (Fig. 11-1A). If the procedure is done on an elective basis to supplement other surgery, then it may be performed under general anesthesia.

Additional Instrumentation

This procedure requires a commercially available tracheostomy tube.

Surgical Technique

The surgical site is variable, but it is generally at the junction of the middle and upper third of the neck. With the operator standing on the right-hand side of the horse (the reverse for a left-handed operator), a 10-

cm incision is made through the skin and subcutaneous tissue; this is facilitated by tensing the skin at the proximal end of the incision with the left hand and making the skin incision with the right hand (Fig. 11-1B). Following incision of the skin and subcutaneous tissues, the bellies of the sternothyrohyoideus muscles are visible. These muscle bellies are bluntly divided in the midline with scissors or the tip of a hard-backed scalpel (Fig. 11-1C). Then the tracheal rings are identified. The scalpel is inserted midway between two of the tracheal rings with a sharp thrust. This incision is made in a horizontal direction about 1 cm in either direction from the midline; when the incision is completed, the tracheostomy tube can be inserted. This method is used when a tracheostomy tube will be left in place for a short period of time.

Another method is to remove an elliptical piece of cartilage from each of two adjacent rings (Fig. 11-1D). This involves removal of a semicircular piece of cartilage from the cranial surface of one ring and the caudal surface of the next ring. Before the semicircular piece of cartilage is severed completely, the isolated section should be grasped with a pair of forceps. The latter method is used when a tracheostomy tube is required for long periods. The tracheal rings should not be severed completely. Because the tracheal rings in the horse are incomplete at the dorsal aspect, cutting through the ventral portion would divide each ring into two pieces and result in collapse of the trachea and chondritis.

In both methods, the incision is not closed, and the wound should be allowed to heal by secondary intention when the tracheostomy tube is removed.

Postoperative Management

The tracheostomy site should be cleaned daily with a sterile physiologic solution, such as saline solution. The area can be dressed with a suitable, nonirritating, antibacterial ointment at the same time. When the tracheostomy tube is in place, it should be removed and cleaned once or twice daily, depending on the amount of accumulated secretions. The site will usually heal uneventfully by secondary intention.

Comments

In an emergency situation, such as when the animal is in danger of suffocation, the surgeon may need to forego a complete aseptic preparation. Occasionally, subcutaneous emphysema develops where air is trapped between the wound edges and dissects along fascial planes. This condition is usually self-limiting, and its chances of occurrence are minimized by handling tissues gently and not dissecting around either side of the trachea. Tracheal stenosis is a potential complication of this surgery, and its likelihood depends on the length of time the tracheostomy tube is left in place.

References

1. Gabel, A. A.: A method of surgical repair of the fractured mandible in the horse. J. Am. Vet. Med. Assoc., *155*:1831, 1969.

2. Moore, J. N., et al.: Tracheostomy in the horse. Arch. Am. Coll. Vet. Surg., *7*:35, 1977.

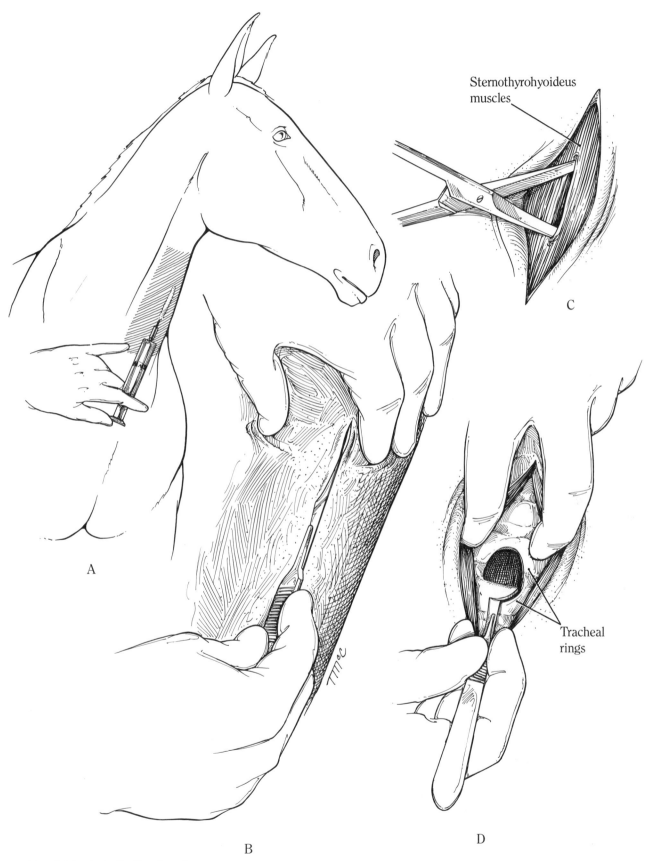

Sternothyrohyoideus
muscles

C

Tracheal
rings

A

B

D

FIG. 11-1. A *to* D, *Tracheostomy*.

Laryngotomy and Laryngeal Ventriculectomy

Laryngeal ventriculectomy is indicated in the treatment of laryngeal hemiplegia and consists of the removal of the mucous membrane lining the laryngeal ventricle. The success rate for this procedure varies with the individual's definition of a satisfactory result. One author believed that over 80% of patients improved after ventriculectomy, but fewer than 10% of the operations could be considered "completely successful."[2] His definition of complete success was "the result obtained when the obstruction is relieved and renders the horse's breathing audibly indistinguishable, to the critical ear, from an unaffected horse at all paces."[2] Another noted surgeon believed that, if after a ventriculectomy the horse can perform its work in a manner satisfactory to the owner, the operation has been successful.[5] Using this criterion, his success rate was 60 to 70%.

In severe cases of laryngeal hemiplegia, additional surgical insertion of a laryngeal prosthesis to abduct the arytenoid cartilage and vocal cord is indicated.[3] Most surgeons perform this second, more involved, surgical procedure when endoscopic examination shows that the arytenoid cartilage is displaced medially from the normal resting position. In these cases, ventriculectomy does not produce sufficient abduction of the vocal cord. In animals in which the arytenoid cartilage is not adducted beyond the normal resting position, so the larynx appears symmetric at rest, ventriculectomy as a sole procedure is justified. If economics are not a consideration and the owner wants the best result possible, we will insert a laryngeal prosthesis in any equivocal case. Details of this procedure are described in our other textbook.[4]

Ventriculectomy is accomplished by performing a laryngotomy through the cricothyroid membrane. The technique of laryngotomy described here is also used for partial resection of the soft palate,[1] arytenoidectomy,[6] and the surgical treatment of epiglottic entrapment,[1] pharyngeal cysts,[1] or lymphoid hyperplasia.[1]

Anesthesia and Surgical Preparation

Laryngotomy and ventriculectomy may be performed with the horse under general anesthesia and in dorsal recumbency or with the standing animal sedated and injected with local analgesic at the surgical site. When the procedure is performed on the standing horse, the ventriculectomy is performed blindly, but it is the same procedure that is performed under general anesthesia. Prior to surgery (ideally, 4 hours prior to surgery), patients are given 2 g of phenylbutazone intravenously to minimize postoperative laryngeal edema. The surgical area is clipped and prepared aseptically.

Additional Instrumentation

This procedure requires a self-retaining retractor (Gelpi, Weitlaner, or Hobday's roaring retractor), a laryngeal bur, and a tracheostomy tube.

Surgical Technique

A skin incision approximately 10 cm long is made from the surface of the cricoid cartilage to beyond the junction of the thyroid cartilages (Fig. 11-2A). In some instances, the triangular depression between the thyroid cartilages and cricoid cartilage can be felt before the skin incision is made. When this is not possible, the central area of the skin incision is located by placing a horizontal line across the area where the rami of the mandible merge with the neck. The skin incision exposes the midline between the sternothyrohyoideus muscles, which are separated with scissors to expose the cricothyroid membrane. After initial separation with scissors, the muscles may be retracted digitally for the length of the skin incision. The cricothyroid membrane is cleared of adipose tissue, and at this stage, it may be necessary to ligate a small vein that commonly is present in the surgical site. The cricothyroid membrane is then incised, commencing with a stab incision, to penetrate the laryngeal mucosa (Fig. 11-2B). The incision is then extended longitudinally from the cricoid cartilage caudad to the junction of the thyroid cartilages cranially. The wings of the thyroid cartilages are retracted with a self-retaining retractor (Gelpi, Weitlaner, or Hobday's roaring retractor).

If a small-diameter, cuffed endotracheal tube is used, ventriculectomy may be performed with the endotracheal tube in place; otherwise, removal of the tube will be necessary for identification of the laryngeal saccule and ventriculectomy. The laryngeal ventricle is identified by sliding the index finger craniad off the edge of the vocal cord and turning the finger laterad and downward toward the base of the ear to enter the ventricle. The laryngeal bur is passed into the ventricle as deeply as possible and twisted to grasp the mucosa (Fig. 11-2C). A sagittal section of the larynx showing the location of the laryngeal ventricle is illustrated in Figure 11-2D. When the operator believes that the mucosa is engaged in the bur, the bur is carefully withdrawn from the ventricle by everting the ventricular mucosa (Fig. 11-2E). At this stage, it is advisable to place a pair of forceps on the everted mucosa to avoid tearing or slippage as the mucosa is fully retracted. The forceps are attached to the mucosa, the bur is untwisted and is removed, and the ventricular saccule is completely everted using traction. With retraction maintained by Ochsner forceps or a similar instrument placed across the saccule, the everted mucous membrane is resected with scissors as close to the base as possible without damaging associated cartilage (Fig. 11-2F). We routinely perform the ventriculectomy bilaterally, but the clinical problem is usually associated with the left side. Following excision of the ventricle, any tags of remaining mucous membrane are removed.

The laryngotomy incision is not sutured, but is left open, because the respiratory tract mucosa cannot be aseptically prepared, and contamination of the incision can occur with subsequent infection and abscessation as potential problems. The laryngotomy wounds heal satisfactorily by secondary

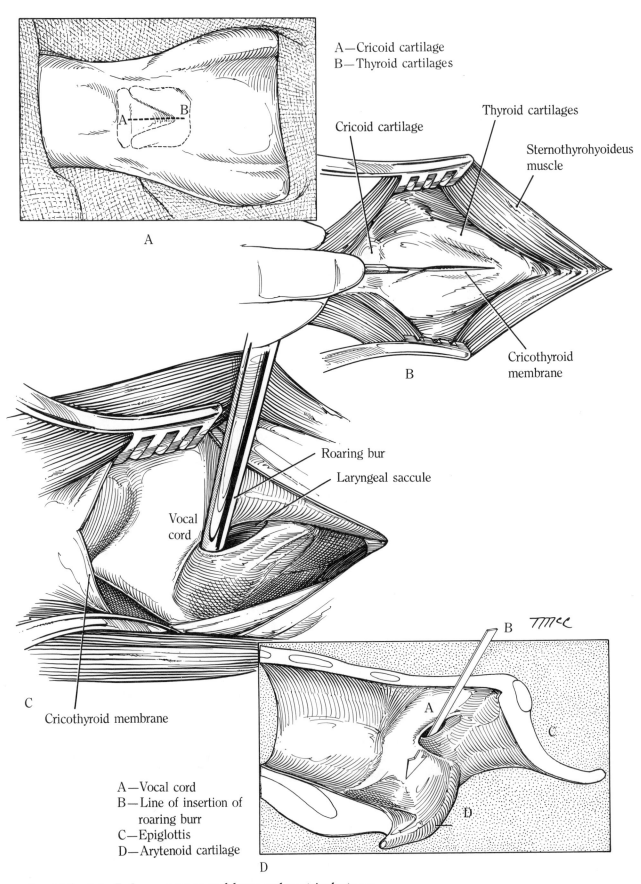

A—Cricoid cartilage
B—Thyroid cartilages

A

Cricoid cartilage

Thyroid cartilages

Sternothyrohyoideus
muscle

Cricothyroid
membrane

B

Roaring bur

Laryngeal saccule

Vocal
cord

C

Cricothyroid membrane

A—Vocal cord
B—Line of insertion of
    roaring burr
C—Epiglottis
D—Arytenoid cartilage

D

FIG. 11-2. A *to* F, *Laryngotomy and laryngeal ventriculectomy.*

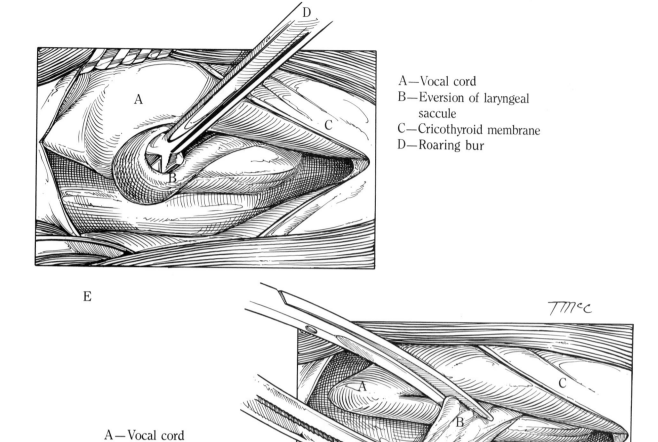

A—Vocal cord
B—Eversion of laryngeal
    saccule
C—Cricothyroid membrane
D—Roaring bur

A—Vocal cord
B—Everted laryngeal saccule
C—Cricothyroid membrane
D—Sternothyrohyoideus muscle

FIG. 11-2. *(continued).*

F

intention; therefore, suturing this wound is not considered justifiable. A tracheostomy tube remains in the laryngotomy site while the horse recovers from anesthesia.

Postoperative Management

Antibiotics are not administered routinely. The laryngotomy wound is cleaned twice daily, and the animal is confined for the 2 to 3 weeks it takes for the wound to heal. After this period, the horse is hand-walked. The horse may be put back to work 8 weeks following surgery.

Comments

The tracheostomy tube is usually left in the laryngotomy opening until the patient recovers from anesthesia. If there is undue trauma during surgery—

more likely with some of the more involved procedures performed by a laryngotomy approach—it may be advisable to leave the tracheostomy tube in place in case laryngeal edema develops. We do not perform a separate tracheostomy without a specific, critical indication.

References

1. Boles, C.: Treatment of upper airway abnormalities. Vet. Clin. North Am. (Large Anim. Pract.), *1*:127, 1979.

2. Marks, D., et al.: Observations on laryngeal hemiplegia in the horse and treatment by abductor muscle prosthesis. Equine Vet. J., *2*:159, 1970.

3. Marks, D., et al.: Use of a prosthetic device for surgical correction of laryngeal hemiplegia in horses. J. Am. Vet. Med. Assoc., *157*:157, 1970.

4. McIlwraith, C. W., and Turner, A. S.: Equine Surgery: Advanced Techniques. Philadelphia, Lea & Febiger, 1987.

5. Raker, C. W.: Laryngotomy and laryngeal sacculectomy. 3rd Annual Surgical Forum: Chicago, 1975.

6. White, N. A., and Blackwell, R. B.: Partial arytenoidectomy in the horse. Vet. Surg., *9*:5, 1980.

Partial Resection of the Soft Palate

Partial resection of the soft palate is indicated in certain cases of dorsal displacement of the soft palate. Dorsal displacement of the soft palate occurs secondary to recognized entities, such as guttural pouch mycosis with secondary involvement of the vagus nerves, and in association with a hypoplastic epiglottis. The most common form of soft palate displacement is intermittent, however, and is usually associated with exercise; factors in the problem are still controversial.[1] It is a clinical impression that the condition may also accompany generalized inflammation of the pharynx. In these cases, the soft palate displacement may resolve itself on resolution of the inflammatory problem. Both so-called paresis and elongation have been postulated as causes, but not proved. Some horses with intermittent dorsal displacement of the soft palate above the epiglottis respond to tongue-tying, which prevents complete retraction of the tongue. Cook has postulated that the basis of the condition is a temporary subluxation of the larynx, which becomes displaced in relation to the soft palate.[3]

Partial resection of the soft palate is not a panacea for dorsal displacement of the soft palate, but it has been the classic method of treatment in horses that do not respond to conservative therapy.[2] Surgical patients should be selected carefully. Other primary causes of the problem should be eliminated, and caution must be used because tranquilizers increase the tendency for soft palate displacement. A flexible endoscope in the caudal portion of the pharynx may interfere with the normal act of deglutition and may lead to an erroneous diagnosis. When the condition is the result of a hypoplastic epiglottis or guttural pouch mycosis with nerve involvement, soft palate surgery is not indicated.

Anesthesia and Surgical Preparation

The horse is prepared for laryngotomy as previously described. In this case, the surgery is always performed with the horse under general anesthesia and in dorsal recumbency.

Additional Instrumentation

This procedure requires a self-retaining retractor (Gelpi, Weitlaner, or Hobday's roaring retractor).

Surgical Technique

Laryngotomy is performed as previously described. In some instances, the body of the thyroid cartilage may be sectioned to extend the laryngotomy incision and to provide additional exposure. If the thyroid cartilage is sectioned, one should be careful not to incise the epiglottis, which is in close association with the thyroid cartilage. Splitting the thyroid cartilage is not performed routinely in this procedure.

When laryngotomy is completed, the endotracheal tube must be withdrawn into the mouth, to enable one to visualize the soft palate. The concave, U-shaped free border of the soft palate will be observed rostrally (Fig. 11-3A). Allis tissue forceps are placed on each side of the soft palate, approximately 1 cm from the midline, and the positioning is checked for symmetry (Fig. 11-3B). An incision into the soft palate with Metzenbaum scissors is made on the right side beside the forceps; this incision is extended toward the midline in a semicircular fashion so that, at the midline, it is about 1 cm from the central free border of the soft palate (Fig. 11-3C). This procedure is repeated on the left side of the soft palate, so a piece of tissue approximately 2 cm × 1 cm is removed from the central free area of the soft palate. Hemorrhage is negligible, and no attempt is made to suture the soft palate. Alternatively, the resection of tissue can be made in a V-fashion, rather than in crescentic fashion.

Soft palate resection should be conservative. It is better to subject the animal to a second surgical procedure for resection of additional soft palate than to resect excessive tissue initially because excessive resection can result in a bilateral nasal discharge of mucus and food material and, possibly, aspiration pneumonia.

Postoperative Management

The horse is confined to a stall until the laryngotomy incision is completely healed and should rest for 4 weeks before being placed into work. Approximately two-thirds of horses undergoing resection of the soft palate have improved sufficiently for racing purposes.[3]

Comments

Based on his theory of the pathogenesis of dorsal displacement of the soft palate, Cook has advocated sternothyrohyoideus myectomy.[3] A preliminary study of this treatment in 21 race horses showed that 17 of them (71%) benefited from this operation. This operation is simple to perform, has fewer potential complications, and requires less convalescence than other procedures. It is described in our other textbook.[4]

References

1. Boles, C.: Abnormalities of the upper respiratory tract. Vet. Clin. North Am. (Large Anim. Pract.), 1:89, 1979.

2. Boles, C. L.: Treatment of airway abnormalities. Vet. Clin. North Am. (Large Anim. Pract.), 1:727, 1979.

3. Cook, W. R.: The biomechanics of choking in the horse. In Proceedings of the 40th Annual Conference for Veterinarians. Fort Collins, Colorado State University, 1979, p. 129.

4. McIlwraith, C. W., and Turner, A. S.: Equine Surgery: Advanced Techniques. Philadelphia, Lea & Febiger, 1987.

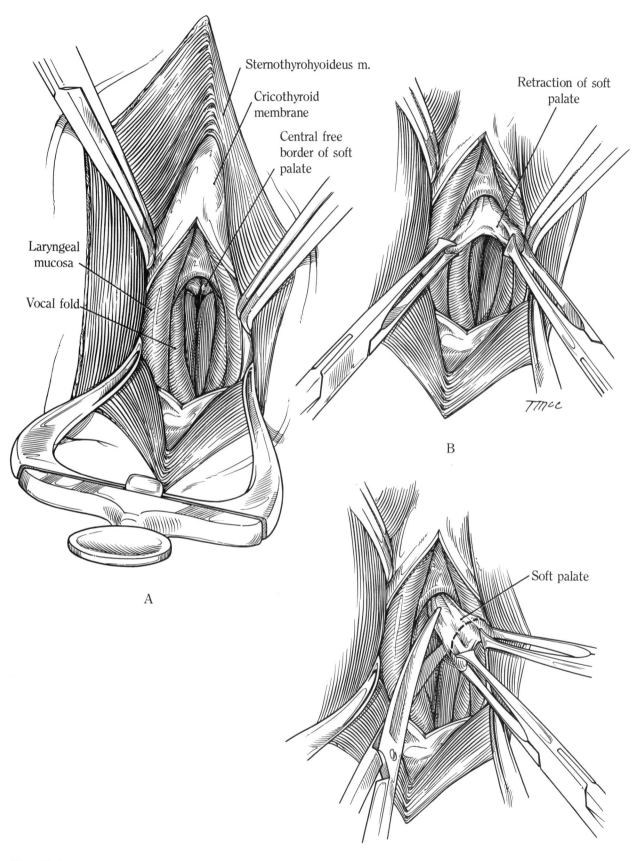

Sternothyrohyoideus m.

Cricothyroid
membrane

Central free
border of soft
palate

Laryngeal
mucosa

Vocal fold

A

Retraction of soft
palate

B

Soft palate

C

Fig. 11-3. A *to* C, *Partial resection of the soft palate.*

Surgical Entry and Drainage of the Guttural Pouches

Each of the three surgical approaches to the guttural pouches has particular uses, advantages, and disadvantages. Viborg's triangle approach is used mainly for drainage of the guttural pouch in cases of empyema. It may also be used for the treatment of guttural pouch tympany.[1] The hyovertebrotomy approach, also known as Chabert's approach, provides access through the dorsolateral aspect of the guttural pouch and is used for the removal of chondroids and inspissated pus. It is commonly combined with Viborg's triangle approach in the treatment of chronic guttural pouch empyema. A drain or seton may be placed through both incisions postoperatively. The hyovertebrotomy approach may also be used to ligate the internal carotid artery in the treatment of guttural pouch mycosis. Further details of the technique of internal carotid artery ligation are described in our other textbook.[5]

The third approach is the ventral or Whitehouse approach (there is also a modified Whitehouse approach). This provides the best surgical exposure to the dorsal aspect of the guttural pouch for procedures such as ligation of the internal carotid artery within the pouch in the treatment of guttural pouch mycosis associated with epistaxis.[4] The Whitehouse approach may also be used to treat guttural pouch tympany.[2] Although the Whitehouse approach seems a logical choice for ventral drainage of the guttural pouch, temporary and permanent dysphagia has been experienced following the use of this procedure for the treatment of empyema. The dysphagia is presumably associated with compromise of the pharyngeal branches of the glossopharyngeal and vagus nerves that pass ventral to the guttural pouch. Because of the thickened nature of the guttural pouch in this inflammatory condition, these nerves may be difficult to identify, and the associated cellulitis may also compromise the nerves. Consequently, we are hesitant to recommend it as a drainage technique for guttural pouch empyema (details of the technique are available elsewhere[1,3]).

If the response to medical treatment of guttural pouch empyema is poor, then surgical drainage of the guttural pouch will be indicated. Surgery is also indicated when the purulent material becomes inspissated or when chondroids have formed. In such cases, the hyovertebrotomy incision combined with ventral drainage through Viborg's triangle is the approach of choice.

Anesthesia and Surgical Preparation

Viborg's triangle approach may be performed using local analgesia, but general anesthesia is preferred. General anesthesia is recommended for the hyovertebrotomy approach. The surgical sites, illustrated in Figure 11-4A, are clipped and prepared in a routine manner.

Additional Instrumentation

This procedure requires retractors.

Surgical Technique

VIBORG'S TRIANGLE

Viborg's triangle is the area defined by the tendon of the sternomandibular muscle, the linguofacial (external maxillary) vein, and the caudal border of the vertical ramus of the mandible. A 4- to 6-cm skin incision is made just dorsal to and parallel with the linguofacial vein from the border of the mandible caudad. The subcutaneous tissue is separated, and the base of the parotid gland is reflected dorsad if necessary (Fig. 11-4B). Care should be taken to avoid trauma to the parotid gland and duct, the lingofacial vein, and the branches of the vagus nerve along the floor of the guttural pouch. This procedure exposes the guttural pouch. Localization of the guttural pouch is facilitated by its distention when it is in a pathologic state. The guttural pouch membrane is grasped with forceps and is incised with scissors (Fig. 11-4C). The wound is left open for drainage, or a drain is inserted. The surgical wound heals by granulation (secondary intention).

HYOVERTEBROTOMY APPROACH

This approach, which gives access to the dorsolateral aspect of the guttural pouch, is more difficult. Care should be taken because of the vessels and nerves within the surgical site. An 8- to 10-cm incision is made parallel and just cranial to the wing of the atlas (Fig. 11-4A). The skin incision exposes the parotid salivary gland and the overlying parotidoauricularis muscle. The ventral part of the parotidoauricularis muscle is incised, and a dissection plane for the parotid gland is established by incising the fascia on its caudal border (Fig. 11-4D). The parotid gland is reflected craniad. The caudal auricular nerve crosses obliquely in the dorsal aspect of the surgical field and is reflected caudad if necessary. Reflection of the parotid gland reveals the occipitohyoideus and digastricus muscles craniodorsally and the rectus capitis cranialis muscle caudodorsally (Fig. 11-4E). The mandibular salivary gland may be identified ventrally. Blunt dissection through areolar tissue exposes the dorsolateral wall of the guttural pouch. The direction of dissection is caudal and then medial to the occipitohyoideus-digastricus muscle group.

The exact site of entry into the guttural pouch may vary, depending on the anatomic placement of the nerve branches overlying the surface. The position of the nerves seems variable and may also be influenced by pathologic distortion of the guttural pouch. Entry is usually made between the glossopharyngeal nerve rostrally and the vagus nerve caudally (Fig. 11-4E). The internal carotid artery runs beneath the vagus nerve in this region and should be avoided. The guttural pouch is incised with scissors.

The hyovertebrotomy incision may be closed primarily if contamination is not excessive and if a drain or seton is not going to be placed in the guttural pouch. The guttural pouch membrane is closed with simple interrupted sutures of synthetic absorbable suture material. One must be

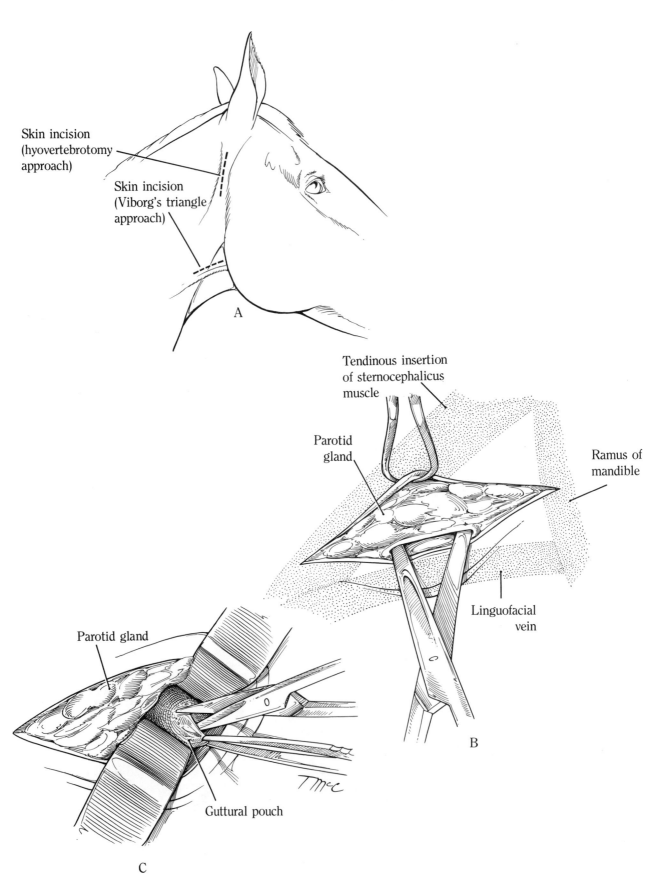

Skin incision
(hyovertebrotomy
approach)

Skin incision
(Viborg's triangle
approach)

A

Tendinous insertion
of sternocephalicus
muscle

Parotid
gland

Ramus of
mandible

Linguofacial
vein

B

Parotid gland

Guttural pouch

C

FIG. 11-4. A *to* E, *Surgical entry and drainage of the guttural pouches.*

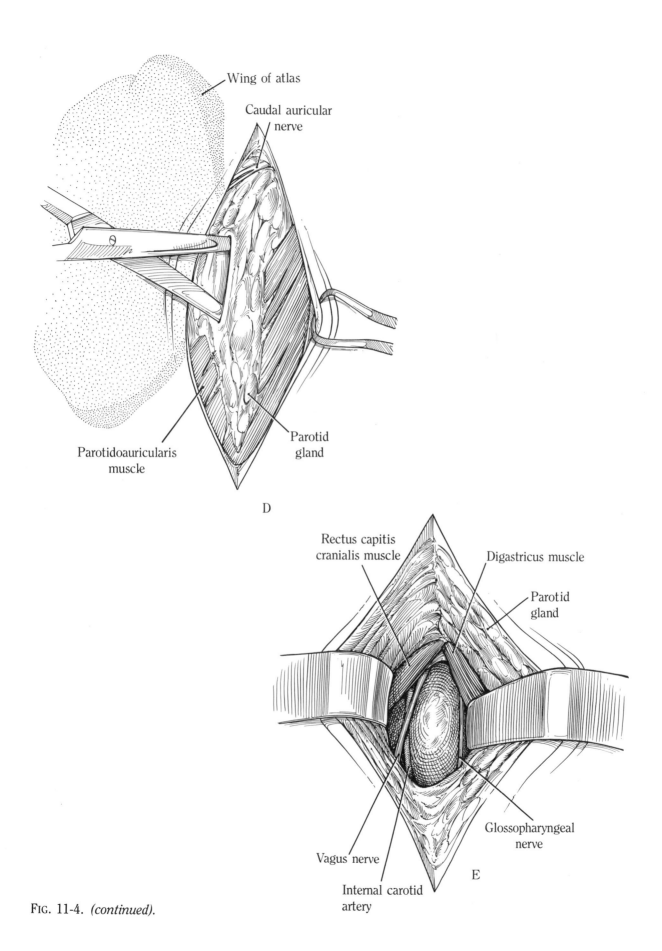

Wing of atlas

Caudal auricular
nerve

Parotidoauricularis
muscle

Parotid
gland

D

Rectus capitis
cranialis muscle

Digastricus muscle

Parotid
gland

Vagus nerve

Internal carotid
artery

Glossopharyngeal
nerve

E

Fig. 11-4. *(continued).*

careful to avoid the adjacent nerves. The fascia associated with the parotid gland is also apposed with synthetic absorbable sutures. The skin is closed with nonabsorbable sutures. In the contaminated wound that typically occurs with guttural pouch empyema, both the hyovertebrotomy incision and Viborg's triangle incision are left open, and a drain or seton is placed in the pouch. The drain typically passes out of the hyovertebrotomy incision dorsally and Viborg's triangle incision ventrally.

An alternative is to close the hyovertebrotomy incision, primarily after preplacing a fenestrated tube drain for postoperative flushing of the pouch. The Viborg's triangle incision is left open to drain.

Postoperative Management

Daily flushing of the pouch may be performed postoperatively. In some instances, removal of additional particulate debris may be necessary, and this can be performed by a combination of flushing and digital manipulation. When pus and debris are evacuated completely from the pouch, flushing is discontinued, any drains are removed, and the incisions are left to heal by secondary intention.

Comments

Some cases of guttural pouch empyema can be treated with the insertion of indwelling catheters to provide local therapy and to assist in drainage. Irritating solutions, however, including certain iodine compounds, should not be infused into the guttural pouches because of severe inflammatory changes. Even povidone-iodine diluted to a 10% solution (1% available iodine) causes considerable reaction.[6] We believe that the mechanical drainage of the contents of the pouch is more important than the antibacterial activity of the solutions placed in them. We advocate early surgical drainage, rather than extended periods of flushing using indwelling catheters.

References

1. Boles, C.: Treatment of upper-airway abnormalities. Vet. Clin. North Am. (Large Anim. Pract.), *1*:143, 1979.

2. Cook, W. R.: Clinical observations on the anatomy and physiology of the equine respiratory tract. Vet. Rec., *79*:440, 1966.

3. Freeman, D. E.: Diagnosis and treatment of diseases of the guttural pouch. Part II. Compend. Contin. Educ. Pract. Vet., *2*:525, 1980.

4. McIlwraith, C. W.: Surgical treatment of epistaxis associated with guttural pouch mycosis. VM/SAC, *73*:67, 1978.

5. McIlwraith, C. W., and Turner, A. S.: Equine Surgery: Advanced Techniques. Philadelphia, Lea & Febiger, 1987.

6. Wilson, J.: Effects of indwelling catheters and povidone-iodine flushes on the guttural pouches of the horse. Equine Vet. J., *17*:242, 1985.

12

EQUINE DENTAL AND GASTRO-INTESTINAL SURGERY

Repulsion of Cheek Teeth

Cheek tooth repulsion is performed when a tooth cannot be extracted through the mouth with forceps. Repulsion of both upper and lower cheek teeth involves trephining a hole to gain access to the base of the tooth and driving the tooth from its socket into the mouth using a dental punch and mallet.

Tooth removal is indicated in cases of infundibular necrosis, fractures, or abscesses of teeth, periodontal disease, chronic ossifying alveolar periostitis, and tumors of the teeth. Infection of the teeth of either the upper or lower arcade may be secondary to fractures of the bones of the skull (mandible and maxilla) that involve the roots of the teeth.

When the maxillary cheek teeth are involved (usually the fourth premolar or the first molar), signs of purulent nasal discharge are present because of secondary maxillary sinusitis. When the disease involves the mandibular teeth, swelling of, or chronic drainage from, the ventral border of the mandible is usually present. The teeth to be removed are ascertained by oral and radiographic examinations. In this chapter, we discuss repulsion of the first molar in the upper arcade and the third premolar in the lower arcade.

Anesthesia and Surgical Preparation

Repulsion of teeth in the horse should be performed with the horse under general anesthesia. The horse is positioned with the affected tooth (teeth) uppermost. A mouth speculum is placed on the horse and is opened sufficiently to allow admission of the surgeon's hand. The hair is clipped over the surgical site, and routine surgical preparation is performed.

Additional Instrumentation

This procedure requires a mouth speculum, molar forceps, mallet or hammer, trephine, molar cutters, straight and curved dental punches, umbilical tape, gauze roll, and a mild antiseptic solution.

Surgical Technique

For the upper teeth, a curved incision should be made through the skin, with the apex pointing dorsad. The exact location of the incision depends on which tooth is to be repelled. The skin flap is reflected back, and the periosteum is incised and reflected from the bone, to expose sufficient area to accept the trephine. A three-quarter-inch trephine should be used for the upper teeth. For the repulsion of lower teeth, a straight incision is made directly over the proposed site of trephination, and the edges of the skin are undermined to allow the trephine to be positioned on the lower border of the mandible. The periosteum is incised and reflected from the mandible. A half-inch trephine should be used for the lower teeth.

The trephine hole is begun by extending the center bit of the trephine 3 mm beyond the end of the trephine and fixing it to the bone. The trephine is turned back and forth in a rotary motion until it has cut a distinct groove in the bone. The center bit on the trephine is retracted, and cutting is continued until a disc of bone is detached (Fig. 12-1A).

LOCATING THE TREPHINE OPENING FOR UPPER CHEEK TEETH

A line from the medial canthus of the eye to the infraorbital canal that continues forward past the roots of the first cheek tooth is the line of maximum height at which any trephining may be done for superior cheek teeth. This line marks the course of the osseous nasolacrimal canal. The trephine openings for all superior cheek teeth should be placed just below this line. In the case of old horses in which the teeth have grown out, it is permissible to drop down nearer to the facial crest. For the first and second upper cheek teeth, which are straight, a line is drawn through the center of each tooth, and a trephine opening is made along each line. For the third, fourth, and fifth upper cheek teeth, which have a caudal curvature, the trephination is made below the nasolacrimal canal, along a line directed over the posterior margin of the table surface of each tooth.

For repulsion of the sixth cheek tooth, a trephine hole must be made through the frontal sinus 4 cm lateral to the midline on a transverse line between the cranial margins of the orbits. It is necessary to go through the frontal sinus and the frontomaxillary opening into the maxillary sinus. The dental punch is passed lateral to the infraorbital canal to the root of the tooth. It is necessary to use a curved punch because the tooth has a tendency to lie under the infraorbital canal. The punch is seated on the base of the tooth, and the tooth is repelled. If the vein that lies above the infraorbital canal is severed, the area will have to be packed. This operation is difficult in young horses because of the marked caudal curvature of the tooth. Fortunately, this tooth does not require removal as frequently as other upper cheek teeth. Figure 12-1A and B shows trephination and repulsion of the fourth upper cheek tooth (first molar).

LOCATING THE TREPHINE OPENING FOR LOWER CHEEK TEETH

The trephine holes for repulsion of the lower cheek teeth are made on the ventrolateral border of the mandible. The inner and outer alveolar plates rest directly on the tooth, so it is necessary to align the punch with the long axis of the tooth, to avoid punching toward the medial alveolar plate and fracturing it. For repelling the first cheek tooth, the trephine is centered

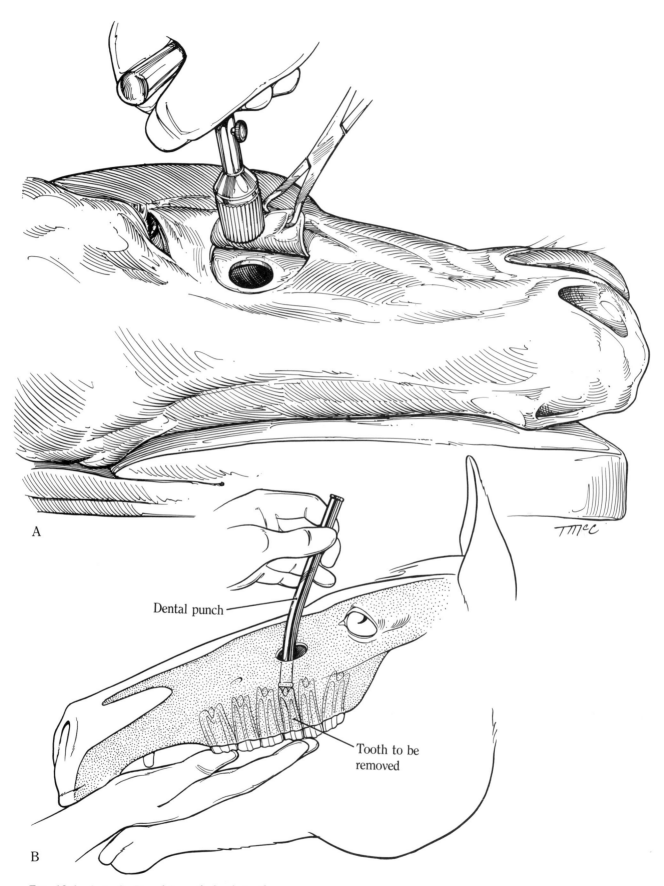

Dental punch

Tooth to be
removed

A

B

Fig. 12-1. A *to* C, *Repulsion of cheek teeth.*

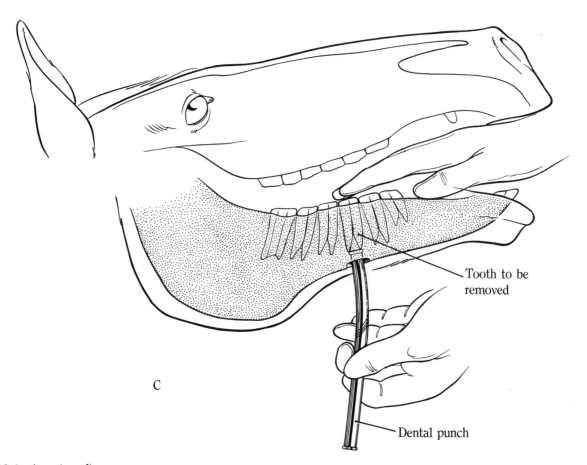

Tooth to be removed

Dental punch

Fig. 12-1. *(continued)*.

directly below the table surface; for the second to fifth cheek teeth, the opening is made below the caudal borders of the teeth because of their caudal curvature (Fig. 12-1C); for horses older than 12 years, the opening can be made directly under the center of the table surface. Exposure of the trephine site for the fourth and fifth lower cheek teeth is complicated by the parotid duct and linguofacial artery and vein, which should be identified and retracted caudad. When a dental fistula is present on the lower border of the mandible, the trephine is positioned directly over the center of it because the fistula usually occurs opposite the affected alveolus.

The location of the sixth lower cheek tooth necessitates trephination over the lateral surface of the mandible. A line is drawn from the center of the table surface of the tooth to the point of greatest curvature of the ramus of the mandible. An incision is made on this line through the skin and masseter muscle over a bulging prominence where the two plates of bone that form the mandible are separated to accommodate the tooth. The muscle is separated from the bone by spreading it with wound retractors. The trephine opening is made and is elongated dorsad with a chisel to give better direction for the punch and to lessen the chances of fracturing the medial bony plate of the mandible. The skin-and-muscle incision is terminated at least 4 cm from the border of the mandible, to avoid severing the branches of the facial nerve that spread out over the surface of the masseter muscle from above, ventrad, and rostrad. Further details of this technique are available in our other textbook.[1]

The surgeon's hand is introduced into the patient's mouth, the diseased tooth is located, and the tooth's path in the sinus or jaw is determined. The punch is directed onto the root of the tooth, and an assistant begins to tap the punch with a mallet. The first few blows with the mallet should be sufficient to seat the punch into the root of the tooth. The trephine hole may have to be enlarged to allow the punch access to the diseased teeth.

Once the punch is seated, the assistant delivers steady blows to the punch. The mallet blows produce a characteristic ringing sound when the punch is seated properly, and the surgeon feels the vibrations of these blows transmitted through the tooth to his hand. If the punch slips off the tooth into alveolar tissue, it will need to be repositioned. After some time, the surgeon will feel the gradual loosening of the tooth with the hand that is in the patient's mouth. Subsequent blows with the mallet should be less forceful as the tooth is driven from the alveolus.

Following tooth repulsion, any fragments should be removed from the alveolus with forceps. The alveolus may require curettage if diseased bone surrounds the tooth. To prevent the socket from becoming packed with food, it should be filled with a suitable material until the socket is almost filled with granulation tissue. Dental wax, dental acrylic, gutta-percha, or gauze rolls may be used, depending on individual preference. If gauze rolls are used, a roll that will fit snugly into the hole is made and is tied around the center with umbilical tape, leaving two long ends. The ends are passed through the socket and trephine hole, the gauze is wedged firmly into the cavity, and the umbilical tape is brought to the exterior. The umbilical tape is then secured to the skin by tying it to another gauze roll. The ends should be kept long, so the gauze roll in the alveolus can be replaced without having to thread the new piece of umbilical tape back through the trephine hole.

Postoperative Management

The horse should be placed on antibiotics preoperatively and for approximately 1 week following surgery. During the first few days, if a gauze pack is used, the pack is changed daily, and the sinus is flushed with a mild antiseptic solution if suppuration is present. The material used to pack the socket remains until the cavity is almost filled with granulation tissue. After a week, the material used to pack the socket can be changed every 2 or 3 days (if gauze is used).

Possible untoward sequelae of this procedure include punching out the wrong tooth, puncturing the hard palate by incorrect positioning of the punch over the tooth, rupturing the palatine artery, and breaking the alveolar plates of an adjacent tooth with the punch, which may lead to alveolar periostitis.

Reference

1. McIlwraith, C. W., and Turner, A. S.: Equine Surgery: Advanced Techniques. Philadelphia, Lea & Febiger, 1987.

Ventral Midline Laparotomy and Abdominal Exploration

The ventral midline approach provides the greatest single incision exposure of the peritoneal cavity of the horse; it is also the quickest approach. It is particularly indicated for surgical management of acute equine abdominal disorders, although some surgeons use the paramedian technique.[4] This approach may also be used for bilateral ovariectomy or for removal of an ovarian tumor. Fears regarding the risk of dehiscence are not justified, and it is a practical approach that avoids both muscles and blood vessels. Although the scope of this text does not extend to detailed surgical management of patients with acute abdominal disorders, a basic discussion of exploratory laparotomy in the horse is appropriate.

Anesthesia and Surgical Preparation

This surgical procedure is performed with the patient in dorsal recumbency under general anesthesia. The ventral abdomen is clipped from the area of the pubis to the area of the xiphoid process extending at least 30 cm from the midline (this may be performed prior to the induction of anesthesia). The area of incision is shaved, and routine aseptic preparation is performed. Draping includes the use of hock drapes over the limbs, to prevent contamination if the laparotomy sheet is displaced. An impervious rubber sheet is also used, so the bowel can be placed over it, to minimize soaking of the cloth drapes underneath.

Additional Instrumentation

This procedure requires long sterile gloves for abdominal exploration and manipulation and special instruments for intestinal surgery.

Surgical Technique

The incision begins over the umbilicus and extends craniad; its length depends on the procedure, but it is generally 30 to 40 cm long (Fig. 12-2A). Such an incision is used in patients with acute abdominal disorders, but cystotomies and ovariectomies require a more caudal incision. The skin incision extends through a layer of subcutaneous tissue, which is thin in most animals. When hemorrhage has been controlled, the linea alba is incised (it is preferable to maintain the incision within the linea alba) (Fig. 12-2B). Slight divergence from the midline will result in entry into the rectus abdominis muscle, particularly in the cranial portion of the incision, but this event is generally of no consequence. Incision of the linea alba reveals the retroperitoneal adipose tissue deeply (Fig. 12-2B). The retroperitoneal adipose tissue is cleared with a sponge to reveal the peritoneum, with the round ligament of the liver demarcating the midline (Fig. 12-2C).

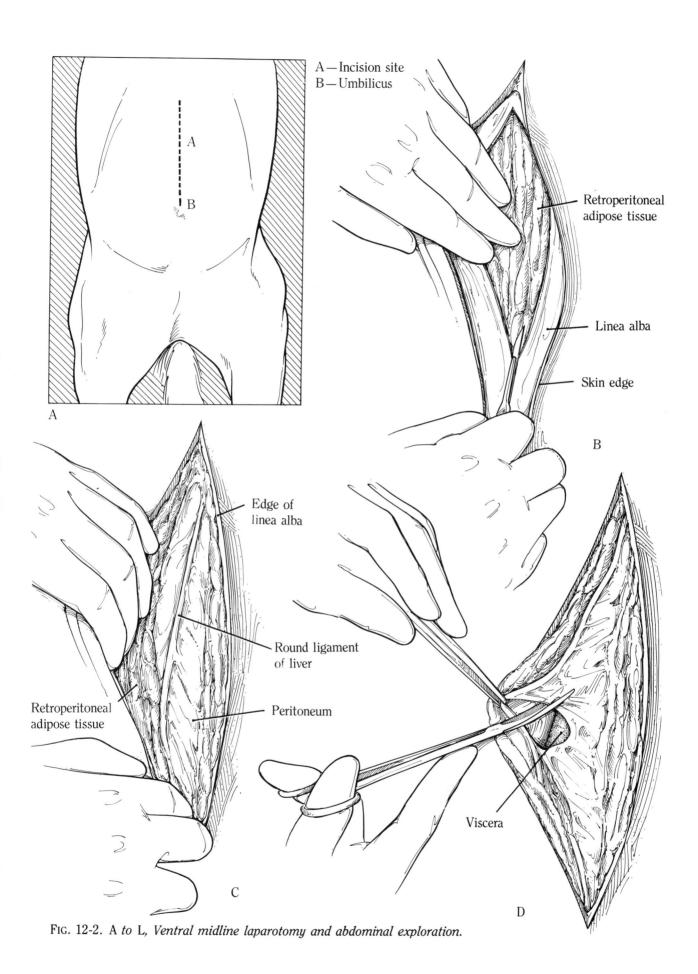

A—Incision site
B—Umbilicus

Retroperitoneal
adipose tissue

Linea alba

Skin edge

Edge of
linea alba

Round ligament
of liver

Retroperitoneal
adipose tissue

Peritoneum

Viscera

FIG. 12-2. A *to* L, *Ventral midline laparotomy and abdominal exploration.*

The peritoneum is picked up and is incised with Metzenbaum scissors, and the incision may either be extended with the scissors (Fig. 12-2D) or torn by hand. Retractors are not used routinely in exploratory laparotomy. Any exteriorized bowel is kept moist while systematic exploration of the abdomen is performed.

Upon opening the abdomen, the problem may be immediately obvious or may be determined quickly on cursory examination. In many instances, however, a systematic examination should be performed prior to closure of the abdomen. The systematic identification of normal, undisplaced viscera only is presented here.

If the cecum is not displaced (it lies ventrally, on the right side of the midline, with the apex directed craniad), it should be identified quickly after entering the peritoneal cavity (Fig. 12-2E). The cecum is a reference point for systematic exploration of both the small and large intestine. The lateral band of the cecum is continuous with the cecocolic fold, which leads into the right ventral portion of the large colon. From this point, the large colon can be explored. The right ventral colon runs craniad and leads into the left ventral colon at the sternal flexure. The left ventral and left dorsal portions of the colon are the mobile parts and bend sharply at the pelvic flexure, which is located near the pelvic inlet (Fig. 12-2F). The left dorsal colon passes forward from the pelvic flexure to the diaphragmatic flexure and becomes the right dorsal colon. This runs caudad in a dorsal position and, on reaching the medial surface of the base of the cecum, turns to the left, becomes narrower, and leads into the transverse colon. It joins the small colon ventral to the left kidney.

The small colon is characterized by two longitudinal bands, one within the mesentery and the other on the opposite (antimesenteric) side. It has two rows of sacculations and is attached to the sublumbar region by the colic mesentery (Fig. 12-2G). The proximal small colon is also attached to the distal duodenum by the narrow duodenocolic fold of peritoneum. This fold is an identification point for the junction of the terminal duodenum and the proximal jejunum.

The small intestine is examined routinely by first locating the ileum. To do this, one retracts the cecum caudad to expose the dorsal band. This thin, avascular band runs into the ileocecal fold, which continues into the antimesenteric border of the ileum (Fig. 12-2H). Using these landmarks, the surgeon can palpate the ileocecal junction deep in the abdomen; the junction cannot be exteriorized. The thin membranous fold called the antimesenteric border is 180° opposite the ileal mesentery and allows one positively to identify the ileum. Once the ileum is located, the small intestine may be examined systematically. Moving proximad, the entire length of the jejunum is explored until the duodenocolic fold, which is the junction between jejunum and duodenum, is reached. The jejunum has a mobile mesentery and is characterized by a lack of bands or sacculations (Fig. 12-2I). The root of the mesentery may be palpated at this stage. The duodenum also may be explored manually, not visually, because the duodenum's lack of mobility makes visualization difficult. The duodenum leads to the pylorus.

At this stage, the epiploic foramen should be palpated. It is most easily examined by standing on the patient's left side and using the left hand. If one holds the duodenum loosely between fingers and thumb with the dorsal surface of the fingers against the caudate lobe of the liver and moves laterad,

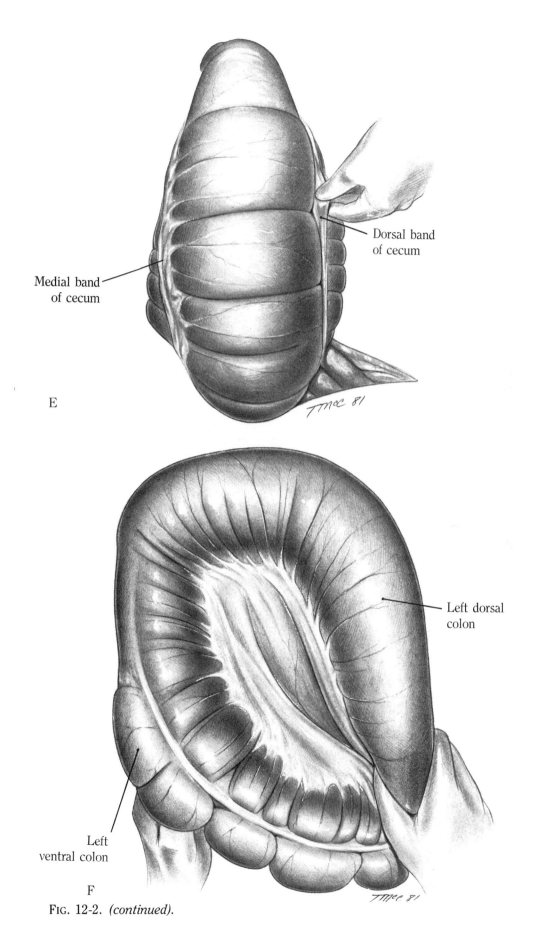

Medial band
of cecum

Dorsal band
of cecum

E

Left dorsal
colon

Left
ventral colon

F

FIG. 12-2. *(continued).*

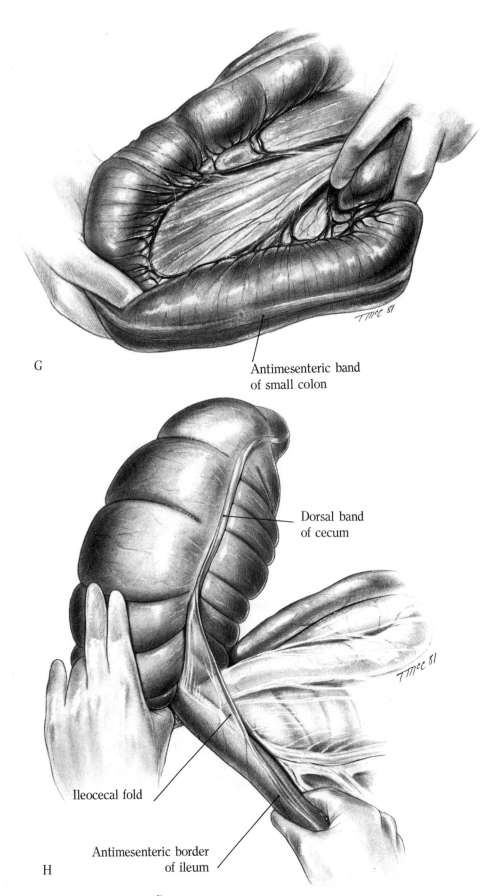

G

Antimesenteric band
of small colon

Dorsal band
of cecum

Ileocecal fold

Antimesenteric border
of ileum

H

FIG. 12-2. *(continued)*.

the fingertips will locate the small opening of the epiploic foramen. This opening is larger in older horses.

The stomach and the spleen, which is in the left lateral quadrant, should be palpated. In a stallion, the internal inguinal rings that are ventrolateral to the femoral canals are palpated; in the mare, the uterus and ovaries are examined.

Further descriptions of how to deal with the various displacements and abnormalities of the equine gastrointestinal tract are presented in our other textbook.[2]

The ventral midline incision is closed in three or four layers. A separate closure of the peritoneum is not necessary, but it is preferred by some surgeons to help keep the bowel in a position to minimize accidental perforations during closure.[3] The peritoneum is thin and tears easily when sutured. Longitudinal splitting of the round ligament of the liver will aid in its closure; when the abdomen is opened, care should be taken not to tear the peritoneum, and retroperitoneal fat should be carefully separated to leave the round ligament of the liver intact. If this layer is closed, a simple continuous suture of no. 1 chromic catgut or no. 2 polyglactin 910 (Vicryl) with a round bodied needle is used.

The linea alba is closed with a simple interrupted or a simple continuous pattern. Simple interrupted sutures should be placed 1 cm apart (Fig. 12-2J). If a simple continuous pattern is used, the suture should commence and should be tied beyond the extremities of the incision in the linea alba.[3] Five or six throws should be used in each knot. If the incision is less than 20 cm (8 in. approx), one length of doubled commercially available suture material is usually sufficient. If the incision is longer, two separate strands should be started beyond the commissure of the linea alba incision and directed to the center of the incision. Bites in the linea alba should be placed 0.75 to 1.00 cm apart (Fig. 12-2K).

The choice of suture material depends on personal preference, but we have been most satisfied with synthetic absorbable materials such as polyglycolic acid (Dexon) or polyglactin 910. The multifilament, nonabsorbable sutures have superior strength, but suture sinuses may be formed, depending on technique and degree of contamination. The subcutaneous tissue is closed with a simple continuous layer of 0 or 2-0 synthetic absorbable material (Fig. 12-2L). The main purpose of this layer is to cover the ends of the suture material, especially when an interrupted pattern is used. A continuous closure has fewer knots to cover with the subcutaneous layer and less chance that the ends of the sutures will protrude into the skin incision. Generally, the skin is closed with a Ford interlocking continuous suture pattern using polymerized caprolactam (Vetafil) (Fig. 12-2L). In most abdominal surgical procedures, speed is important; this suture pattern offers satisfactory closure as well as speed. An even faster and more convenient alternative is the use of skin staples (see Chap. 4).

Peritoneal drainage is not used routinely following abdominal surgery. The routine use of Penrose drains, in particular, is to be discouraged because of the risk of retrograde infection. If contamination is suspected or if bowel anastomosis has been performed, the abdomen should be irrigated and a heparinized plastic drain (Redi-Vacette Perforated Tubing) should be inserted, mainly to drain the irrigation fluid. Generally, the drain is removed within 24 hours.

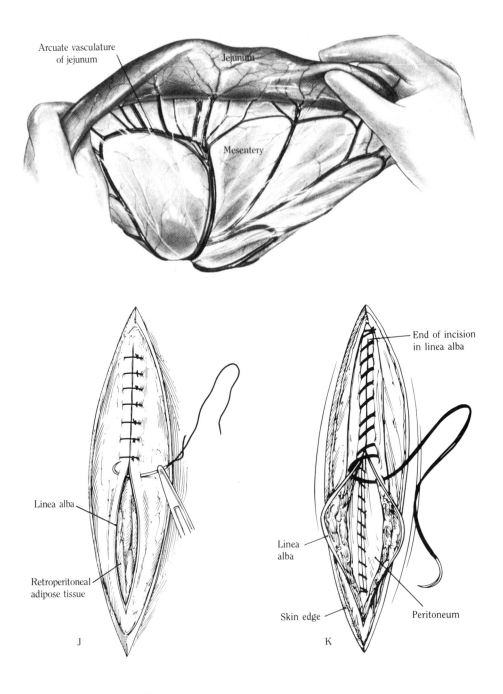

Arcuate vasculature
of jejunum

Jejunum

Mesentery

Linea alba

Retroperitoneal
adipose tissue

J

End of incision
in linea alba

Linea
alba

Skin edge

Peritoneum

K

Fig. 12-2. *(continued).*

Postoperative Management

Phenylbutazone (2 g) is administered at the end of surgery to decrease the immediate incisional (parietal) pain. Antibiotics are used, the type and dosage depending on the particular surgical procedure. Additional drugs and supportive therapy may be necessary in patients with acute abdominal disorders. If a drain has been inserted, its patency must be checked regularly by applying negative suction to its end using a syringe. Bandaging is not used routinely, but a stent bandage may be indicated. Skin sutures or staples are removed in 12 to 14 days.

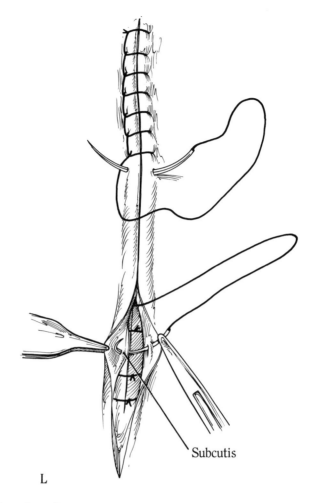

Subcutis

L

FIG. 12-2. *(continued).*

References

1. McIlwraith, C. W.: Complications of laparotomy incisions in the horse. *In* Proceedings of the 24th Annual Convention of the American Association of Equine Practitioners in 1978:1979, p. 209.

2. McIlwraith, C. W., and Turner, A. S.: Equine Surgery: Advanced Techniques. Philadelphia, Lea & Febiger, 1987.

3. Turner, A. S., et al.: Experience with continuous absorbable suture pattern in the closure of ventral midline abdominal incisions in horses. Equine Vet. J. *20*, 1988.

4. Vaughan, J. T.: Surgical management of abdominal crisis in the horse. J. Am. Vet. Med. Assoc., *161*:1199, 1972.

Standing Flank Laparotomy

The flank approach still is useful for some procedures. Although it is not recommended for patients with acute abdominal pain because it provides only limited exposure, it has been used in some instances. For example, the flank approach may be used for a standing exploratory laparotomy in a debilitated animal suspected of having neoplasia. In this instance, identification of a problem is all that is required, and complicated surgical manipulation is not performed. It is also a convenient approach for intestinal biopsies. For correction of other intestinal problems, except typhlectomy, we favor the ventral midline approach. The standing flank approach can be used successfully for the correction of uterine torsion,[5] but it is not recommended for mares with a poor disposition because torsion on the ovarian pedicle is painful and may cause the horse to go down. Although the flank approach can also be used for removal of enteroliths, ovariectomy,[1] and cryptorchidectomy,[3,7] we generally do not favor it for these procedures.

The procedure is not recommended for patients with large ovarian tumors or if their size cannot be determined on rectal examination.[2] For large ovarian tumors, a ventral midline approach is preferable.[6] The method is described in our other textbook.[4] A right flank laparotomy has been performed to diagnose choleliths in horses,[8] and in smaller horses, choledolithotripsy is possible.[9]

Anesthesia and Surgical Preparation

Tranquilization of the patient is optional. The paralumbar fossa area is clipped, and the immediate area of the skin incision is shaved. The surgical area is prepared for aseptic surgery in a routine manner. Local analgesia is instituted by either a line block or an inverted L block; refer to Chapter 2 for these techniques. The surgical area is then given a final preparation before surgery. With the standing procedure, aseptic preparation of a wide area and limited draping are preferred.

Additional Instrumentation

This procedure requires long sterile gloves for abdominal palpation and manipulation and special instruments for intestinal surgery.

Surgical Technique

A 20-cm skin incision is made midway between the tuber coxae and the last rib (Fig. 12-3A). The dorsal limit of the incision is below the longissimus dorsi muscle and level with the tuber coxae. The incision is continued through the subcutaneous tissue, and any hemorrhage is controlled.

At this stage, there are two techniques for dividing the muscle layers. In the "grid" technique, all three layers may be divided along the direction of the muscle fibers. With the exception of the external abdominal oblique muscle, the fascial components of the flank muscles are weak, and splitting the muscles is preferred to transecting them. The grid technique, however, decreases the exposure. One of us (C.W.M.) routinely uses a modified grid technique with a vertical incision through the fascia and muscle of the external abdominal oblique (the two alternate incisions in the external abdominal oblique muscle are illustrated in Figure 12-3B). The grid incision between the muscle fibers in a caudoventral direction is started with scissors and is completed with fingers (Fig. 12-3C). In the modified grid approach, the fascia and muscle are incised with a scalpel (Fig. 12-3D).

The remainder of the procedure is illustrated in a situation in which the external abdominal oblique muscle has been separated using the grid approach. In Figure 12-3E, the dotted line shows the line of cleavage in the internal abdominal oblique muscle where the fibers run cranioventrad. This layer is split to reveal the transverse abdominal muscle deeply (Fig. 12-3F). A vertical split is made in the layer (line of cleavage is indicated in Figure 12-3F). For this layer, the muscle should be tented with thumb forceps and knicked with scissors. The opening is enlarged to reveal retroperitoneal adipose tissue (Fig. 12-3G), and the peritoneum is opened to expose the viscera (Fig. 12-3H).

The surgeon should then don a sterile rubber sleeve to explore the peritoneal cavity. It is possible to exteriorize the small intestine, small colon, and the pelvic flexure of the large colon. In addition, it is feasible to palpate the spleen, kidney(s), liver, stomach, cecum, large colon, cranial mesenteric artery, rectum, pelvic inlet, bladder, aorta, and reproductive tract.[10] The peritoneal surface is also examined.

The flank incision is closed in five layers. The peritoneum and transverse abdominal muscle are closed with simple interrupted sutures of 0 synthetic absorbable material. The internal abdominal oblique muscle is apposed with four or five simple interrupted sutures of 0 synthetic nonabsorbable material (Fig. 12-3I). A negative suction drain may be placed between the internal and external abdominal oblique muscles, and the last layer is closed with no. 1 or no. 2 synthetic absorbable material in a simple interrupted pattern. Care is taken to ensure firm apposition of the fascia in the external abdominal oblique muscle. The suction drain, rather than a Penrose drain, is used to prevent seroma formation.

The subcutis is closed with a simple continuous pattern using synthetic absorbable sutures. The skin is closed with nonabsorbable sutures in a simple interrupted or Ford interlocking pattern (Fig. 12-3J).

Postoperative Management

Whether or not antibiotics are used and which type of antibiotics are used depend on the individual case. The negative suction syringe is taped over the patient's back and is emptied regularly. The drain is removed when the volume of aspirated contents decreases (2 to 3 days). The skin sutures are removed in 12 to 14 days.

References

1. Blue, M. G.: Enteroliths in horses: a retrospective study of 30 cases. Equine Vet. J., *11*: 76, 1979.

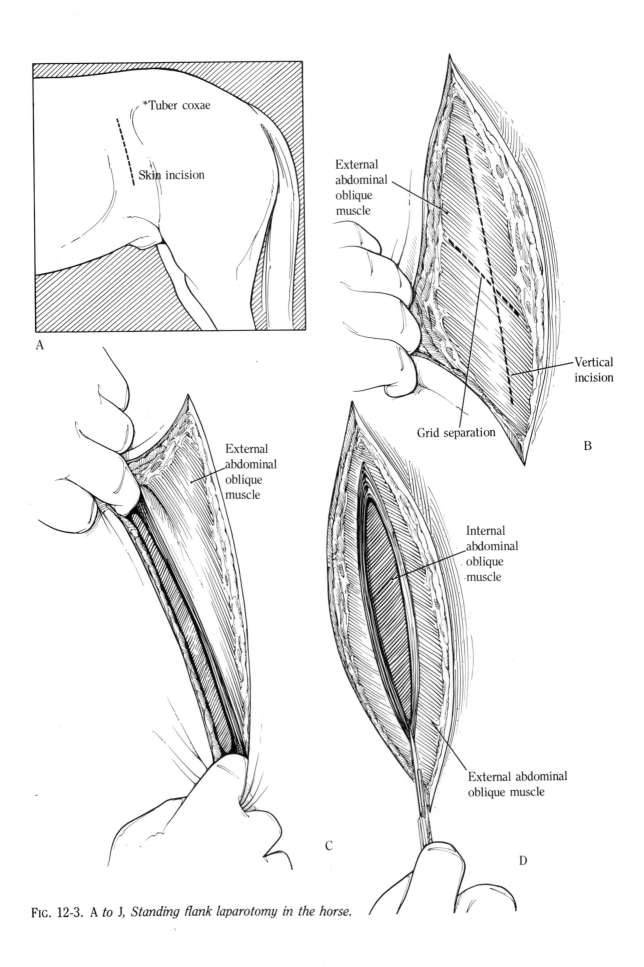

FIG. 12-3. A *to* J, *Standing flank laparotomy in the horse.*

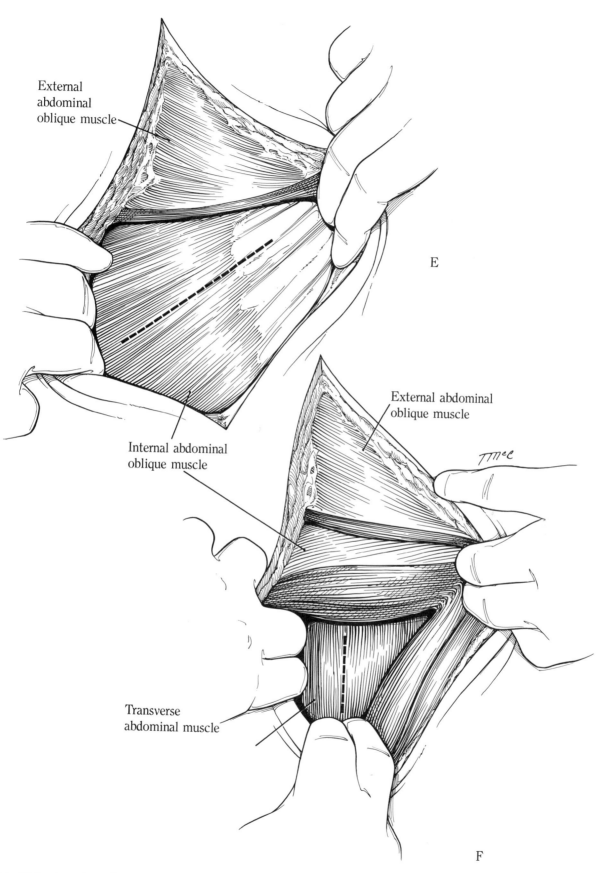

External
abdominal
oblique muscle

E

Internal abdominal
oblique muscle

External abdominal
oblique muscle

Transverse
abdominal muscle

F

Fig. 12-3. *(continued).*

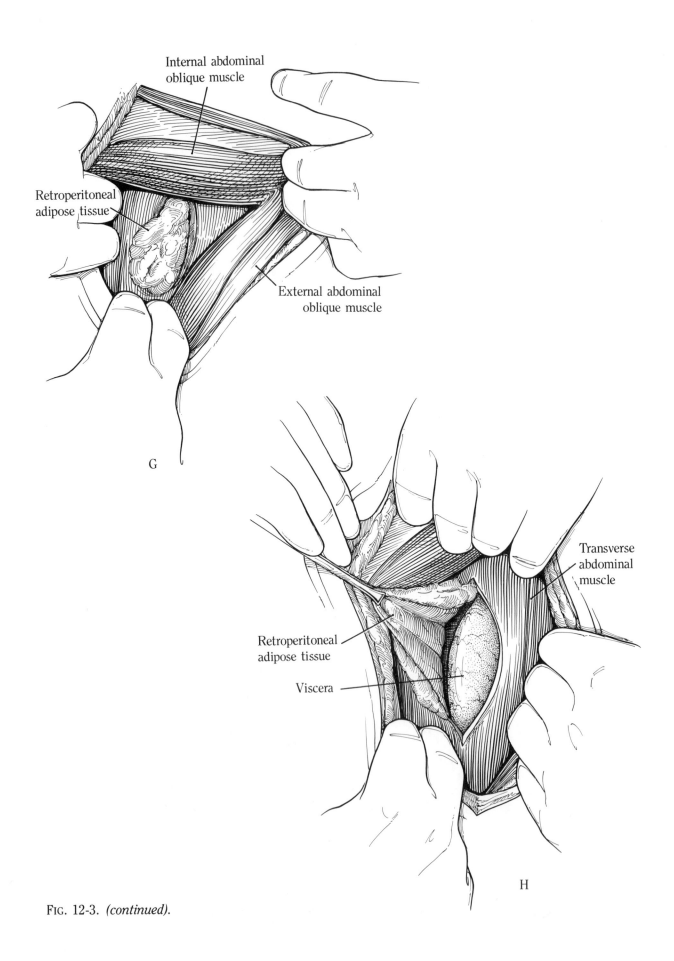

Internal abdominal
oblique muscle

Retroperitoneal
adipose tissue

External abdominal
oblique muscle

G

Transverse
abdominal
muscle

Retroperitoneal
adipose tissue

Viscera

H

Fig. 12-3. *(continued).*

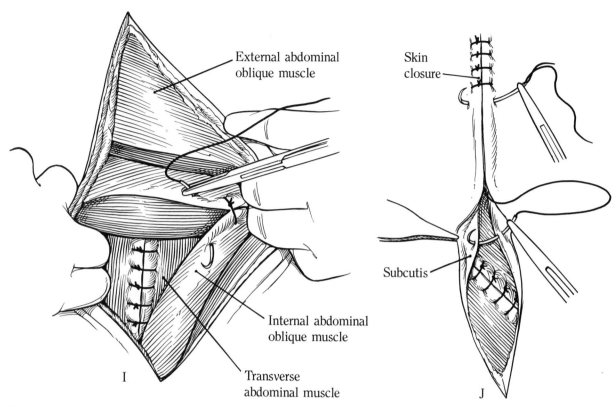

External abdominal
oblique muscle

Skin
closure

Internal abdominal
oblique muscle

Subcutis

Transverse
abdominal muscle

I

J

Fig. 12-3. *(continued).*

2. Bosu, W. T. K., et al.: Ovarian disorders: clinical and morphological observations in 30 mares. Can. Vet. J., *23*:6, 1982.

3. Burger, C. H.: The standing position for abdominal cryptorchidectomy in the horse. J. Am. Vet. Med. Assoc., *135*:102, 1959.

4. McIlwraith, C. W., and Turner, A. S.: Equine Surgery: Advanced Techniques. Philadelphia, Lea & Febiger, 1987.

5. Pascoe, J. R., Meagher, D. M., and Wheat, J. D.: Surgical management of uterine torsion in the mare: a review of 26 cases. J. Am. Vet. Med. Assoc., *179*:351, 1981.

6. Pugh, D. G., and Bowen, J. M.: Equine ovarian tumors. Symp. Contin. Educ., *7*:710, 1985.

7. Scott, E. A., and Kunze, D. J.: Ovariectomy in the mare: presurgical, surgical and postsurgical complications. J. Equine Med. Surg., *1*:5, 1977.

8. Traub, J. L., et al.: Surgical removal of choleliths in a horse. J. Am. Vet. Med. Assoc., *182*:714, 1983.

9. Traub, J. L.: Personal communication, 1987.

10. Vaughan, J. T.: Surgical management of abdominal crisis in the horse. J. Am. Vet. Med. Assoc., *161*:1199, 1972.

Umbilical Herniorrhaphy
in the Foal

Umbilical hernias may be congenital or acquired and are seen in foals, calves, and pigs. Many small umbilical hernias may appear to resolve spontaneously, but large or strangulated umbilical hernias require surgical correction. Various methods are described in the literature for treatment of umbilical hernia: counterirritation, clamping, transfixation sutures, and even safety pins and commercially available rubber bands. The most popular of these techniques is the wooden or metal clamp technique (the clamps are illustrated in the discussion of instruments used in large animal practice in Chapter 3). This method may result in infection, loss of clamps, or premature necrosis of the hernial sac. The last complication can lead to an open wound and, possibly, evisceration or formation of an enterocutaneous fistula. These methods are obviously unsuitable for the occasional strangulated hernia.

Ideally, surgery should be performed after one is sure that apparent external resolution is not going to occur and before the animal is too big (a typical hernia is represented in Figure 12-4A). Generally, the hernial sac is lined with peritoneum and contains some bowel (usually jejunum or ileum) or omentum. The technique we describe is applicable to calves and pigs, as well as foals. Naturally, in food animal species, one should consider the economic factor before attempting surgery. Another factor that the surgeon should always consider is possible heritability of hernias.

If the patient has large defects in the body wall or incisional hernias from previous abdominal surgery, it may be a candidate for the insertion of a prosthetic mesh. The application of this technique is described in our other textbook.[1]

Anesthesia and Surgical Preparation

Inhalation anesthesia is preferable. Anesthesia in small foals can generally be induced with halothane administered by mask. Anesthesia in yearlings is induced intravenously and is maintained with an inhalation anesthetic. The animal is placed in dorsal recumbency and is prepared for aseptic surgery in a routine manner.

Surgical Technique

An elliptical skin incision, pointed at both ends, is made around the hernial sac (Fig. 12-4B). This shape avoids puckering or "dog ears" at the end of the wound at the time of skin closure. The shape of the incision should be such that sufficient skin remains at the wound edges to allow apposition without undue tension. Using either sharp dissection or blunt-tipped scissors, the surgeon dissects the subcutaneous tissue down to the hernial sac and ring (Fig. 12-4C). The portion of skin over the hernial sac is discarded, and bleeding points are ligated or cauterized as they are encountered. Further sharp dissection around the base of the hernial sac delineates the hernial ring; this dissection should extend around the ring and outward for about 1 cm (Fig. 12-4D). When the bowel has been incarcerated in the hernial sac, it is generally necessary to enter the sac carefully to replace the offending piece of bowel into the abdominal cavity. When opening the hernial sac, one must be careful not to cut through any adherent bowel because gross contamination of the surgical site will occur. If the surgeon cannot cut into the hernial sac without incising the bowel, the abdomen should be opened carefully along the linea alba, cranial to the hernial ring. This will allow the surgeon to identify the incarcerated portion of the bowel and to decrease the chance of inadvertent incision of the bowel.[1]

When the hernial sac and ring have been freed of fascia, the sac is inverted into the abdomen, and the hernial ring is closed with the modified horizontal mattress pattern, or Mayo overlap technique, also called "vest-over-pants." This suture pattern is essentially U-shaped. The index finger and middle finger of the left hand are inserted into the hernial ring; this presses the hernial sac against the abdominal wall. Using the index finger as a guide, the needle and suture are introduced about 1.5 to 2 cm from the edge of the ring (Fig. 12-4E). The exit point of the needle is about the middle of the thickness of the hernial ring. For the next portion of the suture, the index finger and middle finger of the left hand are transferred to the other side of the hernial ring. The needle is introduced into the hernial ring about 1 cm from the edge of the ring and directly parallel to the edges of the ring to exit about 1 cm further along the edge of the hernial ring. The final leg of the suture is parallel to the first and enters the hernial ring in the middle of its thickness and exits about 1.5 to 2 cm from the edge of the ring (Fig. 12-4F). Modified horizontal mattress sutures are placed in the hernial ring as they are required (generally 2 to 4 sutures). The ends of each suture should be secured with hemostats (Fig. 12-4G), and the sac should once again be inverted into the abdomen. Steady traction on all the ends of the sutures closes the hernial ring (Fig. 12-4H). The result is an overlap of the two edges of the hernial ring (Fig. 12-4I). While maintaining this traction, the surgeon ties the sutures individually; then the overlapping edge of the hernial ring is sutured to the body wall using a simple interrupted pattern (Fig. 12-4J).

The suture material used for herniorrhaphy is a matter of choice. We prefer a synthetic absorbable suture, such as polyglycolic acid or polyglactin 910 (Dexon or Vicryl). No. 2 polyglycolic acid or polyglactin 910 is generally satisfactory for most sizes of foals. Prior to the introduction of these types of suture materials, we used no. 2 or no. 3 medium chromic catgut (doubled) in many umbilical hernias with satisfactory results. If the hernia is being operated on for the second or third time, we recommend the use of braided, synthetic nonabsorbable sutures placed under aseptic conditions.

After suturing the flap, closure consists of a simple continuous subcutaneous suture using 0 or 2-0 synthetic absorbable material (Fig. 12-4K). Skin closure is performed with a nonabsorbable material of the surgeon's choice (Fig. 12-4L).

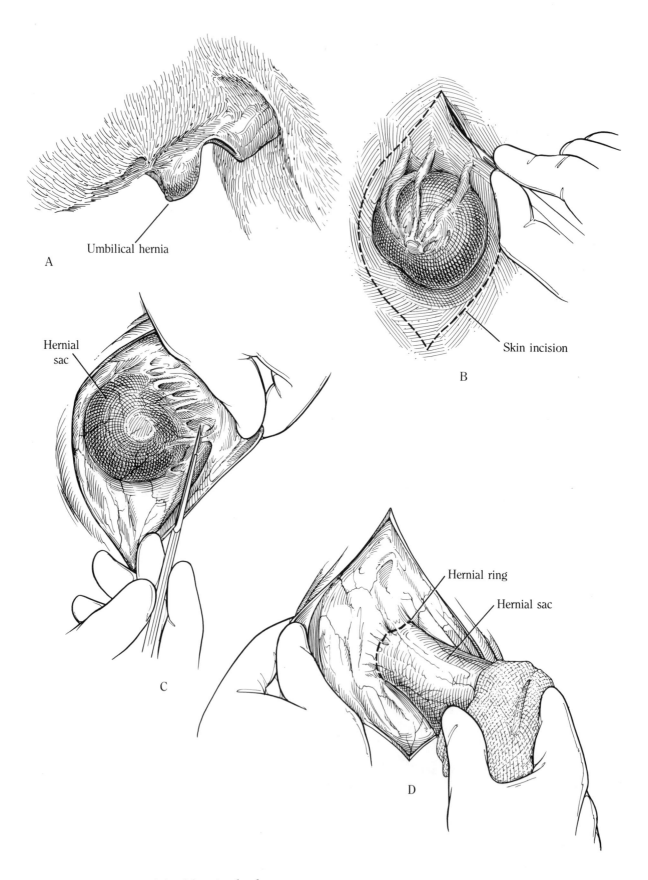

Umbilical hernia

A

Skin incision

B

Hernial sac

C

Hernial ring

Hernial sac

D

FIG. 12-4. A *to* L, *Umbilical herniorrhaphy.*

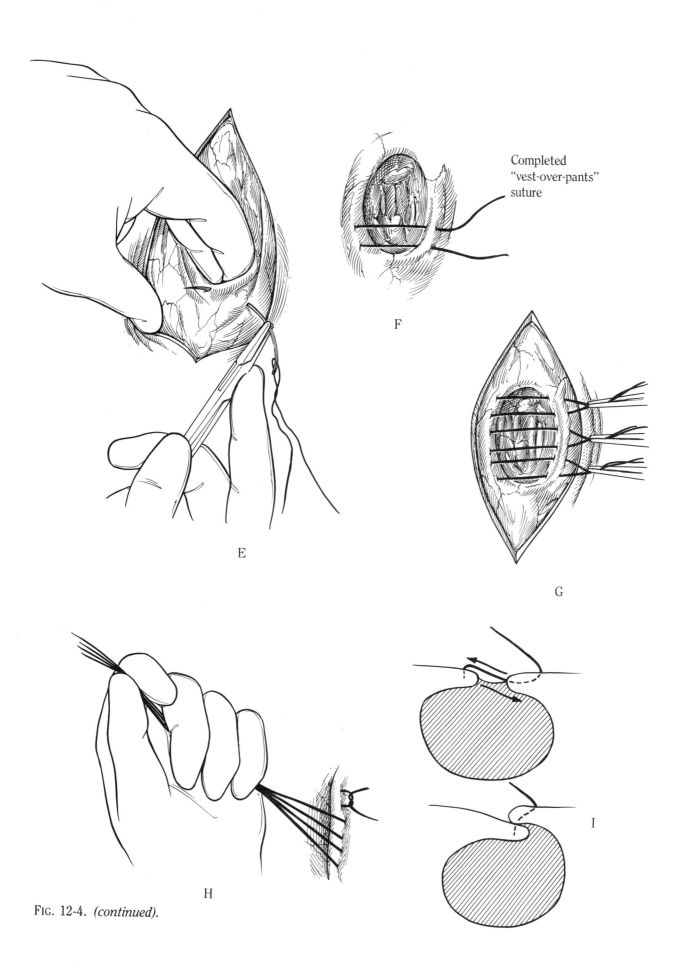

Completed
"vest-over-pants"
suture

E

F

G

H

I

Fig. 12-4. *(continued)*.

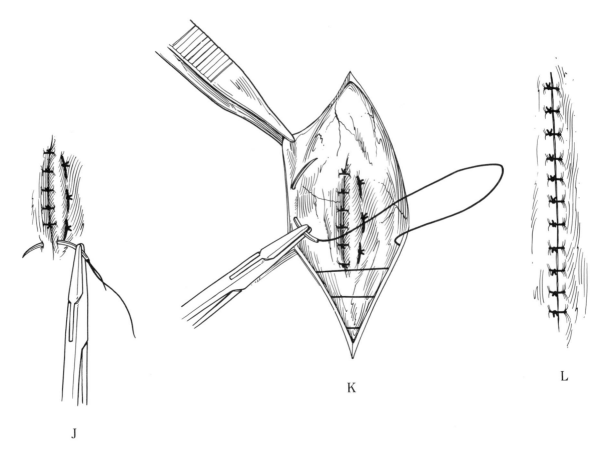

J

K

L

Fig. 12-4. *(continued)*.

Postoperative Management

The decision to use antibiotics is left to the discretion of the surgeon. If the surgery is performed under aseptic conditions, antibiotics generally are not required. We recommend antibiotics if braided, synthetic nonabsorbable suture material is used. Preoperative antibiotics are also indicated if strangulation is suspected or if an enterocutaneous fistula has developed. Postoperative exercise seems to minimize swelling at the surgical site. Generally, a plaque of edema appears on the second or third postoperative day and persists for 2 to 3 weeks. Sutures are removed 10 to 14 days postoperatively. Some surgeons prefer trusses or belly bands to aid in the reduction of edema, but we do not use these routinely on umbilical hernias.

Comments

The incidence of incarceration of an umbilical hernia in foals is low, and signs include increased swelling of the hernia, which becomes firm and warm, and a plaque of edema surrounding the hernia sac. Colic is an inconsistent sign of hernial strangulation. Incarceration of only a portion of the intestinal wall (Richter's hernia) does not produce a complete obstruction of the lumen, but a Richter's hernia may progress to an enterocutaneous fistula.[2]

When entire portions of the intestine are incarcerated, resection and anastomosis of the intestine may be required unless color and motility improve when the segment is freed.

The operation we have described is also suitable for umbilical hernia repair in calves and pigs. Hernias in these species can be large and may be complicated by abscess formation. In such cases, pre- and postoperative antibiotics are indicated. It is also wise to resolve the abscess before attempting repair, especially if the abscess is. large. If an abscess is present, the use of braided, synthetic nonabsorbable material should be avoided.

For umbilical hernia repair in male pigs, the incision should avoid the preputial diverticulum and prepuce.

References

1. McIlwraith, C. W., and Turner, A. S.: Equine Surgery: Advanced Techniques. Philadelphia, Lea & Febiger, 1987.

2. Markel, M. D., Pascoe, J. R., and Sams, E. A.: Strangulated umbilical hernias in horses: 13 cases (1974-1985). J. Am. Vet. Med. Assoc., *190*:692, 1987.

13

BOVINE
GASTRO-
INTESTINAL
SURGERY

Principles of Laparotomy

Laparotomy is commonly performed either for exploratory purposes when a clinical diagnosis is still uncertain or for a specific purpose when a clinical diagnosis has already been made. Flank laparotomy performed on the standing animal under local anesthesia is the most common technique. Flank laparotomy through the left paralumbar fossa is commonly used for exploratory laparotomy if a problem is suspected on the left side, and the procedure is specifically indicated for left-sided abomasopexy, rumenotomy, and cesarean section. The right paralumbar approach is used for exploratory laparotomy if a problem is suspected on the right side, and it is specifically indicated for surgical conditions of the abomasum, including right-sided omentopexy or abomasopexy, small intestine, cecum, and colon. A right-flank approach may also be used for cesarean section when ruminal distention or right-sided positioning of the fetus causes the surgeon to consider the right side a superior approach to the left side. Although flank laparotomy is generally performed on the standing animal, general anesthesia may be indicated when surgery is to be performed through the right flank for a small intestinal or colonic problem because the pain and shock associated with surgery may cause the animal to go down during the procedure.

Ventral paramedian laparotomy is an alternative that necessitates the animal being cast or sedated in dorsal recumbency. The two main indications for this technique are for ventral abomasopexy and cesarean section, in which it offers advantages in the delivery of oversized or emphysematous fetuses and in complicated deliveries, including uterine tears. Another advantage of ventral paramedian laparotomy is less-visible postoperative scarring in feedlot heifers. The paramedian incision is parallel to the midline, between the midline and the subcutaneous abdominal vein. The incision for paramedian abomasopexy extends from the umbilicus craniad to the xiphoid process, as illustrated later in this chapter. The incision for paramedian cesarean section extends from the umbilicus caudad to the udder and is illustrated in Chapter 14.

A third, less common laparotomy approach is the ventrolateral oblique incision, which may be performed on the right or left side and may also be indicated for cesarean section. As with the paramedian approach, fetal and uterine debris can be removed more efficiently, with less potential contamination of the peritoneum than with a flank approach. The ventrolateral oblique incision is considered advantageous to the paramedian incision in the high-producing dairy cow with large subcutaneous abdominal veins and the potential for severe hemorrhage.[1] This technique may be performed conveniently with the cow in lateral recumbency.

Reference

1. Noorsdy, J. L.: Selection of an incision site for cesarean section in the cow. VM/SAC, *75*:530, 1979.

Flank Laparotomy and Abdominal Exploration

The following are indications for left-flank laparotomy: general exploratory laparotomy, particularly if a problem amenable to treatment from the left side is suspected; rumentomy; left-flank abomasopexy; and cesarean section when the viable fetus is only moderately oversized and the cow is capable of enduring the surgery in the standing position. Right-flank laparotomy is indicated in the following instances: exploratory laparotomy when a problem amenable to treatment from the right side is suspected; right-flank abomasopexy and omentopexy; surgical correction of small intestinal, cecal, and colonic conditions; and cesarean section when, because of rumenal distention or fetal positioning, removal of the calf by a left-flank approach would be difficult or when hydrops amnii or allantois is present.

The left-flank laparotomy has an advantage in that intestinal evisceration is generally precluded by the bulk and position of the rumen.

Anesthesia and Surgical Preparation

Typically, this surgical procedure is performed with the animal standing, and anesthesia is provided by a line block, an inverted L block, or a paravertebral block; refer to Chapter 2 for these techniques. For surgery of the small or large intestinal tract, pain and shock associated with both the condition itself and the surgical manipulation may cause the animal to go down during surgery, with obvious compromise to aseptic technique. In such patients, general or high-epidural anesthesia may be used.

The surgical area is clipped and is prepared for aseptic surgery in a routine manner. Draping of the animal is not performed routinely because it is difficult to maintain the position of the drape on the standing animal. Any bars on the stocks adjacent to the operative field are draped.

Surgical Technique

The site of the incision for left-flank laparotomy is illustrated in Figure 13-1A. A vertical incision is made in the middle of the paralumbar fossa extending from 3 to 5 cm ventral to the transverse processes of the lumbar vertebrae for a distance of 20 to 25 cm. For rumenotomy in a large cow, it may be advantageous to make the incision cranial to the midway point. For cesarean section, the incision may begin 10 cm ventral to the transverse processes and may extend 30 to 40 cm.

To incise the skin, reasonable pressure should be exerted on the scalpel to ensure complete penetration. This incision is continued ventrad, so the skin is opened in one smooth motion. Separation of the skin and subcutaneous tissue reveals fibers of the external abdominal oblique muscle (Fig. 13-1B). This layer is incised vertically to reveal the internal abdominal oblique muscle (Fig. 13-1C). A similar incision through the internal abdominal oblique muscle reveals the glistening aponeurosis of the transverse abdominal muscle (Fig. 13-1*D*). Then the muscle is picked up with tissue forceps and is nicked with a scalpel in the dorsal part of the incision to avoid cutting the rumen. The incision through the transverse abdominal muscle and peritoneum may be extended with scissors or a scalpel, for entrance into the peritoneal cavity (Fig. 13-1*E*).

A thorough, systematic examination of the abdomen should always be carried out before specific surgical manipulation is performed on a viscus. Unless a left displacement of the abomasum is present, the rumen will be visible following completion of the left-flank laparotomy incision, and the color of its serosa may be noted (Fig. 13-1*F*). The rumen is palpated to determine the nature of its contents. The left kidney is pendulous and also can be palpated straight in from the incision if the rumen is empty. If the rumen is full, the kidney is located by passing a hand around caudal to the dorsal sac of the rumen. Passing a hand forward on the left side of the rumen, the spleen, reticulum, and diaphragmatic area may be palpated, and the presence of adhesions or abscesses in this area may be ascertained. Moving behind the rumen over to the right side, the viscera within the omental bursa are palpated. Further forward on the right side, it is possible to palpate the caudate lobe of the liver and the gallbladder. The pelvic region, including the uterus (in a cow) and bladder, should also be palpated. It is questionable whether routine palpation of the ovaries and fimbriae of the uterine tubes is appropriate in the cow, especially if peritonitis is present in the abdomen. It is possible that local infection and adhesions could result in problems with reproduction. Following this exploration, any specific procedures indicated, such as rumenotomy or abomasopexy, are performed.

Abdominal exploration may be similarly performed through a right-flank incision. If the viscera are in normal position, the duodenum will be encountered running horizontally across the dorsal part of the incision with the mesoduodenum dorsal and the greater omentum ventral. The pylorus and abomasum can be palpated ventrally. The greater omentum may be reflected craniad to allow examination of the jejunum, ileum, cecum, and colon. The kidneys and pelvic region can also be palpated at this stage. The rumen can be palpated, but examination of the reticulum and diaphragm, as performed with left-flank laparotomy, is not possible. The omasum, liver (the right flank approach allows complete palpation of this organ), gallbladder, and diaphragm can be palpated cranially on the right side. The anatomic peculiarities with abomasal displacements are discussed in the sections of this chapter on abomasopexy and omentopexy.

Routinely, a flank laparotomy incision is closed in three layers. The peritoneum and transverse abdominal muscles are closed together with a simple continuous suture pattern using no. 2 or 3 chromic catgut (Fig. 13-1*G*). Placing this suture layer in a ventral-to-dorsal direction is helpful to maintain the viscera within the incision, particularly on the right side. The internal and external abdominal oblique muscles and subcutaneous fascia may be closed with a second simple continuous layer using no. 3 catgut (Fig. 13-1*H*). This suture line is anchored to the deeper transversus muscle at various intervals to obliterate dead space. It is also desirable to take even bites on either side with the muscle closures, so the muscles will come together without a defect and without wrinkling. If the external and

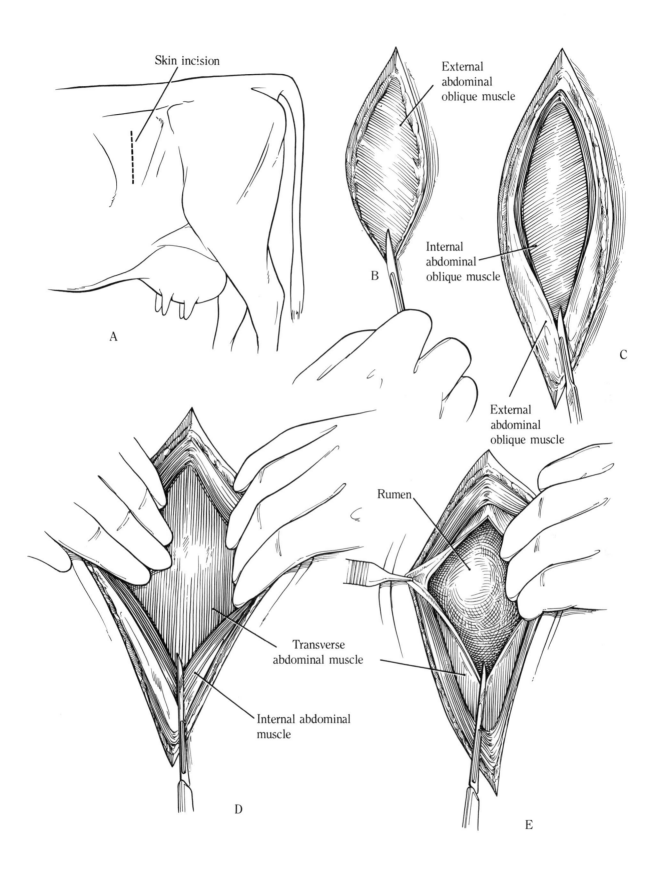

Skin incision

External
abdominal
oblique muscle

Internal
abdominal
oblique muscle

External
abdominal
oblique muscle

A

B

C

Transverse
abdominal muscle

Internal abdominal
muscle

Rumen

D

E

FIG. 13-1. A *to* H, *Flank laparotomy and abdominal exploration.*

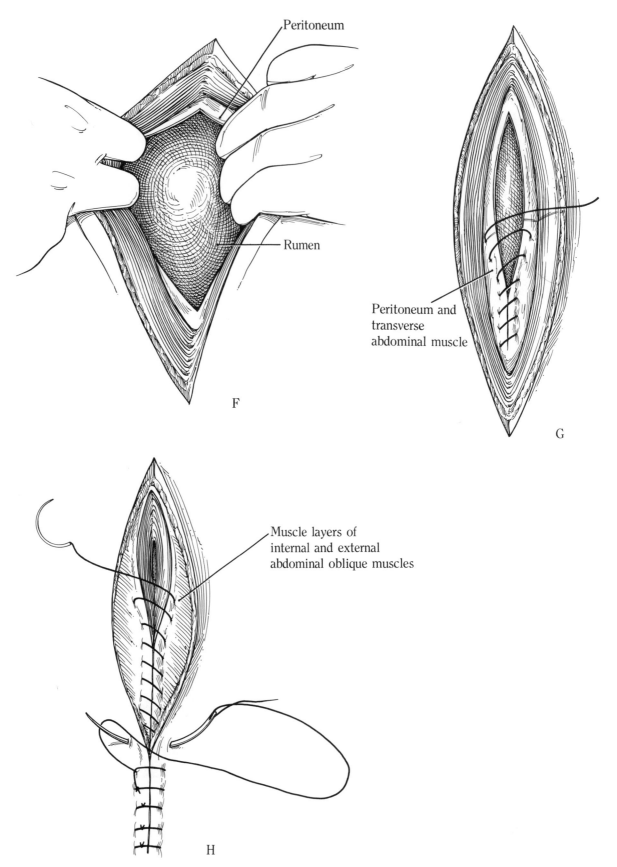

Peritoneum

Rumen

F

Peritoneum and
transverse
abdominal muscle

G

Muscle layers of
internal and external
abdominal oblique muscles

H

FIG. 13-1. *(continued).*

internal abdominal oblique muscle layers are substantial in a large cow, closure should be performed in separate layers. Generally, skin closure is performed with a continuous Ford interlocking pattern using heavy polymerized caprolactam (Vetafil) (Fig. 13-1*H*). The skin sutures are anchored at intervals to the underlying tissue to obliterate dead space. At the surgeon's option, two to three simple interrupted sutures may be placed in the ventral aspect of the incision (Fig. 13-1*H*); this measure allows easy drainage if infection develops in the incision. Such an event is possible in the compromised conditions under which this surgical procedure may have to be performed. If the skin incision has been obviously contaminated, as by the delivery of an emphysematous fetus, an interrupted suture pattern may be more appropriate.

Postoperative Management

Antibiotics are administered, if indicated, depending on the procedure. Supportive management is also instituted in accordance with the animal's condition. Sutures may be removed 2 to 3 weeks after surgery; at 10 to 14 days, the incision is still vulnerable to trauma, and in cattle housed together, a "popped" incision may occur if sutures are removed at this time.

Rumenotomy

Rumenotomy is indicated for the removal of metallic foreign bodies, whose presence may cause traumatic reticulitis or traumatic reticuloperitonitis, materials such as baling twine or plastic bags that are obstructing the reticulo-omasal orifice, and foreign bodies lodged in the distal esophagus or over the base of the heart.

Rumenotomy is also indicated for evacuation of rumen contents in selected cases of rumen overload. Generally, rumenotomy is limited to those cases in which the causative agent is primarily in the rumen. Finely ground feedstuffs readily pass into the omasal-abomasal region, but coarser, more fibrous material remains in the rumen for longer periods. Other indications for rumenotomy include rumen impaction and impaction and atony of the omasum or abomasum.[1]

Anesthesia and Surgical Preparation

The left-flank area is prepared for aseptic surgery in a routine manner, and local anesthesia is instituted by line block, inverted L block, or paravertebral block.

Additional Instrumentation

If one does not suture the rumen to the skin as described here, placement of a rumenotomy board or fixation ring will be necessary.

Surgical Technique

Rumenotomy is performed through a left paralumbar incision (a 20-cm incision generally is sufficient) with the animal standing. The technique for left-flank laparotomy has been described previously. In large cows, the flank incisions for rumenotomies sometimes are made just caudal and parallel to the last rib, to place the incision closer to the reticulum. It is essential, however, to leave sufficient tissue caudal to the last rib for suturing (the incision should be approximately 5 cm (2 in.) caudal to the last rib).

Following opening and systematic exploration of the peritoneal cavity (no attempt is made to break down firm adhesions in the region of the reticulum), it is necessary to anchor the rumen to the incision to avoid contamination of the abdominal musculature and peritoneum during the rumenotomy procedure. A technique for suturing the rumen to the skin prior to rumenotomy is illustrated in Figure 13-2*A* to *D*. A continuous inverting suture pattern is used, to pull the rumen over the edge of the skin incision (Figure 13-2*A* and *B*). This suture should be of heavy-gauge material such as heavy or extra-heavy polymerized caprolactam (Vetafil). Two large, inverting sutures are placed at the ventral aspect of the incision so that the rumen projects well over the skin edge; this avoids contamination in the ventral region (Fig. 13-2*C*). Alternate techniques for isolating the

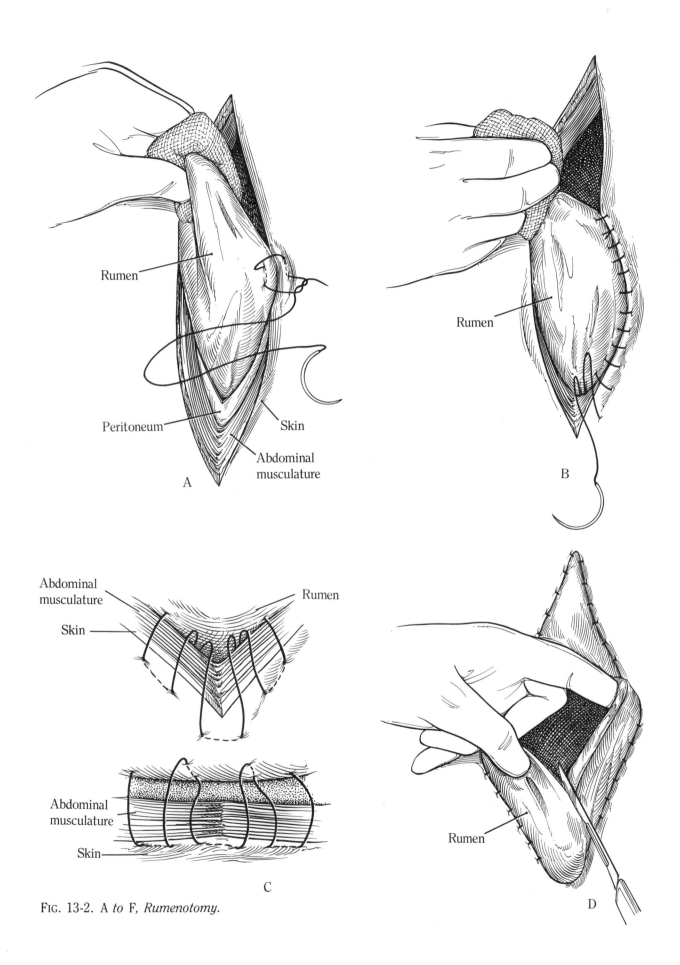

Rumen

Peritoneum

Skin

Abdominal
musculature

A

Rumen

B

Abdominal
musculature

Rumen

Skin

Abdominal
musculature

Skin

C

Rumen

D

FIG. 13-2. A *to* F, *Rumenotomy.*

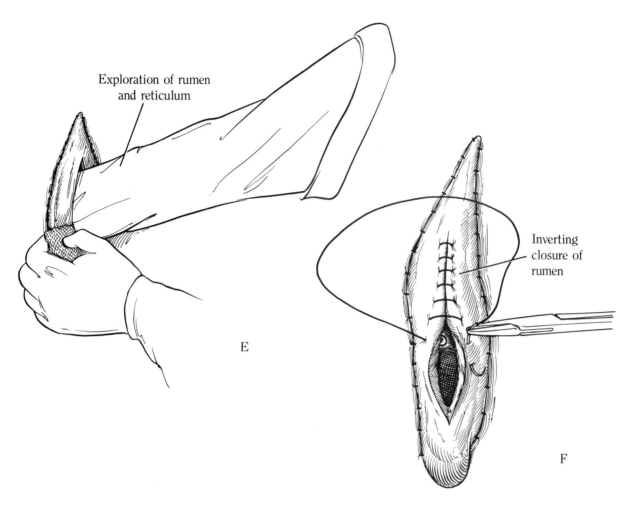

Exploration of rumen
and reticulum

E

Inverting
closure of
rumen

F

FIG. 13-2. *(continued).*

rumen and preventing contamination include the use of stay sutures, a rubber rumenotomy shroud, a fixation ring (Weingart's),[2] or a rumenotomy board. These alternatives are quicker than suturing the rumen, but they are also more easily displaced; the consequent contamination may be disastrous.

The rumen is incised with a scalpel (Fig. 13-2D), and the operator, wearing long rubber gloves, evacuates and explores the rumen (Fig. 13-2E). The inside of the rumen and the reticulum are explored, and if a foreign body is present, it is removed.

To reach the reticulum from the rumenotomy incision, the dorsal wall of the rumen (where a natural air pocket exists) should be followed, until it becomes the ventral wall, at which point one is in the reticulum. Following a direct line from the incision, one encounters ingesta as well as the cranial pillar of the rumen and ruminoreticular fold. To help locate foreign bodies, the reticulum can be gently picked up with the hand. The area where the foreign body is usually has extended adhesions and cannot be picked up. This is an ideal area to look for foreign bodies. Moreover, while exploring the inside of the reticulum, one should also feel for abscesses. Abscesses are frequently found on the medial wall of the reticulum near the reticulo-omasal orifice. If abscesses are found, they should be evaluated. If the cow's economic value justifies the surgeon to proceed, abscesses that adhere to the reticulum should be lanced or drained. This is best accomplished by carrying a scalpel or scalpel blade, attached to a piece of string or polymerized caprolactam (vetafil) in case it is dropped, into the reticulum and lancing the abscess into the reticulum through the adhesion. Following this exploration, the reticulum may be swept with a magnet to pick up additional metallic debris. A magnet is placed (or replaced) in the reticulum, and fresh rumen contents (if available) are placed in the rumen. Alkalinizing products may be inserted at this stage in cases of rumen overload, and mineral oil may also be instilled when indicated. The surgeon's contaminated gloves are then discarded.

The rumen incision is closed with a row of continuous inverting sutures of no. 2 or 3 chromic catgut (Fig. 13-2F). A single layer is usually adequate,[2] but a double row may be necessary in a large, distended rumen. The surgical site is then irrigated with polyionic fluid, with or without dilute povidone-iodine solution, prior to removal of the rumen-fixation suture or apparatus. Closure of the laparotomy incision has been described previously.

Postoperative Management

Postoperative medication varies with the indication for the rumenotomy. Although rumen overload often requires intensive fluid therapy, traumatic reticulitis requires little intensive care. Antibiotics are indicated following the removal of foreign bodies from the reticulum. Oral fluids can be administered following rumenotomy, and mild osmotic laxatives, such as magnesium hydroxide, often promote gut motility.

References

1. Baker, J. S.: Abomasal impaction and related obstructions of the forestomachs in cattle. J. Am. Vet. Med. Assoc., *175*:1250, 1979.

2. Hofmeyr, C. F. B.: The digestive system. *In* Textbook of Large Animal Surgery. Edited by F. W. Oehme and J. E. Prier. Baltimore, Williams & Wilkins, 1974.

Rumenostomy
(Rumenal Fistulation)

The techniques of rumenal fistulation have been developed for experimental purposes, as well as for the relief of chronic bloat. The experimental techniques use various types of cannulas to create a permanent opening, whereas the therapeutic technique provides temporary, symptomatic relief. Chronic bloating results from abnormal function of the parasympathetic nerve supply to the cardia of the stomach and dorsal sac of the rumen. This situation can result from reticuloperitonitis or fibrinous pneumonia-pleuritis involving the vagus nerve. Bloat may also develop secondary to enlarged lymph nodes or liver abscess; it is also observed occasionally in nursing cows and is thought to be associated with disturbed rumen metabolism. Another cause of bloat, especially in feedlot cattle, is altered rumen flora secondary to a rapid change from one feed to another. The technique of rumenostomy that we describe here is used as a therapeutic device in animals with chronic bloat.

Anesthesia and Surgical Preparation

This surgical procedure is performed with the animal standing. If rumenal tympany is present, it is relieved by a stomach tube; this measure will facilitate exteriorization of the rumen later. The left paralumbar fossa area is prepared surgically in a routine manner. A circular area immediately ventral to the transverse processes of the lumbar vertebrae and approximately 10 cm in diameter is infiltrated with local anesthetic.

Surgical Technique

A circular piece of skin, approximately 4 cm in diameter, is removed to expose the underlying abdominal musculature (Fig. 13-3A). The abdominal muscles and peritoneum are bluntly dissected to expose the rumen. It may be necessary to remove some of the external abdominal oblique muscle if it is thick and limits exposure of the rumen. The wall of the rumen is then grasped with forceps, and a portion of it is pulled through to the exterior. In this fashion, a "cone" of rumen is brought to the skin surface, where it is anchored to the skin with four horizontal mattress sutures of polymerized caprolactam (Vetafil) (Fig. 13-3B); these mattress sutures pass through rumen and skin. The central portion of the exposed rumen is removed (Fig. 13-3B), and the incised edge of the rumen is sutured to the skin with simple interrupted sutures of nonabsorbable material (Fig. 13-3C and D). The rumenal fistula that results from this procedure should be no larger than 2 to 3 cm in diameter. The muscle layers perform a valve-like function and help to control seepage of rumenal ingesta while relieving gas accumulation in the rumen.

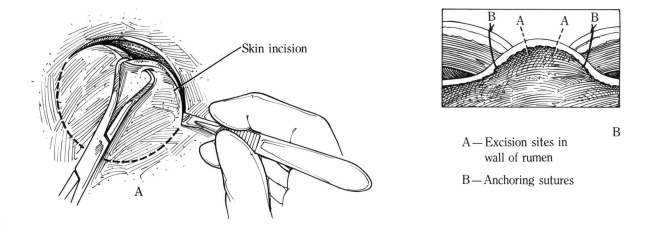

A— Excision sites in
wall of rumen

B— Anchoring sutures

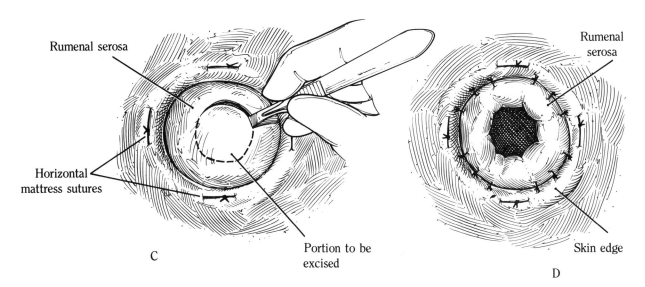

Fig. 13-3. A to D, Rumenostomy.

Postoperative Management

When surgery is performed properly, antibiotics need not be administered, and aftercare is not usually indicated. Many animals with chronic bloat fail to recover normal eructation, so the fistula should be permanent. If the fistula is made with the dimensions we have described, it should remain patent for a sufficient time. A smaller fistula will close earlier. With the valve-like function of the muscle layers, the fistula generally stays open as long as gas is expelled from it; however, it usually closes once the animal regains normal eructation.

Right-flank Omentopexy

Right-flank omentopexy may be used in the treatment of left-sided displacement of the abomasum (LDA) and right-sided dilatation of the abomasum, with or without torsion (RDA or RTA). This technique is one of three described in this text for the fixation of the abomasum following correction of a displacement. It involves suturing the superficial layer of the greater omentum in the region of the pylorus to the abdominal wall in the right flank.

In the hands of experienced operators, right-flank omentopexy for the treatment of LDA has a high success rate.[1] It has also been used successfully in the treatment of RTA.[2] The maintenance of long-term fixation of the abomasum can be questioned, however, particularly with inexperienced surgeons. Adipose tissue is weak, and the trauma of a cow being knocked down could be sufficient to tear or stretch the omental attachment. Right displacement of the abomasum can also occur if the abomasum pivots around an intact omental adhesion.[1] We believe that the techniques of abomasopexy are more reliable and predictable in providing long-term fixation of the abomasum. In addition, that an LDA cannot be visualized prior to correction with this technique may create problems if adhesions are present.

Anesthesia and Surgical Preparation

This surgical procedure is performed with the animal standing. The right paralumbar area is clipped and is prepared surgically. Local anesthesia may be administered using a paravertebral block, an inverted L block, or a line block.

Surgical Technique

The abdomen is entered through a 20-cm vertical incision in the right paralumbar fossa starting 4 to 5 cm ventral to the transverse processes of the lumbar vertebrae (Fig. 13-4A). When the peritoneal cavity is entered in the case of an LDA, the duodenum will be ventrad instead of in its normal horizontal position. Wearing sterile sleeves, the surgeon palpates the left side of the abdomen by deflecting the greater omentum craniad; then he passes his left arm caudal to the omentum and rumen to palpate the abomasum distended with gas on the left side of the rumen. This confirms the diagnosis of LDA. In addition, while palpating the displaced organ, one should feel for any evidence of adhesions.

The abomasum may be deflated using a 12- to 13-gauge needle with a length of sterile tubing attached. The needle is carried caudal to the rumen to the most dorsal part of the displaced abomasum and is inserted obliquely through the abomasal wall. Pressure is applied firmly with the forearm and the hand to release the gas. The needle is withdrawn and is carried back carefully, with the tubing folded to avoid contamination.

The abomasum is returned to its normal position by following the peritoneal surfaces ventrally with the hand between the rumen and the body wall. Once to the left of the rumen, the hand, with the fingers closed, is used to sweep the abomasum back to the right side of the abdomen. Gentle dorsocraniad pulling on the omentum, which has also been displaced to the left, is also helpful in this manipulation. If the rumen is full, it may be necessary to elevate the caudal ventral blind sac of the rumen with the inside of the elbow, to allow the abomasum to be pulled along under the rumen. Once the abomasum is returned to its normal position, the duodenum resumes its normal horizontal position (Fig. 13-4B) and is commonly observed to fill with gas. The greater omentum, which is observed through the abdominal incision, also feels loose (Fig. 13-4B). Unnecessary handling of the duodenum during these manipulations may cause postoperative duodenitis.

If the surgery is performed for the treatment of an RDA or RTA, care should be taken not to incise the dilatated abomasum when entering the peritoneal cavity. The various right-sided malpositions of the abomasum when using a right-flank approach are detailed in the section on right-flank abomasopexy. The abomasum commonly requires evacuation before the displacement can be corrected. An RTA usually has large quantities of fluid. Correct positioning of the abomasum is recognized in the same fashion as in LDA. Once the abomasum has been returned to its correct position, the technique of omentopexy is the same whether it is an LDA, RDA, or RTA.

The omentum is grasped and pulled out through the incision. It is gently retracted dorsad and caudad until the pylorus can be visualized. This fold of omentum may be held by an assistant or attached to the upper part of the skin incision with towel forceps while the anchoring sutures are placed. Two mattress sutures of no. 3 chromic catgut (one cranial to the incision and one caudal to it) are placed through the peritoneum and transverse abdominal muscle and through both layers of the fold of omentum (Fig. 13-4C). The sutures are placed about 3 cm caudal to the pylorus. The peritoneum and transverse abdominal muscle are then sutured in a simple continuous pattern with no. 2 or no. 3 catgut, and the omentum is incorporated into the suture line in the ventral two-thirds of the incision (Fig. 13-4D). The internal and external abdominal oblique muscle layers and the skin are closed as in a routine flank laparotomy.

Postoperative Management

Postoperative management depends on the individual case. Some animals require little or no aftercare; other animals may have septic metritis, mastitis, or ketosis and may also have been deprived of feed and water. Such animals require appropriate fluid therapy. Animals operated on for RTA are in particularly critical condition. These patients should be monitored regularly for clinical signs, milk production, and urine ketones. Propylene glycol should be administered if indicated. Rumenal stimulants may be given, and if the animal's appetite has not returned in 2 days, a rumen inoculation may be appropriate. Cows with metritis or mastitis should be treated appropriately.

Comments

The drawbacks of this technique for the treatment of abomasal fixation were noted in the introduction to this section. Admittedly, some recurrent

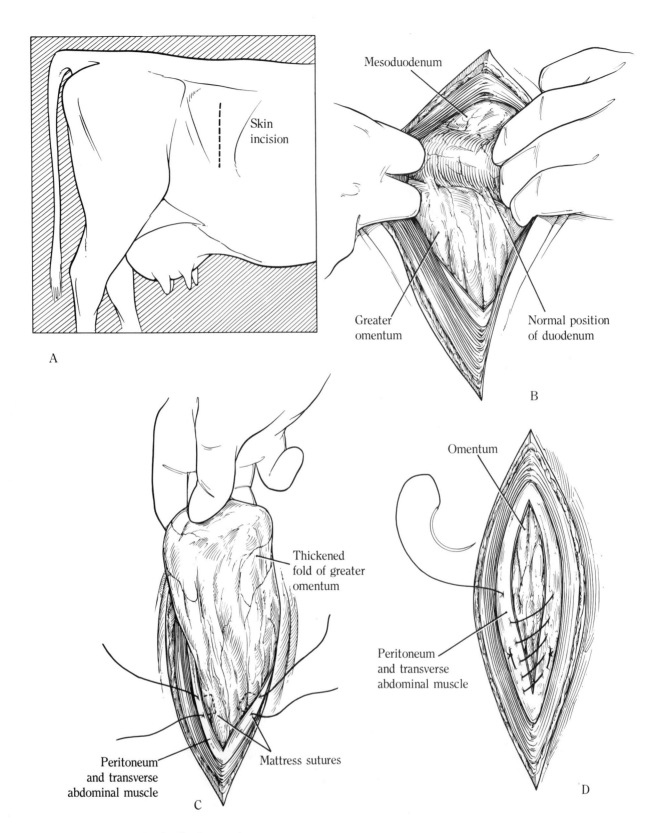

Labels in figure:

A — Skin incision

B — Mesoduodenum; Greater omentum; Normal position of duodenum

C — Thickened fold of greater omentum; Mattress sutures; Peritoneum and transverse abdominal muscle

D — Omentum; Peritoneum and transverse abdominal muscle

FIG. 13-4. A *to* D, *Right-flank omentopexy*.

displacements can be prevented by good technique, by ensuring that the point of omental fixation is not too far dorsal or caudal to the pylorus. Even in the hands of experienced operators, however, redisplacement may occur in the long term. Because of potential rotation of the abomasum around the omental attachment, the technique is certainly questionable for the treatment of RDA or RTA. Right-flank omentopexy was developed when the only alternative was paramedian abomasopexy, which required the patient to be in dorsal recumbency. In some cows, this position was undesirable, so a surgical procedure that could be performed with the animal standing had obvious advantages. The subsequent development of the flank abomasopexy technique offered a third alternative.

References

1. Gabel, A. A., and Heath, R. B.: Correction and right-sided omentopexy in treatment of left-sided displacement of the abomasum in dairy cattle. J. Am. Vet. Med. Assoc., *155*:632, 1969.

2. Gabel, A. A., and Heath, R. B.: Treatment of right-sided torsion of the abomasum in cattle. J. Am. Vet. Med. Assoc., *155*:642, 1969.

Ventral Paramedian Abomasopexy

Ventral paramedian abomasopexy may be used in the treatment of left- or right-sided displacement of the abomasum (LDA or RDA) and in early cases of right-sided torsion of the abomasum (RTA).[1]

Anesthesia and Surgical Preparation

The cow is sedated (chloral hydrate given intravenously to effect is satisfactory and economical) and is cast in dorsal recumbency. Alternatively, 2 oz. chloral hydrate can be administered orally (two no. 10 gelatin capsules filled with chloral hydrate), and the patient may be cast using a rope. Oral administration of chloral hydrate also has some antifermentative effect. The cow's legs are tied, and its body is supported by a trough or weighted side frames. The patient should be tilted slightly to the right, to facilitate later closure of the incision. An area from the xiphoid process to the umbilicus is clipped and is surgically prepared in a routine manner. Local anesthesia is administered by local infiltration along the proposed incision or an inverted L block of the right paramedian area.

Additional Instrumentation

This procedure requires a 12-gauge needle with rubber tubing.

Surgical Technique

A 20-cm incision is made between the midline and the right subcutaneous abdominal vein, starting approximately 8 cm behind the xiphoid process and ending immediately cranial to the umbilicus (Fig. 13-5A and B). The small branches of the subcutaneous abdominal vein that are cut when incising the skin and subcutaneous tissue need to be ligated because the lack of muscle tissue in this region inhibits natural hemostasis, and may result in hematoma and seroma formation. The incision is continued through the external rectus sheath (aponeuroses of external and internal abdominal oblique muscles) (Fig. 13-5C), and the rectus abdominis muscle, to reveal the fibers of the internal rectus sheath (the transverse abdominal aponeurosis) running crosswise in the incision line. The transverse abdominal aponeurosis and peritoneum are incised (Fig. 13-5D). The transverse aponeurosis may be cut separately with a scalpel and the peritoneum may be entered using scissors, or both layers may be opened together with scissors.

In most cases of LDA, the abomasum will have returned to a relatively normal position during the casting procedure. If necessary, the abomasum should be returned to its normal position. Rarely, in the case of an RDA or RTA, it may be appropriate to empty gas with a 12-gauge needle and rubber tubing (Fig. 13-5E). This is probably unnecessary with an LDA. Once

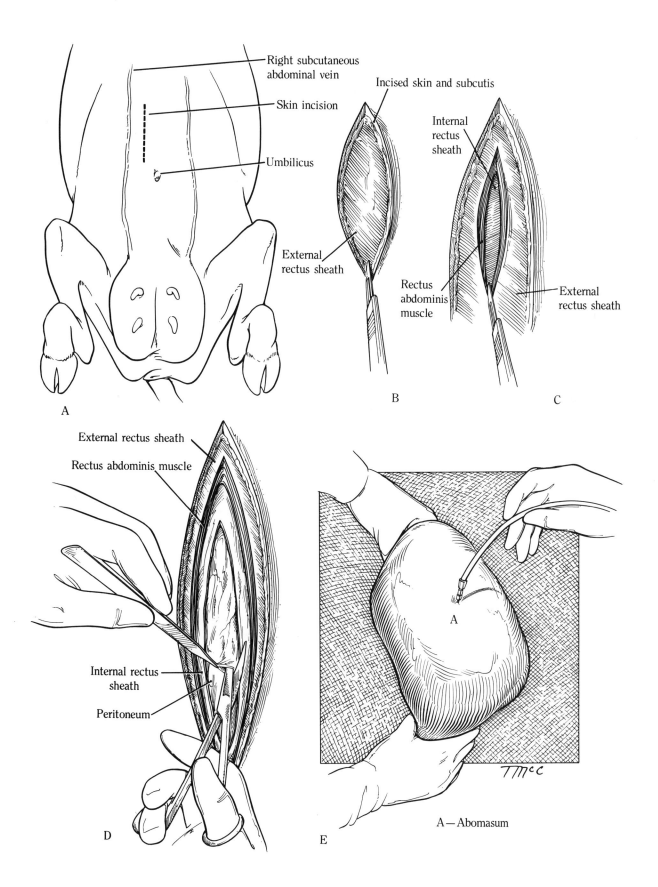

Right subcutaneous abdominal vein

Skin incision

Umbilicus

External rectus sheath

Incised skin and subcutis

Internal rectus sheath

Rectus abdominis muscle

External rectus sheath

A

B

C

External rectus sheath

Rectus abdominis muscle

Internal rectus sheath

Peritoneum

D

A

A—Abomasum

E

FIG. 13-5. A *to* H, *Ventral paramedian abomasopexy.*

the correct position of the abomasum has been ascertained, the lateral aspect of the greater curvature of the abomasum (where it is free of omentum) is sutured to the peritoneum and internal rectus sheath approximately 2 cm lateral to the paramedian incision line using three mattress sutures of no. 2 chromic catgut (Fig. 13-5*F*). The peritoneum and internal rectus sheath are then closed with simple continuous sutures of no. 2 chromic catgut, incorporating the abomasum in the suture line (Fig. 13-5*G*). The heavy, external rectus sheath is closed with horizontal mattress sutures of no. 3 chromic catgut (Fig. 13-5*H*), and the skin is closed with a Ford interlocking suture using 0.6-mm polymerized caprolactam (Vetafil) (Fig. 13-5*H*). The patient is rolled into left lateral recumbency, followed by sternal recumbency.

Postoperative Management

The patient is encouraged to rise to its feet as soon as possible. The use of antibiotics is optional. Some animals require little aftercare; other animals may be dehydrated or have septic metritis, mastitis, or ketosis and should be treated appropriately. Patients should be monitored for clinical signs, milk production, and ketosis and provided with a diet high in crude fiber. If there is a lack of gut motility a day following surgery, neostigmine (Stiglyn) may be administered and repeated hourly if necessary. A rumen inoculation may also be appropriate.

Comments

Some surgeons have used nonabsorbable sutures (passed to the exterior) for fixation of the abomasum, as well as for closure of the external rectus sheath. In our experience, catgut is satisfactory. Nonabsorbable suture is considered by some practitioners to be contraindicated because it may cause fistula formation if it extends full thickness through the abomasum.

The ventral paramedian approach has several advantages: the abomasum is brought into position more easily in most cases, and instantaneous repositioning commonly occurs; the abomasum is easily viewed for detailed examination and detection of ulcers; and strong, positive, long-lasting adhesions can be anticipated.

The following are disadvantages of the ventral paramedian approach: the casting procedure requires more assistance and may be more stressful to the animal; the cow in dorsal recumbency may regurgitate; and the remainder of the abdomen cannot be explored satisfactorily. In a severe case of RTA, this method is considered inappropriate because it is difficult to remove fluid from the abomasum, and it is preferable to operate with the animal in a standing position because of its compromised systemic condition.

Reference

1. Lowe, J. E., and Loomis, W. K.: Abomasopexy for repair of left abomasal displacement in dairy cattle. J. Am. Vet. Med. Assoc., *147*:389, 1965.

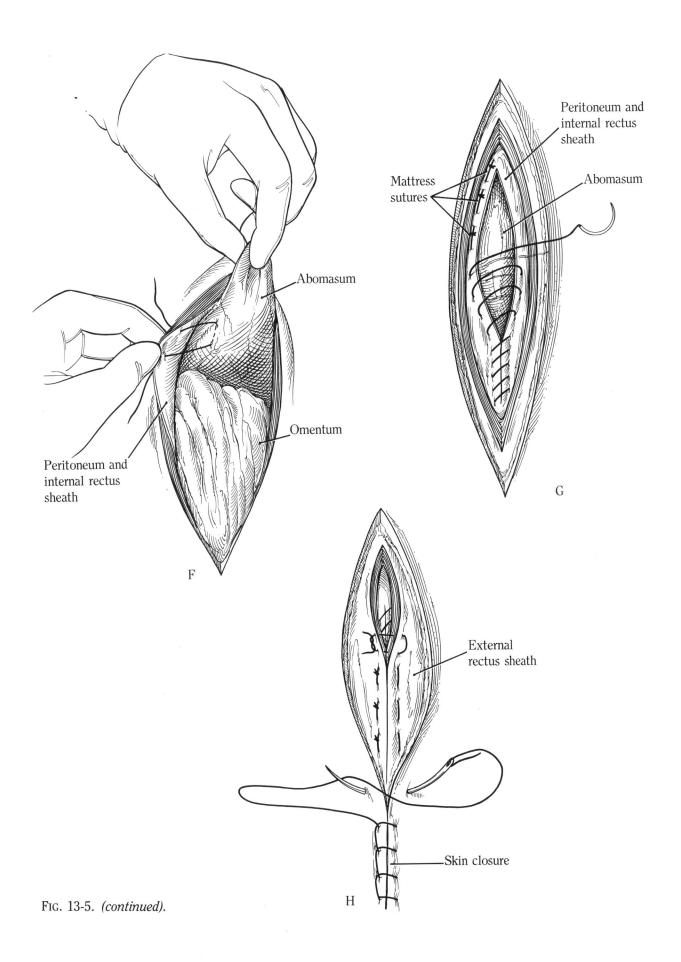

Abomasum

Peritoneum and
internal rectus
sheath

Omentum

F

Peritoneum and
internal rectus
sheath

Mattress
sutures

Abomasum

G

External
rectus sheath

Skin closure

H

Fig. 13-5. *(continued)*.

Left-flank Abomasopexy

Left-flank abomasopexy is indicated for the treatment of left-sided displacement of the abomasum (LDA).[1,2] This technique has the advantage of offering direct fixation of the abomasum to the ventral body wall, and the surgery is performed with the animal in the standing position. In addition, adhesions or ulceration of the displaced abomasum can be visualized and treated, and an exploratory rumenotomy can be performed if indicated. The abomasal anchoring achieved with the left-flank abomasopexy is not considered as secure as that achieved with the ventral paramedian technique.

Anesthesia and Surgical Preparation

The left-flank area is clipped and prepared as for a left-flank laparotomy. An area from the xiphoid process to the umbilicus and from the midline to the right subcutaneous abdominal vein is also prepared surgically. This second area is not anesthetized. The left flank is anesthetized by a paravertebral block, inverted L block, or line block.

Additional Instrumentation

A large, straight, cutting needle or an S-curved cutting needle is required.

Surgical Technique

A left-flank laparotomy is performed using a 20- to 25-cm incision in the paralumbar fossa, as previously described. Caution should be exercised when entering the abdomen because a distended abomasum may lie immediately within the incision area. Usually, the abomasum is visible through the incision. An 8- to 12-cm simple continuous or interlocking suture line of heavy polymerized caprolactam (Vetafil) is placed in the greater curvature of the abomasum 5 to 7 cm from the attachment of the greater omentum (Fig. 13-6A). The suture bites pass through the submucosa, and a meter of suture material should extend from each end of the suture line. Hemostats are placed on these suture ends in such a fashion that the cranial and caudal ends are easily identified. The abomasum may then be deflated using a 12-gauge needle and rubber tubing (Fig. 13-6A) if this is considered necessary. The needle is placed into the dorsal portion of the abomasum and is inserted at an angle to obviate leakage when the needle is withdrawn. It is important that the abomasum not be deflated prior to the insertion of the suture; otherwise, the site for suture placement may be retracted away from the incision.

The cranial end of the polymerized caprolactam is attached to a large, straight, cutting needle or to an S-curved cutting needle; this needle is carried along the internal body wall to a position right of midline, but medial to the subcutaneous abdominal vein and 15 cm caudal to the xiphoid process. The forefinger protects the end of the needle, and the lateral fingers

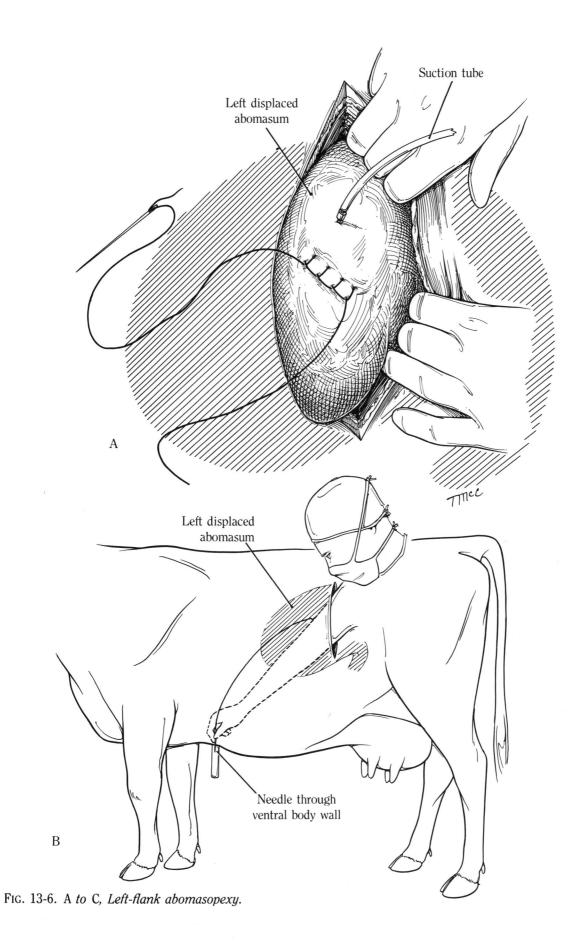

Suction tube

Left displaced
abomasum

A

Left displaced
abomasum

Needle through
ventral body wall

B

Fig. 13-6. A *to* C, *Left-flank abomasopexy.*

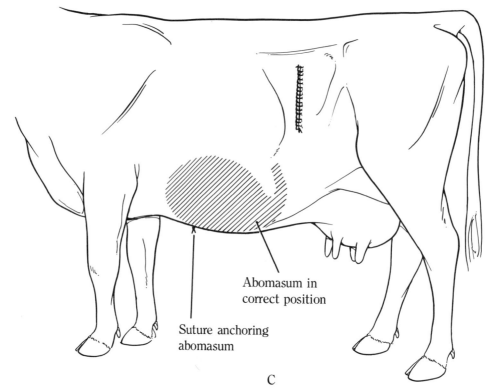

Abomasum in
correct position

Suture anchoring
abomasum

C

FIG. 13-6. *(continued).*

reflect the viscera away from the body wall and ahead of the needle. An assistant can apply upward pressure on the abdominal wall in the area where the needles are to be inserted through the body wall. An empty syringe case works well for this purpose.

The needle is inserted quickly through the ventral body wall (Fig. 13-6B). The assistant grasps the needle, and the caudal suture is placed through the body wall 8 to 12 cm caudal to the cranial suture. The assistant then grasps the two suture ends and applies gentle traction; at the same time, the surgeon pushes the deflated abomasum into its normal position. When the sutured area of the abomasum is lying against the floor of the abdomen, the assistant ties the suture ends together (Fig. 13-6C). The suture is left in place for 4 weeks; the ends are then cut as close to the skin as possible. This time is considered necessary to allow the development of adhesions sufficient to prevent redisplacement. The flank laparotomy incision is closed routinely.

Postoperative Management

The use of antibiotics is optional. Some animals require little aftercare. Other animals may be dehydrated or have septic metritis, mastitis, or ketosis; these animals should be treated appropriately. Patients should be monitored for clinical signs, milk production, and ketosis and provided with a diet high in crude fiber. If there is a lack of gut motility a day following surgery, neostigmine (Stiglyn) may be administered and repeated hourly if necessary. A rumen inoculation may also be appropriate.

Comments

The advantages of left-flank abomasopexy were noted in the introduction to this section. This technique has the following disadvantages: the site for abomasal fixation to the body wall is difficult to reach in large cows if the surgeon has short arms; care is necessary to avoid puncturing viscera as the needle is carried to the floor of the abdomen; and in some cases, the abomasum may be lying in a cranioventral position and may be difficult to expose sufficiently for placement of the suture.[2] Auscultation during the clinical examination prior to surgery should identify the situation, and another approach may be considered.

References

1. Ames, S.: Repositioning displaced abomasum in the cow. J. Am. Vet. Med. Assoc., *153*: 1470, 1968.

2. Baker, J. S.: Displacement of the abomasum in dairy cows: part II. Pract. Vet., Summer/Fall: 1, 1973.

Right-flank Abomasopexy

Right-flank abomasopexy is indicated in the treatment of right-sided displacement and dilatation of the abomasum (RDA) or right-sided torsion of the abomasum (RTA).[1] Animals with RTA generally have more acute clinical signs. In addition, they may have marked electrolyte changes, particularly in the chloride and potassium levels.[6] The severity of RTA has been classified into four grades, on the basis of the volume of sequestered abomasal fluid, and this classification is useful and less subjective than the common clinical means.[6]

Right paramedian abomasopexy is a valid alternative for treating RDA and mild cases of RTA, but right-flank abomasopexy is considered more appropriate in the severely affected cow. Fluid can be removed from the abomasum more easily through a flank incision and there is less risk to a patient in a compromised condition if it is operated on in the standing position. In severe RTA with abomasal compromise, suture material may pull through the abomasal wall, and the use of omentopexy should be considered.[3] In animals that survive the surgery, however, this problem has not been observed.[2]

Anesthesia and Surgical Preparation

The right-flank area is prepared for surgery in a routine manner. Local anesthesia is instituted by performing a paravertebral block, inverted L block, or a line block.

Additional Instrumentation

This procedure requires a sterile, medium-sized stomach tube, a 12-gauge needle and sterile tubing, and a large, straight, cutting needle or S-curved cutting needle.

Surgical Technique

The right-flank approach to the bovine abdomen has been described previously. A 20- to 25-cm incision is made. At this stage, the particular problem needs to be recognized, and certain guidelines can be stated. In a simple RDA, the greater omentum comes into view through the laparotomy wound in the right flank as in a normal animal. The greater omentum may be looser because the distance between the abomasum and the descending duodenum is less than normal. The fundus will typically have moved caudolaterad and will appear uncovered by omentum. Abomasal torsions (volvulus may be a better term) occur counterclockwise when viewed from the rear and counterclockwise when viewed from the right flank. The omentum is usually wrapped in the torsion site, and the abomasum therefore appears at the incision without omentum covering it.

The color of the abomasal serosa is ascertained before one attempts to deflate the abomasum or correct its position. If the serosa appears viable and the organ is tightly distended, a 12-gauge needle with rubber tubing attached is inserted to relieve the gaseous pressure and to facilitate further exploration and manipulation. It is easier to remove gas and fluid before detorsion because the abomasum is closer to the incision. Early or less-severe torsion may not even require fluid removal, but severe torsion may require fluid removal before the torsion can be reduced. Placement of the suture requires careful thought, to ensure correct positioning at the completion of the procedure. An interlocking suture is placed in the middle of the greater curvature of the abomasum near the attachment of the greater omentum in the manner previously described and illustrated for left-flank abomasopexy. When a purse-string suture has been placed in the abomasal wall, a stab incision is made, and a sterile, medium-sized stomach tube is inserted into the abomasum (Fig. 13-7). The fluid within the abomasum is then removed. If the fluid is difficult to drain, lavage may be performed. At the end of abomasal drainage, 2 to 3 L of mineral oil are instilled into the abomasum, the tube is withdrawn, and the purse-string suture is tied. The abomasopexy is completed as described for left-flank abomasopexy.

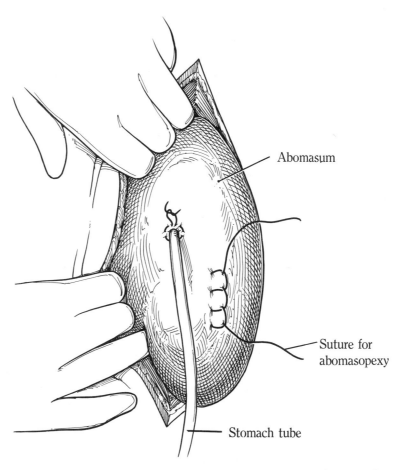

Abomasum

Suture for
abomasopexy

Stomach tube

FIG. 13-7. *The fluid within the abomasum is removed using a medium-sized stomach tube.*

Postoperative Management

Antibiotics are administered postoperatively. Many of these animals need intense fluid therapy with particular emphasis on replacement of the chloride deficit (see Chap. 2). For this purpose, 0.9% sodium chloride solution is generally appropriate; supplementation with potassium chloride may also be indicated. With adequate fluid and electrolyte therapy in the presurgical and early postsurgical periods, the metabolic effects of RTA generally can be controlled. In severely affected cows, the abomasum's inability to regain normal function is often more important. The abomasum becomes filled and impacted if its function is not restored.[6] Typically, cases of abomasal torsion appear to improve in the first 24 to 48 hours and then deteriorate at 48 to 72 hours, with abomasal atony. Motility stimulants, such as neostigmine (Stiglyn), have been recommended, but neostigmine must be used repeatedly to have any effect above the pylorus, and even then its benefit is minimal. Oral supportive therapy, in which sodium chloride and potassium chloride are added to water, can be used in a patient capable of absorbing the fluid.

Comments

Some surgeons believe that their success in treating cows with RTA was due largely to not opening the abomasum prior to surgery.[5] Now this claim generally is considered invalid. That acidic fluid high in chloride is easily absorbed from the abomasum following detorsion is questionable. In addition, any fluid deficit sustained by draining the abomasum can be replaced by intravenous fluid therapy; this is considered more reliable than anticipating reabsorption of the fluid from the abomasum after detorsion. The rationale for removing fluids that potentially contain endotoxins is logical, but its validity is controversial. Whether deposition of mineral oil directly into the abomasum inhibits further toxin reabsorption is uncertain, and its value is equally controversial. One author believes that this measure has contributed to his success,[1] whereas another author does not think that this measure improved the prognosis for severely affected cows.[6]

References

1. Baker, J. S.: Right displacement of the abomasum in the bovine: a modified procedure for treatment. Bovine Pract., *11*:58, 1976.

2. Baker, J. S.: Personal communication, 1980.

3. Boucher, W. B., and Abt, D.: Right-sided dilatation of the bovine abomasum with torsion. J. Am. Vet. Med. Assoc., *153*:76, 1968.

4. Espersen, G.: Dilatation and displacement of the abomasum to the right flank, and dilatation and dislocation of the cecum. Vet. Rec., *76*:1423, 1964.

5. Gabel, A. A., and Heath, R. B.: Treatment of right-sided torsion of the abomasum in cattle. J. Am. Vet. Med. Assoc., *155*:642, 1969.

6. Smith, D. F.: Right-side torsion of the abomasum in dairy cows: classification of severity and evaluation of outcome. J. Am. Vet. Med. Assoc., *173*:108, 1978.

14

BOVINE
UROGENITAL
SURGERY

Calf Castration

Castration of beef calves is a routine management procedure that should be performed early in a calf's life. It is recommended that nursing calves be castrated at 1 to 4 weeks of age. Bucket-reared calves should probably be castrated 3 to 4 weeks later because of their slower start nutritionally and inferior condition. Sometimes it may be necessary to wait longer on an individual calf. Some calves will be held to weaning before castration if progeny testing for weight gain is performed.

Anesthesia and Surgical Preparation

This surgical procedure is generally performed quickly without anesthesia or skin preparation. This apparent lack of attention to normal surgical principles is based on economics, convenience, and the special situations under which the surgery is performed. In defense of the practice, the procedure can be performed quickly, and attention is paid to preventing contaminated hands from coming into contact with exposed tissues that are to remain in the calf.

Additional Instrumentation

This procedure requires emasculators.

Surgical Technique

The scrotum is grasped, and a horizontal incision is made through skin and fascia at the widest part of the scrotum (junction of middle and distal thirds). The entire distal segment of the scrotum is transected (Fig. 14-1A), and the common vaginal tunic is left intact. Traction is then placed on the testes, and the skin is pushed proximad so the fascia is separated from the spermatic cords enclosed in the common tunics (Fig. 14-1B). The operator's hands should not touch the proximal regions of the spermatic cords.

The spermatic cords are emasculated (site of emasculation is illustrated in Fig. 14-1*B*). It is important that the emasculators be pushed proximad and that tension on the cord be relaxed when emasculation is performed (Fig. 14-1*C*). Following removal of the emasculators, any redundant adipose tissue is removed (Fig. 14-1*D*). The incision may be sprayed with a topical antibacterial powder, and at the discretion of the operator, this powder may also be put up inside the incision.

Postoperative Management

Concurrent immunization for black leg and malignant edema is recommended. Prior immunization would be preferable, but it is often not practical. The calves should be watched for hemorrhage for approximately 24 hours. Exercise of the calves is important following castration. Infection may occur 5 to 15 days following castration and often occurs beyond the period in which one would normally expect infection. The infection usually takes the form of severe cellulitis and should be treated with drainage and antibiotics.

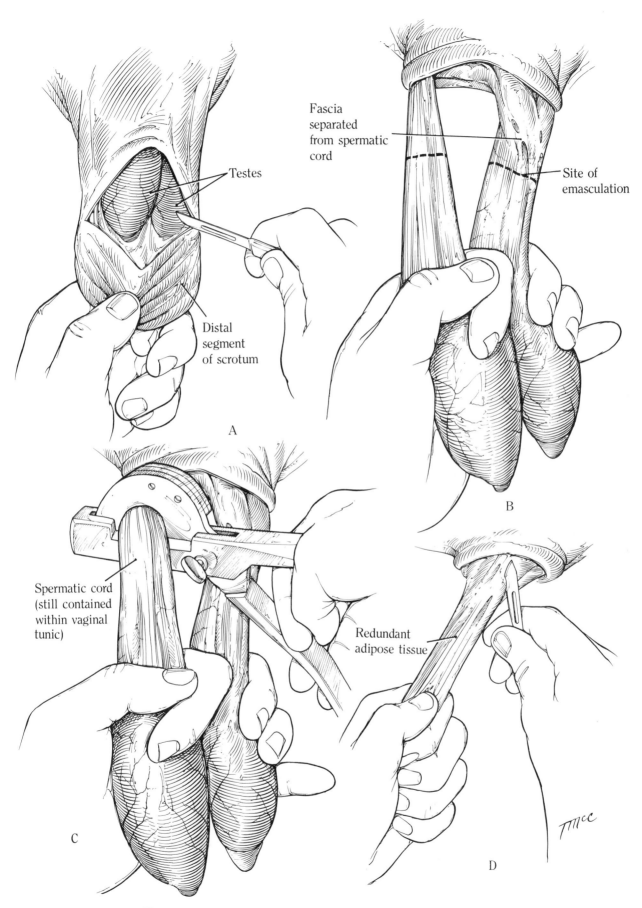

Testes

Fascia
separated
from spermatic
cord

Site of
emasculation

Distal
segment
of scrotum

A

B

Spermatic cord
(still contained
within vaginal
tunic)

Redundant
adipose tissue

C

D

FIG. 14-1. A *to* D, *Calf castration.*

Urethrostomy

Urethrostomy is most commonly performed in steers because of obstruction by urethral calculi. The occurrence of urethral obstruction in steers, as opposed to bulls, is influenced by the smaller diameter of their urethrae. The obstructions may occur at any site, but the most common location is near the distal sigmoid flexure of the penis adjacent to the attachments of the retractor penis muscles.

The chemical composition of the urethral calculi may vary, depending on the steer's diet. Silicate calculi, which are rough and hard, occur in steers grazing stubble and pastures consisting largely of grasses.[1] Phosphate calculi, which are soft, smooth, and often multiple, are more common in steers in feedlots.[2]

Failure to relieve the obstructed urethra results in death from uremia, resulting from rupture of the urinary bladder, or in rupture of the urethra, with attending cellulitis, septicemia, and death. The following technique generally is regarded as a salvage procedure to remove urine. It is usually performed to "buy time" until the animal's condition can be stabilized sufficiently to permit slaughter.

Anesthesia and Surgical Preparation

This surgical procedure is performed using caudal epidural anesthesia with the animal in the standing position or cast in dorsal recumbency. Sometimes xylazine hydrochloride (Rompun) is used for sedation. The positioning of the animal for surgery is determined by the surgeon. The animal may be cast in dorsal recumbency with its legs tied cranially and the surgeon kneeling behind it (Fig. 14-2A). This method may produce unwanted, additional pressure on an already distended urinary bladder. It is preferable to operate on large steers and bulls in the standing position. When the animal is positioned, the surgical site is clipped and is prepared for surgery in a routine manner.

Urethrostomy in steers and bulls may be performed at several sites. If it is performed just ventral to the anus at the level of the floor of the pelvis (high urethrostomy), severe scalding and matting of the escutcheon and medial aspects of the limbs result; generally, the animal is penalized at market with a lower value for slaughter. The other site for urethrostomy is in the region of the distal flexure of the sigmoid flexure of the penis (low urethrostomy). The advantage of the low incision, which we describe, is that the penis can be directed so the urine is forced caudad, away from the medial aspects of the limbs, to reduce damage from urine scald. In addition, an incision in this region is more likely to expose the calculi because they most commonly lodge in this region.

A low urethrostomy may also be performed cranial to the scrotum or scrotal remnant.

Additional Instrumentation

This procedure requires a urinary catheter.

Surgical Technique

The penis is palpated immediately caudal to the remnants of the scrotum (cod). The scrotal remnant is grasped and is stretched craniad, and the distal flexure of the sigmoid flexure is located. A 10-cm skin incision is made on the midline directly over the penis (Fig. 14-2A and B), and blunt dissection is then performed to locate the penis. In Figure 14-2A to G, the patient is in dorsal recumbency. Generally, the penis is deeper than one would anticipate and is a firm fibrous structure about the thickness of the index finger. During the dissection, the surgeon encounters subcutaneous adipose tissue and several layers of elastic tissue surrounding the penis. With traction, a portion of the penis is exposed through the skin incision (Fig. 14-2C). The retractor penis muscles should be identified because they serve as a useful guideline to the location of the ventral surface of the penis. Care should be taken not to twist the penis and thereby to lose the relationship of the retractor penis muscles and ventral surface of the penis. At this point, it may be possible to palpate the calculi in the urethra.

Several options exist at this point, depending on the severity of inflammation of the urethra and surrounding tissues. If inflammation of these structures is minimal and the calculi can be located, a small incision is made directly over the calculus (calculi) on the ventral aspect of the penis (Fig. 14-2D). The calculus (calculi) is then removed. Prior to closure of the urethra, a catheter should be inserted up the urethra, both proximally and distally, to search for further stones and to ensure urethral patency. The urethra may be sutured if there is no urethral necrosis. A catheter may be placed in the urethra to minimize stricture formation during closure. Simple interrupted or simple continuous sutures of an absorbable suture material are inserted. The sutures should go down to, but not through, the urethral mucosa. The penis is replaced into its normal position, and the dorsal third of the skin incision is closed (Fig. 14-2E). The remainder of the incision may be left open to heal by secondary intention.

If there is any necrosis of the urethra and if the urethra's ability to hold sutures is in question, the urethra and skin incisions may be left to heal by secondary intention.

If damage to the penis and surrounding tissues is extensive with rupture of the urethra, transection and extirpation of the penis are performed. The penis is dissected carefully from the dorsal arteries and veins of the penis and is transected to leave an 8- to 12-cm proximal stump (Fig. 14-2F). The length of the penis varies with the size of the patient. From the surgeon's view, the arteries and veins appear ventral to the exposed stump of the penis. These vessels are ligated (some surgeons do not consider this necessary). It is a common error to isolate an insufficient amount of penile stump prior to anchoring it to the skin. The stump should be of sufficient length that when it is sutured to the skin there is no infolding of skin because of excessive tension. The stump of the exposed penis is directed

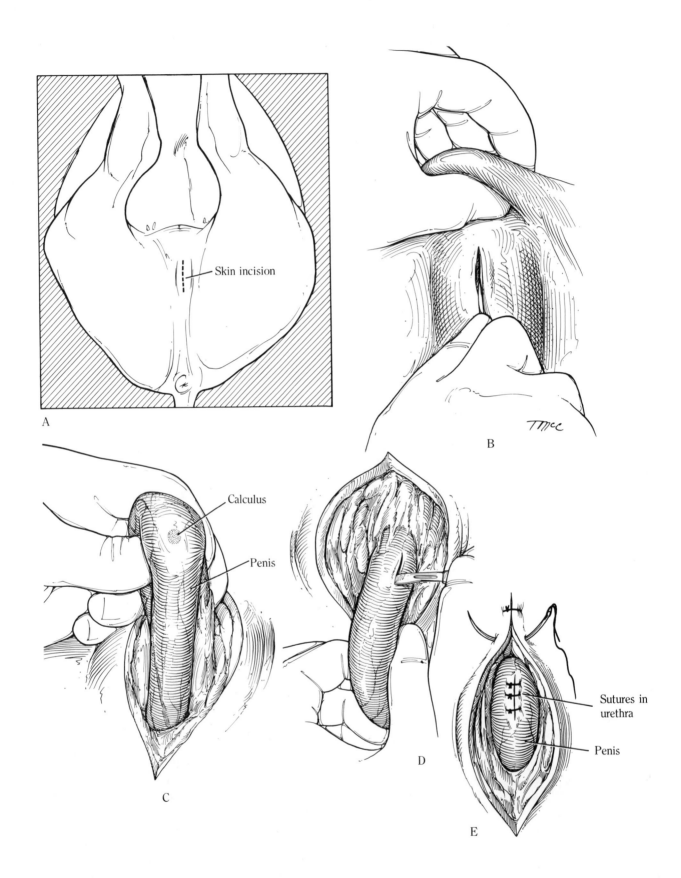

Skin incision

Calculus

Penis

Sutures in
urethra

Penis

A

B

C

D

E

FIG. 14-2. A *to* H, *Urethrostomy.*

caudoventrad and is anchored to the skin and two sutures. The sutures should pass through the skin, tunica albuginea, and corpus cavernosum penis. Care is taken to ensure that the urethral lumen is not compromised. The stump of the penis should not be bent because iatrogenic urethral obstruction may occur. The urethra at the end of the penile stump is split, and the edges are sutured to the lateral aspects of the penis (Fig. 14-2G). This part of the technique is not performed routinely by all surgeons. Figure 14-2H shows a completed urethrostomy with the patient standing.

In animals with urethral obstruction and signs of subcutaneous edema and cellulitis, urethral rupture has usually occurred. The urine accumulation in the tissues causes a violent inflammatory response that may result in sloughing of the skin of the ventral abdomen. To facilitate drainage, the

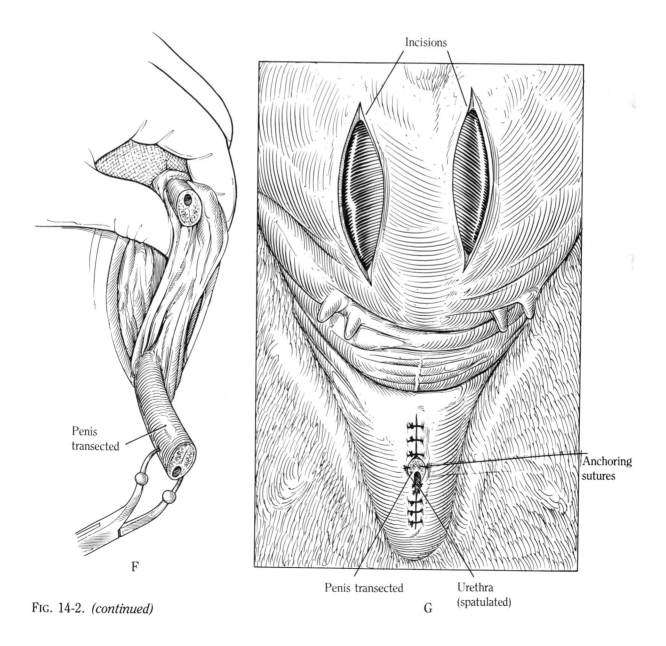

FIG. 14-2. *(continued)*

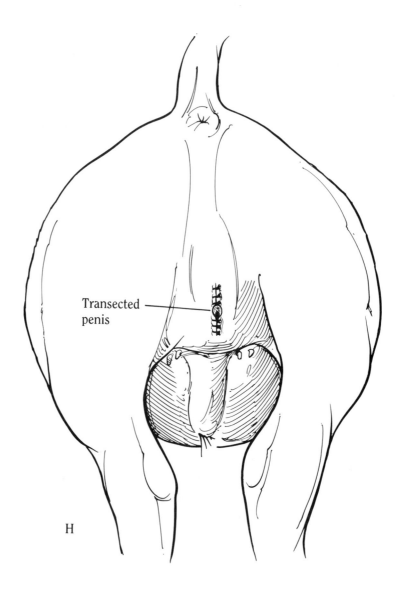

Transected
penis

H

surgeon should make several bold, longitudinal incisions lateral to the prepuce with a scalpel, being careful to avoid the subcutaneous abdominal veins (Fig. 14-2G). This procedure assists in resolution of the inflammatory process.

Postoperative Management

Unless the animal is destined for immediate slaughter, antibiotics should be administered. Other supportive measures, such as intravenous fluids, diuretics, and general therapy for shock, may also be indicated. The animal should be sent to slaughter as soon as it is judged that the carcass would be acceptable.

References

1. Blood, D. C., Henderson, J. A., and Radostits, O. M.: Veterinary Medicine, 5th Ed. Philadelphia, Lea & Febiger, 1980.

2. Walker, D. F.: Penile surgery in the bovine: part I. Mod. Vet. Pract., *60*:839, 1979.

Hematoma Evacuation of the Bovine Penis

The essential defect in hematoma of the penis ("broken penis") is rupture of the tunica albuginea of the penis. The rupture occurs at a predictable location on the dorsal aspect of the distal bend of the sigmoid flexure opposite the insertion of the retractor penis muscles.[3] The size of the defect in the tunica albuginea varies and is probably related to the blood pressure within the corpora cavernosa penis at the time of rupture. The amount of extravasated blood is probably related to the length of time erection is maintained after injury.

The question of whether to treat the hematoma conservatively or surgically is controversial. Generally, the decision for surgery is made on the basis of the size of the hematoma and the length of time elapsed between the accident and treatment. Many patients respond satisfactorily to conservative treatment, and the number of patients now treated surgically is smaller than in previous years. It is believed that, with larger hematomas, more of the peripenile fascial layers are damaged or involved (this may be obvious at surgery); consequently, the incidence of adhesions or the risk of adhesion formation is greater. With a large hematoma, the attachment region of the retractor penis muscles is also involved; if palpation reveals involvement to this extent, surgical treatment will be necessary. Mechanical interference with penile extrusion may be a problem with a large hematoma.

The ideal time for surgery is probably an hour after injury. It is believed that bleeding quickly ceases after relaxation of the penis; therefore, waiting for so-called organization of the hematoma is not necesssary. After 7 to 10 days, extensive granulation and increased fibrosis in the peripenile areas make surgery difficult. Although organization of the fibrous tissue may make the surgery easier after 25 days, as compared to 10 to 25 days, difficulty can still be anticipated.

Anesthesia and Surgical Preparation

The surgery is performed with the animal either sedated with chloral hydrate, cast in lateral recumbency, and with local infiltration (line block) at the surgical site (Fig. 14-3A) or under general anesthesia, if available.

Surgical Technique

A skin incision approximately 13 cm long is made in a cranioventral direction over the most prominent part of the swelling (Fig. 14-3A and B), and this incision is continued through the subcutaneous tissues into the hematoma. Care should be taken not to incise the penis because it may be deflected by the hematoma and may be closer to the skin than anticipated. Care should also be taken to avoid any additional damage to the dorsal nerves of the penis. The clots of the hematoma are removed manually (Fig. 14-3C). In an acute case, the rent in the tunica albuginea is easily identified.

If fibrin deposition and granulation tissue formation have occurred, however, careful dissection through the fascial layers surrounding the penis may be necessary to locate the rent in the tunic (Fig. 14-3D). At this stage, any peripenile adhesions need to be broken down. The penis is grasped firmly, distal to the tunic defect, and all peripenile adhesions are broken down (Fig. 14-3E). With manual rotation of the penis, the retractor penis muscles may be identified, and any adhesions in this area also removed. A nonsterile assistant then grasps the penis through the prepuce and extrudes it, so the surgeon can ascertain the free motion of the penis and can locate any further adhesions.

The edges of the rent in the tunica albuginea are debrided and are sutured with simple interrupted sutures of no. 0 catgut or 0 polyglactin 910 (Vicryl) (Fig. 14-3F). Although secondary-intention healing and fibrous union of the defect would be anticipated without suturing, it is probably preferable to suture the defect because vascular shunts may form between the corpora cavernosa penis and the dorsal vessels.[4] Although a rupture, if it recurs, will probably recur at the same site,[1,3] it is questionable whether suturing the defect will actually reduce the chances of recurrence. Some authors have proposed suturing of the tunica albuginea to be unnecessary.[2] The fascial layers of the penis are not sutured because it is believed that suturing these layers may promote adhesions. The skin is closed with vertical mattress sutures of nonabsorbable material (Fig. 14-3G).

When preputial inflammation, swelling, or prolapse is present and problems with manual retraction of the penis are anticipated postoperatively, an umbilical tape suture is placed through the dorsal aspect of the penis (Fig. 14-3H) and tied. Care should be taken to ensure that the tape is not passed through the urethra. This tape facilitates postoperative manipulation of the penis.

Postoperative Management

Penicillin is administered postoperatively to reduce the possibility of abscess formation after the injury. If extensive swelling of the prepuce is present, it should be reduced by hot packs and bandaging; diuretics may also be appropriate. If the swelling has caused a preputial prolapse, ointment should be applied to the exposed mucosa. The penis is extended daily for 10 days. If the umbilical tape is used for this purpose, care should be taken not to place undue tension on the tape or it may tear out of the penis.

Drainage of a seroma at the surgery site may be necessary, but seromas generally resorb spontaneously. The recommended period of sexual rest appropriate following surgery varies and ranges from 45 days, in the opinion of our contributing author, B. L. Hull, to 6 months.[1] Hull also believes that surgical treatment has a better prognosis (approximately 75% success rate) than conservative treatment (approximately 50% success rate) over a series of cases. That severe cases are selected for surgery more often than mild cases may give an impression of a poorer prognosis, however.

Hematomas may recur when the bulls are returned to service. In this case, the early hematomas are probably associated with tearing of adhesions in the area of the original rupture site; the ones that arise at a later time may be associated with reinjury unrelated to the original rupture. Injury of the dorsal nerves of the penis may cause failure to ejaculate or copulate,

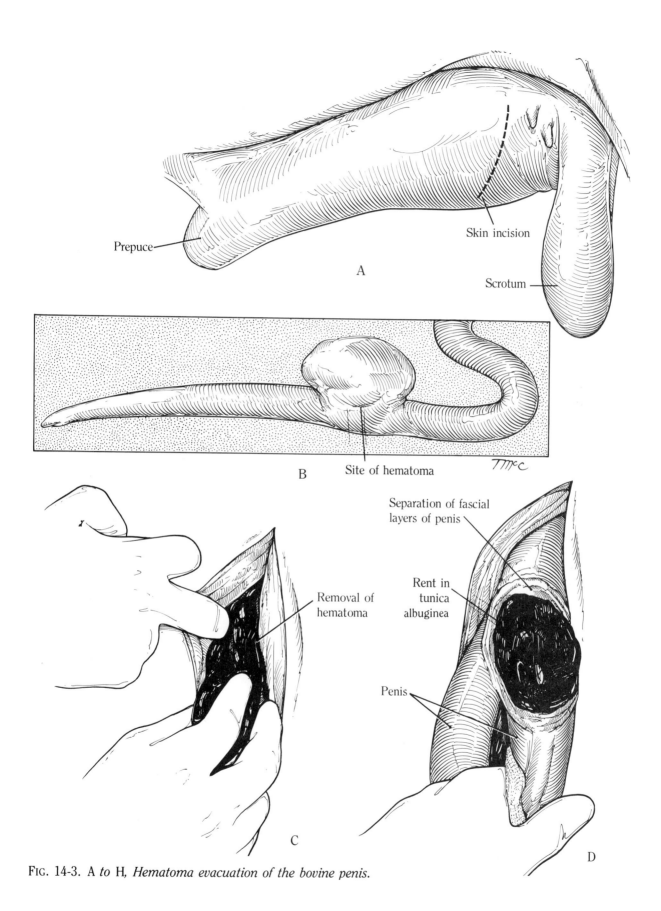

Prepuce

Skin incision

Scrotum

A

Site of hematoma

B

Removal of
hematoma

Separation of fascial
layers of penis

Rent in
tunica
albuginea

Penis

C

D

FIG. 14-3. A *to* H, *Hematoma evacuation of the bovine penis.*

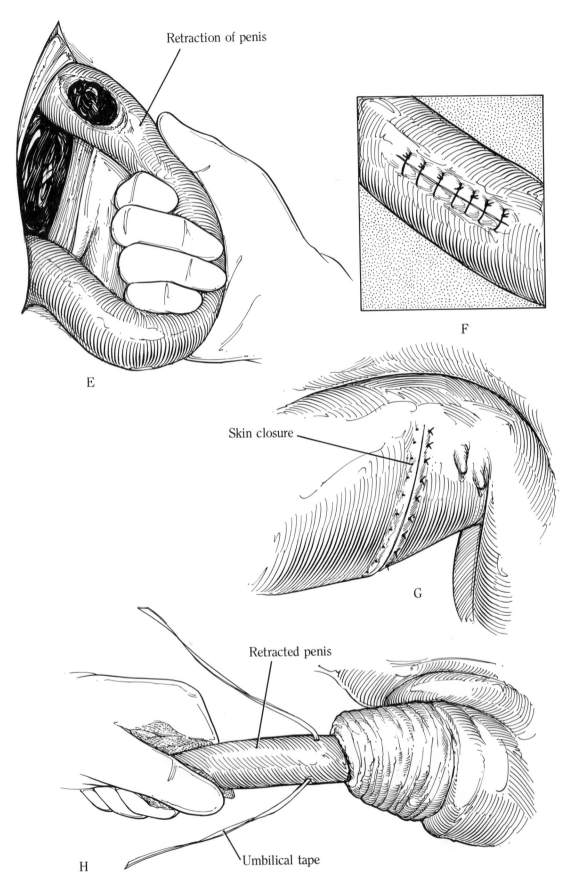

Retraction of penis

E

F

Skin closure

G

Retracted penis

Umbilical tape

H

FIG. 14-3. *(continued)*.

but recoveries up to 18 months later have been observed.[1] Thrombus formation in the corpora cavernosa and formation of vascular shunts have also been proposed as causes of nonerection postoperatively,[3] although these problems also occur following conservative treatment.

References

1. Aanes, W. A.: Personal communication, 1980.

2. Pearson, H.: Surgery of the male genital tract in cattle: a review of 121 cases. Vet. Rec., *91*:498, 1972.

3. Walker, D. F., and Vaughan, J. T.: Bovine and Equine Urogenital Surgery. Philadelphia, Lea & Febiger, 1980.

4. Young, S. L., Hudson, R. S., and Walker, D. F.: Impotence in bulls due to vascular shunts in the corpus cavernosum penis. J. Am. Vet. Med. Assoc., *171*:643, 1977.

Preputial Amputation (Circumcision) in the Bull

Preputial amputation (circumcision) is indicated in selected cases of preputial prolapse with fibrosis and ulceration of the prepuce. The breeds most often affected are the *Bos indicus* breeds (Brahman and Santa Gertrudis) and the polled *Bos taurus* breeds (notably Angus and Polled Hereford).[2] The two reasons advanced for the breed differences are a pendulous sheath and the absence of the retractor muscles of the prepuce in the polled breeds.[1,3] Protrusion of the parietal preputial lining followed by trauma or other irritation may produce inflammatory changes that ultimately prevent retraction of the prepuce.[1] Conservative treatment may be successful, but prolapse frequently recurs and eventually leads to chronic prolapse that requires surgical treatment. Prophylactic circumcision is also practiced in some areas.

Anesthesia and Surgical Preparation

Presurgical conservative treatment is usually necessary to reduce swelling and to improve the condition of the tissue. Prior to surgery, fibrosis and edema are reduced to a minimal level, decreasing the risk of postoperative infection and failure. Feed is withheld from the bull 24 hours prior to surgery. Surgery is performed with the bull in right-lateral recumbency, either under general anesthesia or with a combination of chloral hydrate sedation and local analgesia. The surgical area is prepared for aseptic surgery in a routine manner.

Surgical Technique

The prolapsed portion of the prepuce to be resected is extended with the left hand, the index finger of which is placed inside the prepuce (the line of amputation is indicated in Fig. 14-4A). Note that the amputation line is oblique, rather than transverse, so the resulting orifice is oval, rather than circular. This precaution reduces the danger of phimosis developing during healing. A row of horizontal mattress sutures of no. 2 polyglactin 910 (Vicryl) is placed around the prolapse immediately proximal to the proposed line of amputation (Figs. 14-4A and B). The sutures are placed in such a manner that they overlap one another around the entire circumference and are passed from the exposed preputial membrane completely through to the preputial cavity and back through both layers of the prepuce (Fig. 14-4B). These sutures are tied tightly, and the prepuce is amputated just distal to the suture line (Fig. 14-4C). The preputial edges are then apposed with a simple continuous pattern suture line using 0 polyglactin 910 (Fig. 14-4D).

It is convenient for the surgeon to perform this procedure on half of the prepuce at a time. The completed amputation (circumcision) is illustrated in Figure 14-4E.

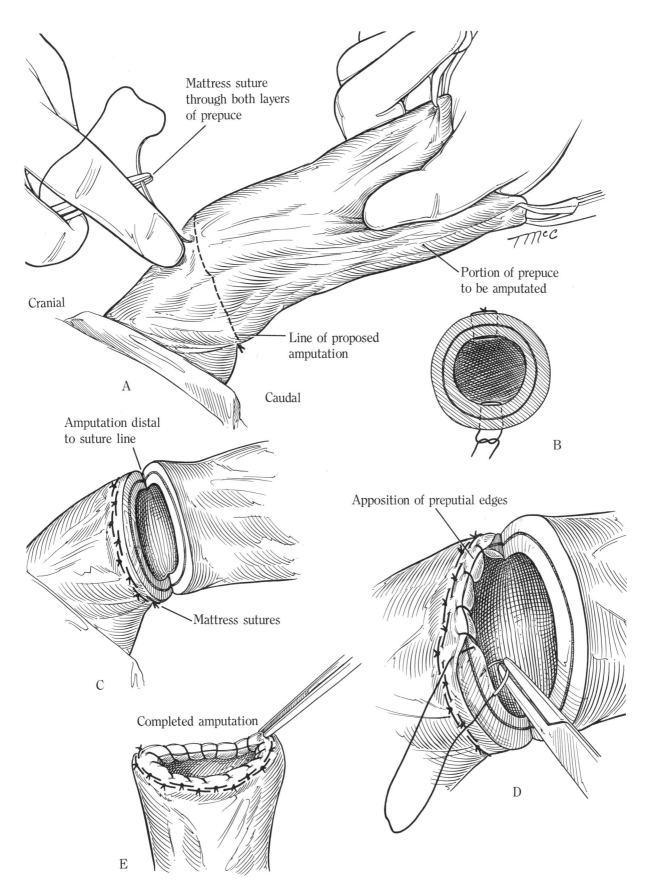

Mattress suture
through both layers
of prepuce

Portion of prepuce
to be amputated

Cranial

Line of proposed
amputation

Caudal

A

B

Amputation distal
to suture line

Apposition of preputial edges

Mattress sutures

C

D

Completed amputation

E

FIG. 14-4. A to E, Preputial amputation (circumcision) in the bull.

Postoperative Management

The bull is placed on antibiotics, and the preputial cavity is infused daily with antibacterial agents until healing is complete. The tissue distal to the encircling mattress sutures ultimately sloughs, but it is believed that the use of a second layer of sutures to close the preputial edges promotes wound healing.

Comments

This technique of amputation is less successful in European (*Bos taurus*) breeds because the preputial membrane is too short. The loss of preputial membrane following surgery may prevent adequate extension of the penis to allow breeding. In less-severe cases, preputial prolapse may be treated by conservative resection of the preputial membrane (reefing) and suturing the healthy internal preputial membrane near the preputial orifice. A V-shaped incision pattern is used to reduce the danger of stenosis. Larsen and Bellenger point out that circumcision results in the loss of equal amounts of the external and internal linings of the prolapsed portion of the prepuce even though the internal lining is frequently not seriously involved in the inflammatory process.[2] These authors advocate conservative resection, to preserve as much of the unaffected inner lining of the prolapsed prepuce as possible and thereby to increase the bull's chances of returning to service.

A technique for amputation of the prolapsed prepuce that is claimed to have advantages for the practitioner with limited facilities involves the insertion of a plastic ring into the preputial cavity.[4] The ring is fixed with sutures and a tourniquet-like effect is produced; the prolapsed portion is sloughed in 1 to 2 weeks.

References

1. Arthur, G. H.: Wright's Veterinary Obstetrics, 4th Ed. Philadelphia, Lea & Febiger, 1975.

2. Larsen, L. H., and Bellenger, C. R.: Surgery of the prolapsed prepuce in the bull: its complications and dangers. Aust. Vet. J., *47*:349, 1971.

3. Long, S. E., and Hignett, P. G.: Preputial eversion in the bull: a comparative study of prepuces from bulls which evert and those which do not. Vet. Rec., *86*:161, 1970.

4. Walker, D. F., and Vaughan, J. T.: Bovine and Equine Urogenital Surgery. Philadelphia, Lea & Febiger, 1980.

Teaser Bull Preparation by Penile Translocation

The role of teaser bulls for the detection of heat in cattle is uncertain. It is possible to use steers that have had testosterone administered to them; in addition, the increased use of prostaglandins may obviate the need for teaser bulls in an artificial breeding program. In the meantime, various techniques have been developed to render the bull sterile or incapable of coitus. The techniques that render the bull incapable of coitus seem to be more acceptable. In this chapter, we describe two popular techniques, penile translocation and penile fixation. As a precaution, these techniques should be accompanied by a sterilization procedure, such as bilateral caudal epididymectomy, which is also described in this chapter.[1]

Anesthesia and Surgical Preparation

This surgical procedure is performed with the animal under general anesthesia or heavy sedation and local analgesia. The bull is placed in dorsal recumbency and is tilted with its left side uppermost. A large area of the midline and ventral left-flank area, including the preputial orifice, is clipped and is prepared for aseptic surgery in a routine manner.

Additional Instrumentation

This procedure requires sponge forceps, a sterile rubber glove, a plastic sleeve, and a tube for insertion within the prepuce to prevent urine contamination.

Surgical Technique

The incision sites are illustrated in Figure 14-5A. A skin incision is made around the preputial orifice approximately 3 cm from the opening, and a ventral midline skin incision is extended caudad from this. The midline incision extends to the base of the penis (Fig. 14-5A). This incision is continued through the subcutaneous tissue, and the penis, prepuce, and surrounding elastic tissue are dissected free from the abdominal wall in preparation for translocation (Fig. 14-5B). A tube placed within the preputial orifice helps to delineate the prepuce during dissection and may also help to prevent urine contamination of the surgical area during surgery. During the dissection, it is important to maintain the integrity of the blood supply of the penis. Bleeding is controlled by ligation.

A circular skin incision is then made in the ventral left-flank area where the preputial orifice is to be moved (Fig. 14-5B). Using a pair of sponge forceps, a tunnel is made from the circular incision through the subcutaneous tissues to the caudal end of the midline incision (Fig. 14-5C). This tunnel must be large enough to permit the relocation of the penis and prepuce without restriction. A sterile rubber glove or plastic sleeve is placed over the preputial orifice (Fig. 14-5D). This prevents contamination of the subcutis from the preputial orifice as it is drawn through the tunnel. If a tube had been positioned previously within the preputial orifice, it is removed at this stage. The penis and prepuce are drawn through the tunnel, and the skin of the preputial orifice is sutured to the circular skin incision (Fig. 14-5E). Two layers of sutures are placed here: one in the subcutaneous tissue, and one in the skin. Before suturing is performed, it is also important to ascertain that no twisting has occurred during the translocation process. This possibility can be prevented by preplacing an identifying suture in the skin of the prepuce prior to its removal (Fig. 14-5B). The ventral midline incision is then closed with nonabsorbable sutures. Although closely placed simple interrupted sutures are illustrated in Figure 15-5E, an argument can be made for bringing the edges together with widely spaced sutures and allowing drainage. It is believed that the latter technique eliminates the problem of postoperative edema.

Because of the excess skin and pendulous sheath in Indian breeds of cattle, it is possible to transpose the penis and prepuce along with the encircling skin, rather than to dissect the penis and prepuce free from the skin.

Postoperative Management

Antibiotics may be administered at the discretion of the surgeon, and the skin sutures are removed in 10 days. The animals are not put into work for 4 to 6 weeks.

Comments

The long-term results of most techniques for teaser bull preparation have been criticized. The various charges against different techniques generally have not taken into account the probability of varying libido among bulls, however.

Reference

1. Walker, D. F., and Vaughan, J. T.: Bovine and Equine Urogenital Surgery. Philadelphia, Lea & Febiger, 1980.

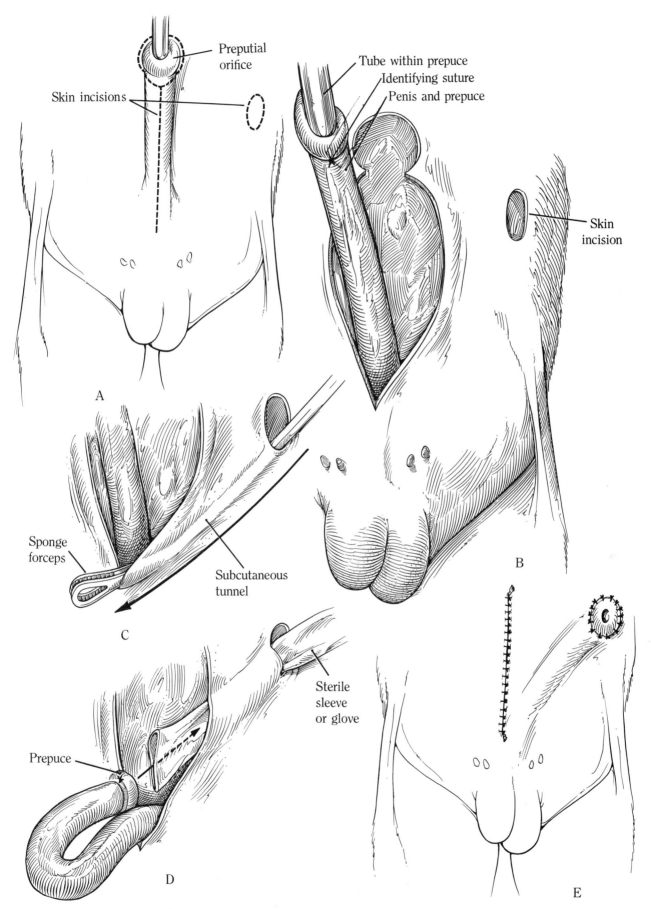

Preputial orifice

Skin incisions

Tube within prepuce
Identifying suture
Penis and prepuce

Skin incision

A

Sponge forceps

Subcutaneous tunnel

B

C

Prepuce

Sterile sleeve or glove

D

E

FIG. 14-5. A *to* E, *Teaser bull preparation by penile translocation.*

Teaser Bull Preparation by Penile Fixation

It has been reported that teaser bulls prepared by penile translocation can occasionally serve a cow. Considering this possibility, we also describe the method of penile fixation, which produces an adhesion of the penis to the lower abdominal wall that prevents protrusion of the penis.[1]

Anesthesia and Surgical Preparation

This surgical procedure is usually performed with the animal tranquilized and under local anesthesia. The surgery can be done on a commercially manufactured operating table, if one is available, or it can be done with the animal cast in lateral recumbency. If done on the floor with the animal in lateral recumbency, the patient's feet must be tied for the safety of the surgeon. The ventral abdominal wall from the end of the sheath to the base of the scrotum is clipped and is prepared for aseptic surgery. A line block of local anesthesia (about 30 ml) is placed along a line where the sheath joins the body wall and about midway between the end of the sheath and the base of the scrotum (Fig. 14-6A).

Surgical Technique

A 10-cm longitudinal incision is made midway between the end of the prepuce and the base of the scrotum at the junction of the prepuce and the ventral body wall (about 2 cm lateral to the midline) (Fig. 14-6A). This incision is made through the skin, subcutaneous tissue, and cutaneous trunci muscle. Blunt dissection through the loose connective tissue brings one to the dorsal surface of the penis. At this point, it is important to identify the urethra (urethral groove) within the penis. If the penis has not been rotated during the surgery, the urethral groove should be on the ventral surface of the penis. Because one must always be aware of the urethra during this procedure, it is often helpful to place a towel clamp around the urethra and its adjacent portion of the penis. This serves to identify the urethra and also as a traction device.

The penis is exteriorized through the incision, and the preputial reflection is identified. The dorsal surface of the penis is cleared of its elastic tunics commencing at the preputial reflection and extending caudad for about 10 cm. This exposes tough fibrous tunica albuginea. Once tunica albuginea has been exposed, the linea alba is cleared of all of its loose connective tissue. The tunica albuginea of the dorsal surface of the penis is now apposed to the linea alba. Before placing the sutures, one should be sure that the glans penis and prepuce are not protruding through the preputial orifice. No. 3 multifilament synthetic sutures (Braunamid) are placed through the dorsal third of the penis (Fig. 14-6B) and then through the linea alba. This suture apposes the linea alba and tunica albuginea (Fig. 14-6C). Figure 14-6D illustrates in cross section the placement of the sutures.

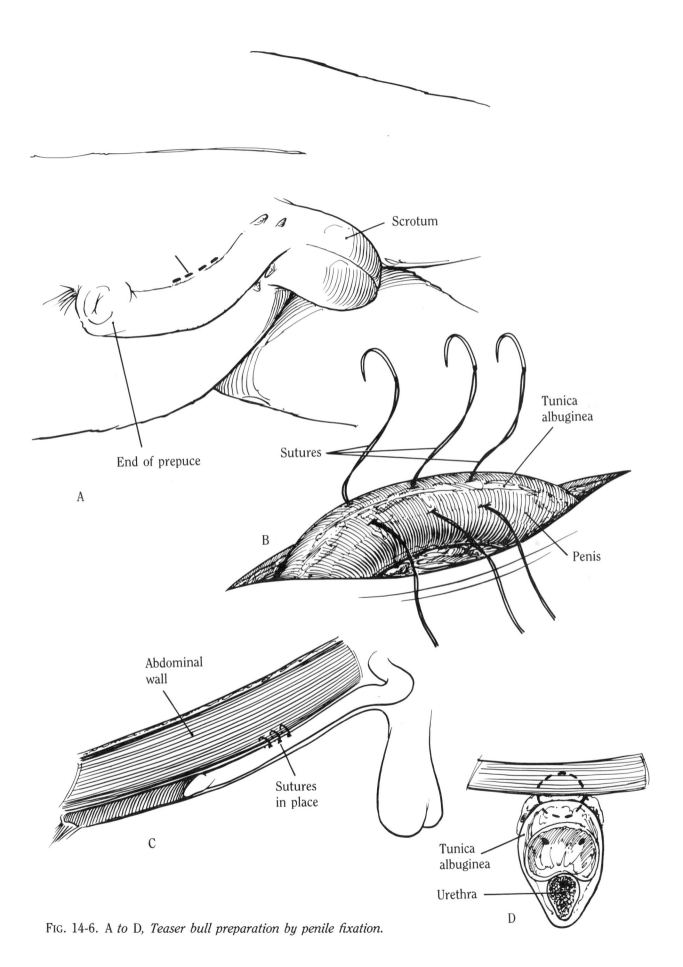

Scrotum

End of prepuce

A

Sutures

Tunica
albuginea

Penis

B

Abdominal
wall

Sutures
in place

C

Tunica
albuginea

Urethra

D

FIG. 14-6. A *to* D, *Teaser bull preparation by penile fixation.*

Care should be taken not to enter the preputial reflection and not to involve the urethra, to avoid iatrogenic urethral obstruction. Usually, three interrupted sutures are adequately placed about 1 to 2 cm apart. It is helpful to preplace these sutures and then to tie them simultaneously. The skin is closed with no. 3 multifilament synthetic suture.

This technique results in a permanent adhesion between the tunica albuginea and the linea alba. Ideally, the bull should have 2 to 3 weeks of sexual rest before use, to allow this adhesion to develop.

Postoperative Management

Antibiotics may be administered at the discretion of the surgeon, and the skin sutures are removed in 2 to 3 weeks.

Comments

Successful results using this technique have been reported.[2] Potential complications include suture breakdown (if catgut is used), seroma formation, and insufficient retraction of the penis. Weight loss is also observed.[2]

The long-term results of many techniques of teaser bull preparation have been criticized. If the economics of wintering a nonproductive unit (teaser bull) and the higher libido of the younger animal are considered, however, one should consider making a new teaser bull every year about 30 days before the breeding season.

References

1. Belling, T. H.: Preparation of a "teaser" bull for use in beef cattle artificial insemination program. J. Am. Vet. Med. Assoc., *138*:670, 1961.

2. Hoffsis, G., and Maurer, L. M.: Evaluation of the penis tie-down method to prepare teaser bulls. Bovine Pract., *11*:78, 1976.

Epididymectomy for Teaser Bull Preparation

Caudal epididymectomy is a technique to sterilize teaser bulls. In the past, it was commonly used as a sole procedure. It has been claimed, however, that these bulls often develop seminal vesiculitis or infections of the accessory genitalia, and they still ejaculate fluid from these glands during copulation. At present, the technique is used more often as insurance for one of the techniques that render the bull incapable of copulation.

Anesthesia and Surgical Preparation

Generally, this surgical procedure is performed with the animal standing in a chute. The distal area of the scrotum is clipped and is prepared for surgery in a routine manner. Local infiltration of analgesia is administered over the tail of the epididymis.

Surgical Technique

The testis is forced manually to the distal segment of the scrotum, and a 3-cm skin incision made over the tail of the epididymis. This incision is continued through the common vaginal tunic until the tail of the epididymis is extruded (Fig. 14-7A). The tail of the epididymis is dissected free from its attachment to the testis using scissors (Fig. 14-7B). The ductus deferens is identified, clamped with forceps, and a ligature of nonabsorbable suture material is placed proximal to the forceps (Fig. 14-7C). The ductus deferens is then transected at the level of the clamp. This procedure is repeated in the body of the epididymis so that the tail of the epididymis may be removed (Fig. 14-7C).

The common vaginal tunic is closed in a separate layer using simple interrupted sutures of absorbable material, so the remaining part of the epididymis is retained within the tunic, but the transected end of the ductus deferens protrudes through the suture line (Fig. 14-7D). The technique is an added precaution against reanastomosis of the reproductive tract. The skin is closed with two to three interrupted sutures of nonabsorbable material. The procedure is repeated on the other testis.

Postoperative Management

Antibiotics are not administered routinely. The bull may be placed in work in 3 weeks if epididymectomy is the only procedure performed. If placed in work earlier, however, the bull should be ejaculated prior to this for semen evaluation, to ensure the bull is sterile before use. Such measures are advised as liability precautions.

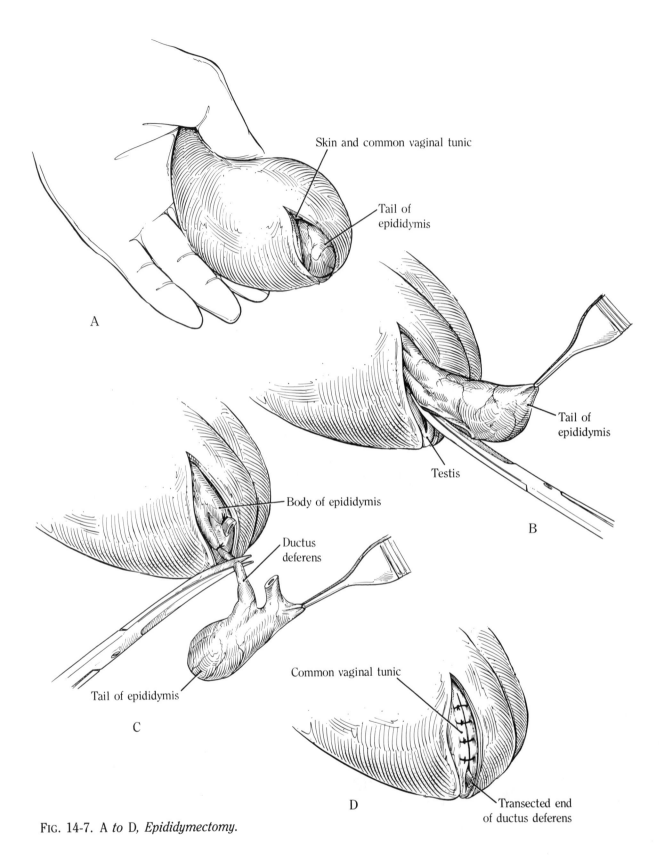

Skin and common vaginal tunic

Tail of
epididymis

A

Tail of
epididymis

Testis

B

Body of epididymis

Ductus
deferens

Tail of epididymis

C

Common vaginal tunic

Transected end
of ductus deferens

D

FIG. 14-7. A *to* D, *Epididymectomy.*

Inguinal Herniorrhaphy in the Mature Bull

The condition must be distinguished from adipose tissue, which occupies the inguinal canal of bulls in good condition, including those prepared for show purposes.[3] The hernia, which usually contains small intestine, occasionally omentum, or both, can be verified by rectal palpation of intestine and omentum passing through the ring. A definitive diagnosis of inguinal hernia cannot be made simply by palpating the scrotum, because many bulls have external deposits of adipose tissue in this region. Sometimes, deposits of adipose tissue are seen with inguinal hernia, and the hernia itself is initiated by a protrusion of subperitoneal adipose tissue through the inguinal ring.[3] Some form of trauma may also be responsible for initiation of an inguinal hernia.[1]

Inguinal hernias in the bull occur with greater frequency on the left side and are generally unilateral (Figure 14-8A shows the external appearance of a left-sided inguinal hernia). If the hernia involves a loop of bowel that does not extend down to the level of the testis, it is termed an inguinal hernia. If the bowel extends down to a position beside the testis, it is termed a scrotal hernia. An indirect hernia occurs when the intestinal loops are contained within the tunica vaginalis, whereas a direct hernia occurs when the hernial sac is separate and cranial to the vaginal ring. Most hernias in the bull are indirect, but direct hernias are also seen.[1]

Additional Instrumentation

This procedure requires sterile umbilical tape 3 mm wide.

Anesthesia and Surgical Preparation

This surgical procedure is best performed with the animal under general anesthesia and in lateral recumbency, with its hind quarters slightly elevated to aid in reduction of the hernia (Fig. 14-8B). The uppermost hind limb is secured in an upward direction and caudad, to improve exposure of the surgical area. A less-satisfactory alternative is sedation with chloral hydrate or xylazine hydrochloride supplemented with local anesthesia (see Chap. 2). The inguinal area is clipped and is prepared for aseptic surgery in a routine manner. The surgical site is draped.

Surgical Technique

A 15- to 25-cm horizontal incision is made through the skin and subcutaneous tissue over the external ring at the base of the scrotum, and hemostasis is maintained by ligation of blood vessels. A blood-free field assists progression of the surgery. Blunt dissection is performed down to the external inguinal ring, to free the common vaginal tunic from the surrounding tissue. The boundaries of the ring are isolated.

If the hernia has reduced itself when the bull is positioned for surgery, then it is not necessary to incise the common vaginal tunic (Fig. 14-8C). If adhesions of the viscera have occurred within the scrotum, then it is necessary to incise the common vaginal tunic to reduce the hernia. An incision is made through the common vaginal tunic parallel to the spermatic cord and cranial to the external cremaster muscle. The hernial contents are examined, and any adhesions are broken down. Occasionally, adhesions are so severe that circulation to intestines has been compromised and intestinal resection is required. These bulls are usually presented to the surgeon on an emergency basis for intestinal obstruction. The bowel is replaced into the abdominal cavity once one has ensured that no adhesions are present at the external inguinal ring.

If the hernia is direct, located cranial to the neck of the scrotum, the subcutaneous tissue is separated, revealing the hernial contents. Adhesions are broken down to enable reduction of the hernia.

The hernial ring is repaired using sterile double 1/8-in. umbilical tape (or any heavy, nonabsorbable suture material) in a simple interrupted pattern. The aim of suturing is to reduce the size of the external inguinal ring so reherniation does not occur. Generally, two or three sutures in the cranial aspect of the ring are required. The sutures are tied, but are not placed under excessive tension. The spermatic cord should be positioned in the caudomedial part of the canal. The remaining ring should be of sufficient size to allow the contents of the spermatic cord to pass freely, yet prevent recurrence of the hernia. As a rule of thumb, there should be enough room for the spermatic cord and one finger. Naturally, hooking any portion of the spermatic cord with the sutures should be avoided. The first suture to be placed is the one closest to the spermatic cord, and it is generally placed about 1 cm from the spermatic cord through the medial and lateral edge of the external inguinal ring (Fig. 14-8D). The sutures, which do not penetrate the peritoneum, are all preplaced by leaving the ends long and clamping the free ends with forceps. Then the sutures are tied (Fig. 14-8E).

If the common vaginal tunic is entered to reduce the hernia, it is closed using fine (0 or 00) absorbable suture material in a simple continuous pattern.

Subcutaneous closure is performed using no. 1 or 2 chromic catgut (Fig. 14-8F). The use of a Penrose drain is indicated because of the considerable amount of dead space. The skin is closed using a synthetic monofilament suture in a simple interrupted pattern (Fig. 14-8G).

Postoperative Management

Generally, antibiotics are not indicated unless there is a break in aseptic technique or intestinal resection is performed. Considerable postoperative swelling generally occurs within 24 to 48 hours. Swelling is more severe if adhesions were present. This swelling usually responds to hydrotherapy (hot) and exercise.

The bull is confined to a clean stall for 4 weeks following surgery, and exercise should be limited for about 8 weeks. The bull should not be used for breeding for 3 to 6 months, pending the result of semen evaluation.

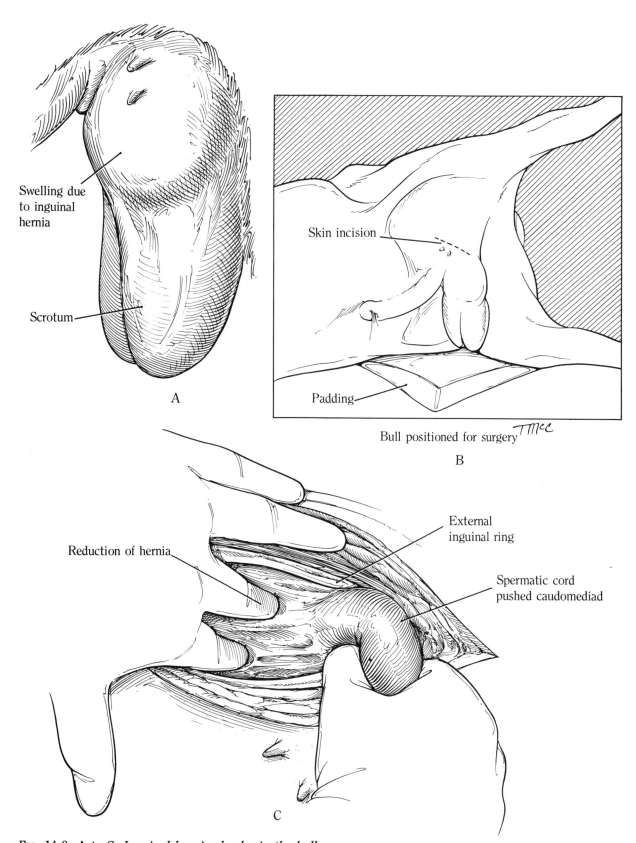

Swelling due to inguinal hernia

Scrotum

A

Skin incision

Padding

Bull positioned for surgery TMcc

B

Reduction of hernia

External inguinal ring

Spermatic cord pushed caudomediad

C

FIG. 14-8. A *to* G, *Inguinal herniorrhaphy in the bull.*

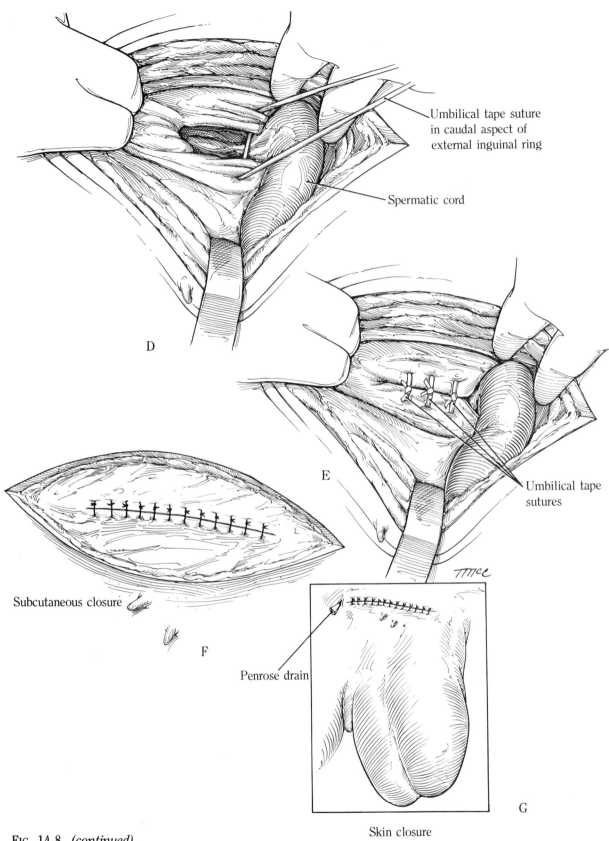

Umbilical tape suture
in caudal aspect of
external inguinal ring

Spermatic cord

D

E

Umbilical tape
sutures

Subcutaneous closure

F

Penrose drain

Skin closure

G

FIG. 14-8. *(continued)*.

Comments

The most outstanding advantage of this method is that, if adhesions are present, they can be broken down and the affected bowel freed. A small survey of nine bulls admitted to the Colorado State University Veterinary Teaching Hospital for inguinal hernia repair showed that five of the nine had adhesions. These five bulls required incisions into their common vaginal tunics to reduce the hernias.

Another method of repair of inguinal hernia in the bull involves a flank laparotomy.[2] The hernia is reduced by the removal of viscera from the vaginal ring, and long, sterile, nonabsorbable suture material, such as umbilical tape, is introduced into the abdominal cavity and is placed in the inguinal ring. Care is taken not to strangulate the spermatic cord as it passes through the vaginal ring. If adhesions are present, this method will not be successful. Moreover, placing sutures is awkward because of the constant presence of abdominal viscera at the surgical site.

References

1. Aanes, W. A.: Personal communication, 1980.

2. Frank, E. R.: Veterinary Surgery, 7th Ed. Minneapolis, Burgess, 1964.

3. Walker, D. F., and Vaughan, J. T.: Bovine and Equine Urogenital Surgery. Philadelphia, Lea & Febiger, 1980.

Cesarean Section in the Cow

Cesarean section is indicated in various types of dystocia, including those caused by relative fetal oversize when the pelvic inlet in young heifers is too small to allow delivery, deformities of the maternal pelvis, fetal monsters, induration of the cervix, fetal malposition, hydrops amnii and allantois, uterine torsion, and emphysematous fetuses. In many cases, the choice between fetotomy or cesarean section may depend on the operator's relative experience with either technique. Case selection is also important. The cow that has suffered a long period of fetal manipulation or attempts at fetotomy and is systemically compromised is not a candidate for cesarean section.

Different approaches are indicated in various dystocia situations.[2] The left paralumbar or flank approach is the standard incision for a viable or recently expired, uncontaminated fetus and a cow capable of tolerating surgery while standing. In some situations, right-flank laparotomy is indicated if there is marked distention of the rumen or when clinical examination dictates that removal from the right side would be more convenient. For example, an oversized fetus situated in the right side of the abdominal cavity would be difficult to remove by left-flank incision. In the routine case, however, the left-flank incision is more convenient because fewer problems with encroaching intestines are encountered.

In the case of a dead and emphysematous fetus, a ventral approach should be used. A ventral paramedian incision, the most common ventral approach, requires the cow to be placed in dorsal recumbency. An alternative is the ventrolateral oblique approach, which may be performed with the animal in lateral recumbency. Both techniques reduce contamination of the peritoneum, which may occur during removal of the emphysematous, contaminated fetus and its associated debris. The ventral approaches are also indicated if the animal is recumbent and is considered incapable of standing during surgery or if the animal is so unmanageable that it is too dangerous for the operator to stand beside the patient during surgery.

Anesthesia and Surgical Preparation

Cesarean section in the cow is performed with the animal under local analgesia. If the flank approach is used, a paravertebral block, inverted L block, or a line block may be used. For the paramedian approach, a high epidural, inverted L block, or line block may be used. Casting with a rope, with or without sedation, is a supplementary restraint for cows in which a ventral approach is used. The surgical area is clipped and is prepared for aseptic surgery in a routine manner.

Surgical Technique

The approaches for flank laparotomy and ventral paramedian laparotomy are described in Chapter 13. Cesarean section has its peculiarities, however.

In the flank approach, the incision is usually made more ventrally in the flank (Fig. 14-9*A*). The ventral paramedian incision for cesarean section (Fig. 14-9*B*) is midway between the midline and the subcutaneous abdominal vein and extends from the umbilicus caudad to the mammary gland (compared to the ventral paramedian incision for abomasopexy, which extends from the umbilicus craniad to the xiphoid process).

Following entrance into the peritoneal cavity, the surgeon manipulates a portion of the uterine horn containing the fetus and attempts to exteriorize an area for hysterotomy (exteriorization is often not possible). Often it is helpful to grasp a leg within the uterus and to use it as a handle to lift the uterus. The uterine incision is usually made over a limb, but in certain malpositions, the area over the head may be incised. The uterus should not be incised over a limb that is in the body of the uterus, but rather, as close to the tip of the horn as possible. This technique allows the uterine horn to be exteriorized for suturing (incisions near the body of the uterus must be sutured within the abdominal cavity).

Figure 14-9*C* depicts exteriorization of an appropriate part of the uterus through a flank incision. Such exteriorization would not be possible with a swollen, emphysematous fetus. In these cases, the need for a ventral approach in which the uterus can be apposed more closely to the incision is obvious. When the uterus is positioned satisfactorily, it is incised (Fig. 14-9*C*). The incision needs to be long enough to allow removal of the fetus without further tearing or extending of the uterine incision. The incision should be made parallel to the long axis of the uterus and on its greater curvature because this area has the fewest large vessels. An attempt should also be made to avoid incising caruncles. The fetus is then removed; the surgeon attempts to retain the uterus so the fetal fluids do not fall back into the peritoneal cavity (Fig. 14-9*D*). Although not depicted in Figure 14-9*D*, chains are commonly attached to the limb(s) of the calf to assist in its delivery from the uterus.

Antibiotic boluses are inserted into the uterus prior to its closure. The uterus is closed with a continuous inverting pattern and absorbable suture material. The Utrecht method of uterine closure is presented here and is illustrated in Figure 14-9*E* to *N*. This technique was developed at the University of Utrecht, the Netherlands, as part of a study to improve the fertility of cattle following cesarean section.[1] It was noted that adhesions often developed between the uterus and visceral organs and originated most often at the ends of the incision where exposed knots were tied; adhesions also developed along the suture line when suture patterns were exposed. Moreover, uterine healing occurred across the wound edges, rather than on the apposed peritoneal surfaces, and the inflammatory response varied with the suture material. The Utrecht method of suturing was developed as a result of these findings.

The starting knot is made using oblique bites (Fig. 14-9*E* and *F*), to bury the knot within the inverted suture (Fig. 14-9*G*). Similarly, the continuous suture pattern is inserted using oblique bites (Fig. 14-9*H* to *J*), so there is minimal exposure of suture material but close apposition of the wound edges. Figure 14-9*K* to *N* depicts the insertion and tying of the final knot so that it is not exposed. Using the Utrecht method, fertility rates improved from 75 to 92%. One surprising feature was that no. 6 nonchromic catgut

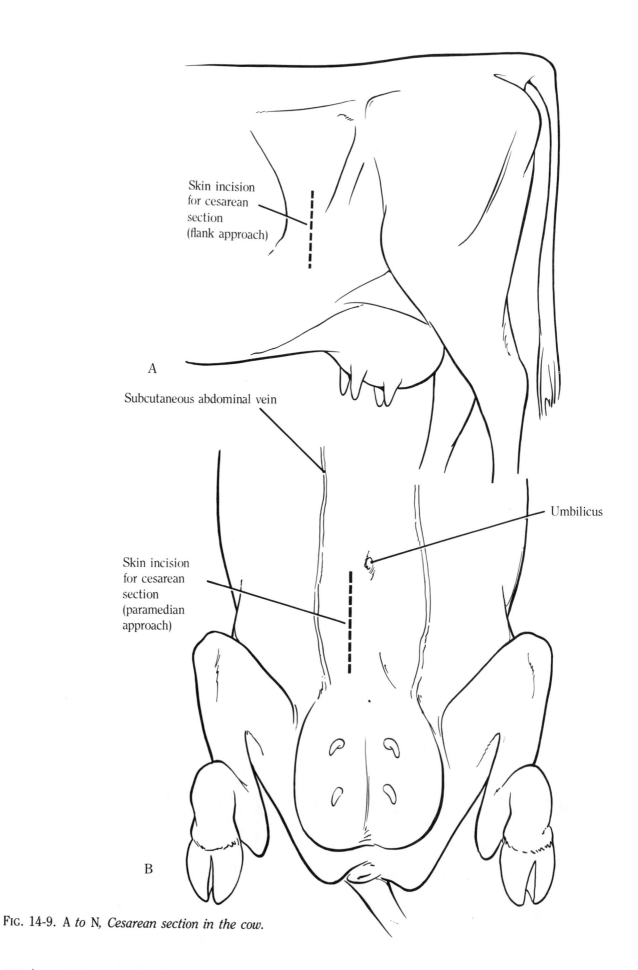

Skin incision
for cesarean
section
(flank approach)

A

Subcutaneous abdominal vein

Umbilicus

Skin incision
for cesarean
section
(paramedian
approach)

B

FIG. 14-9. A *to* N, *Cesarean section in the cow.*

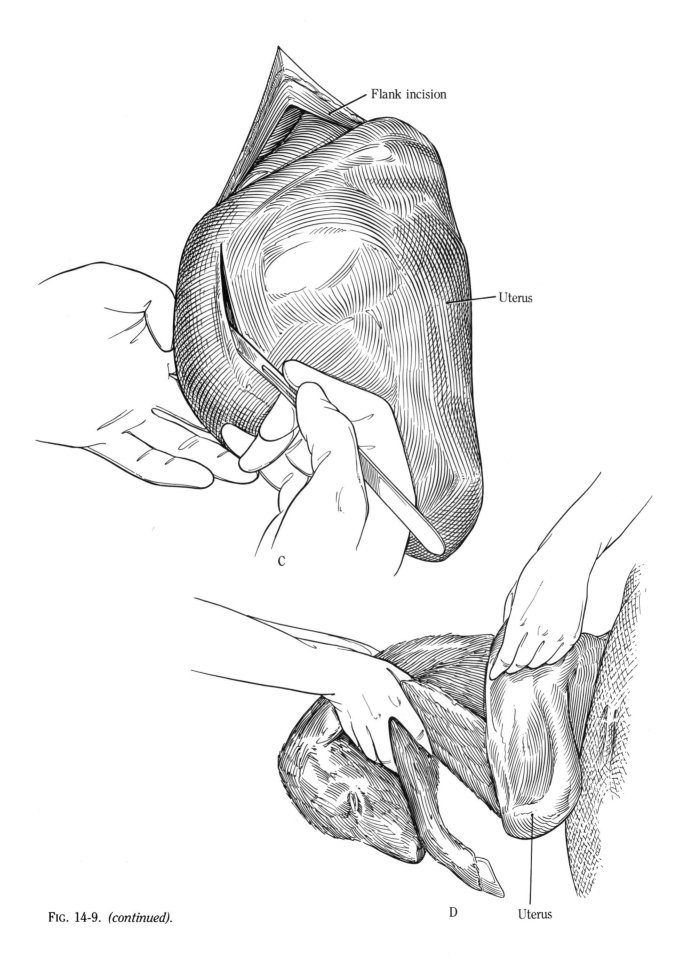

Flank incision

Uterus

C

Uterus

D

FIG. 14-9. *(continued).*

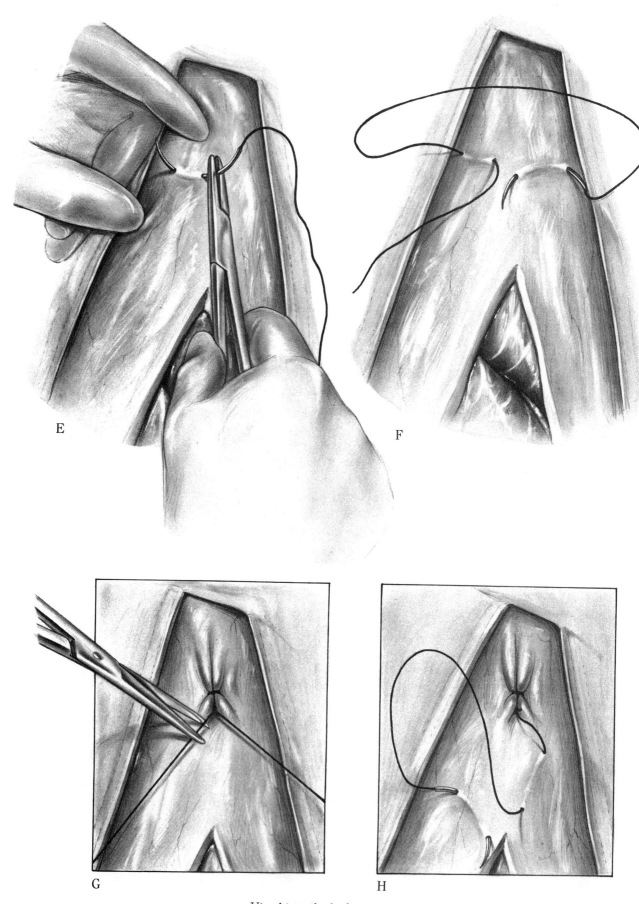

E

F

G

H

Utrecht method of uterine closure

Fig. 14-9. *(continued)*.

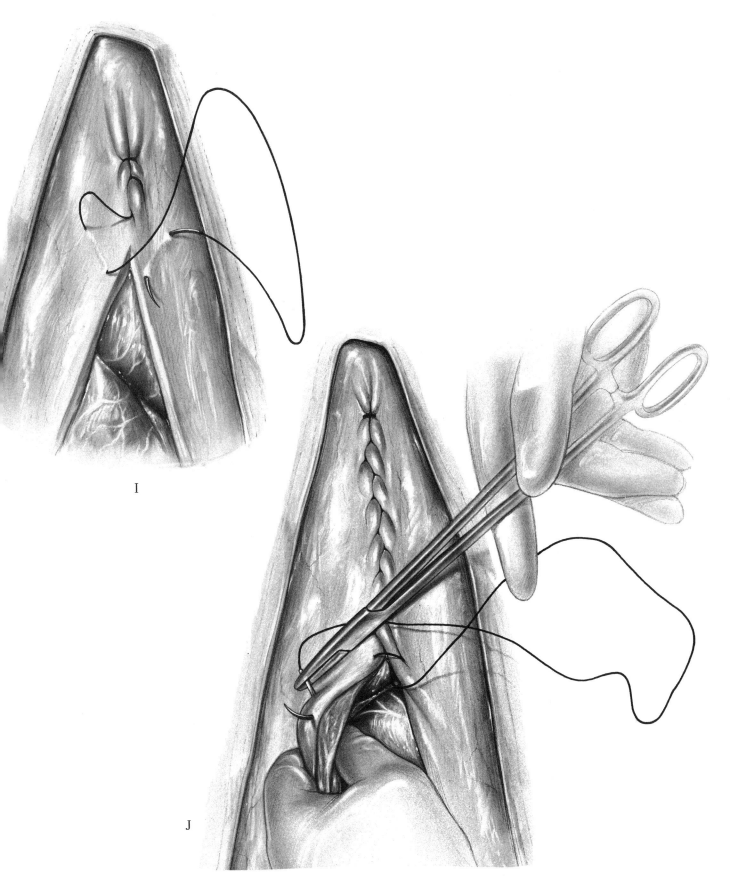

I

J

FIG. 14-9. *(continued)*.

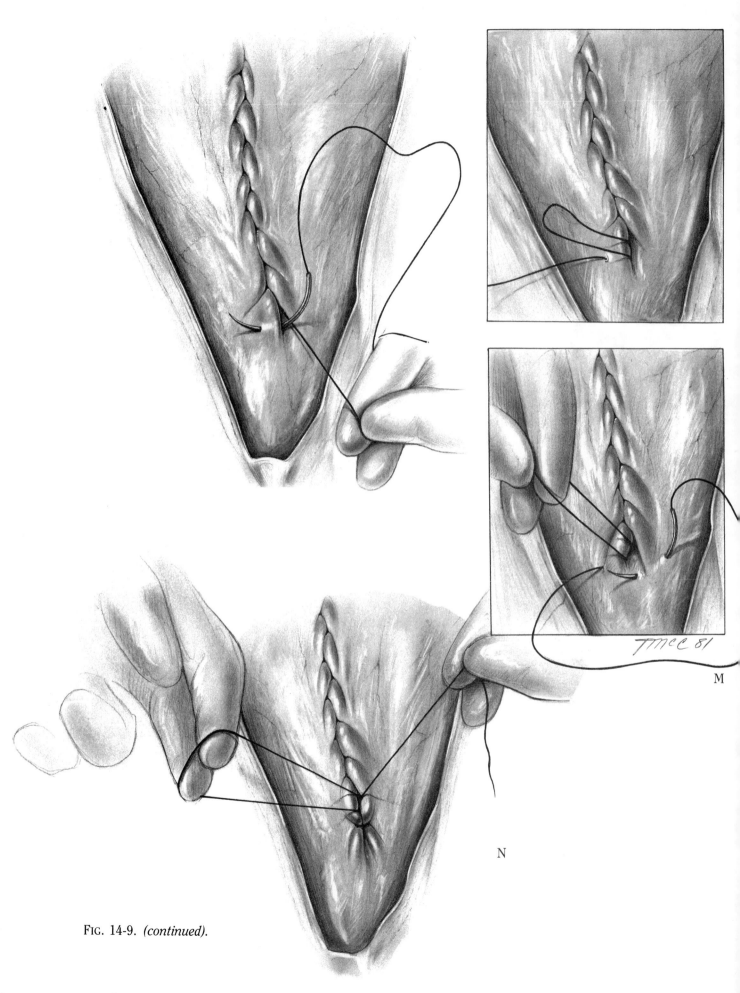

M

N

FIG. 14-9. *(continued)*.

produced the best results.[1] With this technique, it is important that each suture be pulled tightly following its insertion; otherwise, the wound edges may gap, and the contents of the uterus may leak. Regardless of the suture pattern used, the rapidly shrinking uterine wall will leave less tissue in each bite of the suture material and may thereby loosen the suture. Once the uterus is closed, it is replaced in position. The laparotomy incision is closed as described in Chapter 13.

Postoperative Management

Antibiotics are administered, and oxytocin may be administered any time after uterine closure, to enhance uterine involution. Fluid therapy may be indicated in certain cases.

Comments

We have questioned the rationale behind the use of large-diameter plain catgut suture material because it is more reactive than chromic catgut or one of the synthetic absorbable materials. One of the reasons that adhesions may be fewer with this material is the time factor. With the abundant blood supply to the involuting uterus, the suture material is probably absorbed so quickly that adhesions have less chance to form than when suture materials remain in situ for long periods of time. As an alternative to nonchromic catgut, chromic catgut or one of the synthetic absorbable materials such as polyglycolic acid (Dexon) or polyglactin 910 (Vicryl) may be used.

The knots are the last portion of the suture line to be absorbed, probably because cellular invasion is more difficult. Therefore, burying the knots at each end of the incision should always be the goal with this suture pattern.

The fetal membranes should only be removed if they can be separated from the uterus without undue traction or if they are lying free within the uterus.

References

1. Ball, L.: Personal communication, 1979.

2. Noorsdy, J. L.: Selection of incision site for cesarean section in the cow. VM/SAC, *75*: 530, 1979.

Retention Suturing of the Bovine Vulva (Buhner's Method)

The buried purse-string suture (Buhner's method) is a simple and effective way to retain vaginal or uterine prolapse in the cow.[1-3] The method consists of a deeply placed circumferential suture that effectively simulates the action of the constrictor vestibulae muscle.[2]

Anesthesia and Surgical Preparation

The cow should be restrained in a chute or crush, and some cows may be recumbent during the procedure. The surgery is performed with the animal under caudal epidural analgesia (see Chap. 2). Following administration and onset of the epidural analgesic, the perianal area and prolapsed tissues are cleaned and treated with an antiseptic. Osmotic agents and massage may then be used to reduce the size of the prolapse.

Additional Instrumentation

This procedure requires Buhner's or Gerlach's perivaginal needle, and perivaginal suture tape, or sterile, 1-cm (half-inch) umbilical tape.

Surgical Technique

A typical prolapse is depicted in Figure 14-10*A*. The prolapse is reduced, the vagina is returned to its correct anatomic location, and the perianal area is scrubbed once again. A transverse skin incision about 1 cm long is made midway between the dorsal commissure of the vulva and the anus. Another horizontal incision is made about 3 cm below the ventral commissure of the vulva. The perivaginal needle is introduced into the ventral skin incision and is driven perivaginally through the deep subcutaneous tissues parallel to the vulva. One hand is placed in the vagina to guide the needle. The needle should be driven as deep as possible (about 5 to 8 cm) and directed out the dorsal skin incision (Fig. 14-10*B*). A piece of sterile perivaginal suture tape (or sterile umbilical tape) soaked in a suitable antibiotic solution, is threaded through the eye of the needle and is drawn down to emerge through the ventral skin incision (Fig. 14-10*C*). At the same time, the tape is held at the dorsal incision, so the end is not lost in the tissue. The tape is then removed from the needle, and the needle is threaded up the contralateral side of the vulva (about 5 to 8 cm) to emerge through the dorsal incision. The tape is threaded into the eye of the needle once again (Fig. 14-10*C*), and then the needle is withdrawn ventrally, resulting in two free ends of tape emerging from the ventral skin incision.

The two free ends of the tape are tied, ensuring that the loop of tape at the dorsal incision is buried (Fig. 14-10D). The tape is tied so the resulting suture encircling the vulva will admit two to three fingers. If a square knot is used to anchor the tape, the knot will bury itself. This minimizes the chances of contamination of the suture material and thereby avoids a wicking effect with the suture and secondary infection. The dorsal and ventral incisions

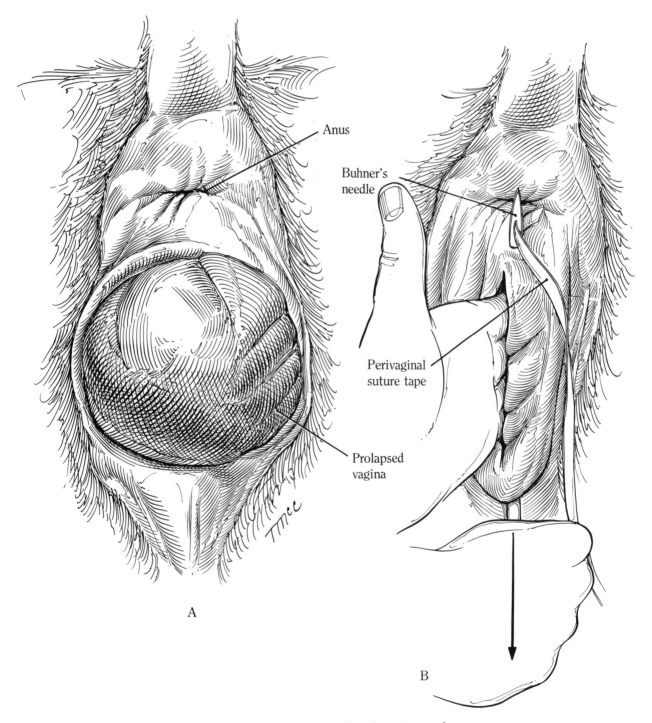

Anus

Buhner's
needle

Perivaginal
suture tape

Prolapsed
vagina

A

B

FIG. 14-10. A *to* D, *Buried purse-string suture for vaginal and uterine prolapse.*

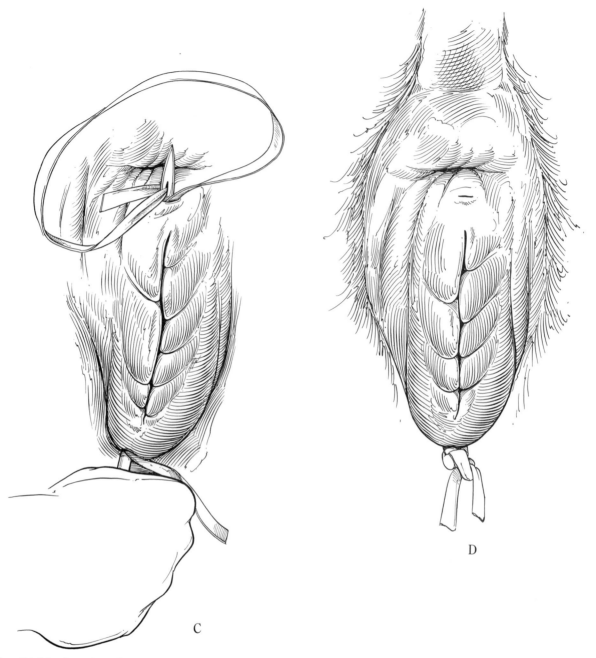

FIG. 14-10. *(continued).*

may be closed with a simple interrupted suture of nonabsorbable material, to decrease further the chances of secondary infection around the umbilical tape. If the cow is close to calving, we recommend that the tape be secured in the ventral incision with a bow knot. This knot allows the suture to be removed or, at least, undone to reduce tension at the time of parturition. One of the other methods to retain the prolapse may also be used.

Postoperative Management

The cow requires close observation, to time removal or loosening of the suture correctly in relationship to parturition. The knot should be untied, and the vulva should be gently dilated, to reduce tension on the suture.[2]

Comments

The purse-string suture may be permanent or temporary. It is strong and does not tear out as frequently as externally placed suture patterns (lacing, Halsted, and quill).[1] These methods promote infection along the suture line, although this infection generally is of minor significance. The Buhner perivaginal suture tape is more expensive than umbilical tape, but it does have advantages.[1] Umbilical tape tends to become twisted and form a string, and it is more likely to cut through the edematous tissues of the vulva. The Buhner perivaginal tape, made of nylon, lies flat and is tolerated better by the tissues. It can remain as a permanent suture, whereas umbilical tape may disintegrate if left in the tissues. Moreover, when the tape has been removed or has disintegrated, the fibrous connective tissue produced by the cow in response to the tape is often sufficient to prevent future prolapse. Infrequently, the scar tissue may be strong enough to result in dystocia.[2]

References

1. Bennett, B. W.: Personal communication, 1980.

2. Hudson, R. S.: Genital surgery of the cow. *In* Current Therapy in Theriogenology. Vol. 2. Edited by D. A. Morrow. Philadelphia, W. B. Saunders, 1986, p. 348.

3. Sloss, V., and Duffy, J. H.: Handbook of Bovine Obstetrics. Baltimore, Williams & Wilkins, 1980.

Cervicopexy For Vaginal Prolapse (After Winkler)

Another method for retaining a prolapsed vagina in the cow is a technique in which the external os of the cervix is sutured to the prepubic tendon. The main advantage of the technique is that postoperative treatment is minimal.[1-3]

Anesthesia and Surgical Preparation

This procedure is performed using epidural anesthesia. Following restraint of the cow in a chute or crush, an epidural anesthetic is given, and the prolapsed tissues are cleaned, treated with the appropriate medication, and replaced.

Additional Instrumentation

This procedure requires an 8.0-cm half-circle cutting needle that has been bent into a U-shape. At least 1.2 m of nonabsorbable suture material, such as polymerized caprolactam (Vetafil) are required.

Surgical Technique

The prepared needle is carried into the vagina by hand. The attachment of the prepubic tendon just cranial to the pelvic symphysis can be palpated through the floor of the vagina. It extends ventrad and craniad from its attachment at an angle of about 90° to the horizontal plane (Fig. 14-11A). The urethra and bladder are located (preferably by inserting a urinary catheter, rather than by simple palpation), to ensure placement of the suture lateral to these structures.

The point of the needle is directed through the floor of the vagina below the vaginal end of the cervix. As originally described, the needle is directed through a triangular area toward the midline back up through the tendon and vaginal floor. This triangular area is formed by a short band of the prepubic tendon that extends caudolaterad, attaching to the iliopubic eminence of the pubis (Fig. 14-11B). To decrease the possibility of breaking the needle, however, it is recommended to pass the needle down through the prepubic tendon and up through the triangular space in a medial-to-lateral direction. A bite of 1.8 cm in the prepubic tendon and 3.5 to 5.0 cm in the vaginal floor is usually adequate. The needle and suture are pulled through the prepubic tendon and vaginal wall sufficiently to continue the suture through the intravaginal part of the cervix. Tension should be applied to the suture, to see whether it is adequately anchored in the prepubic tendon. A urinary catheter should be reintroduced into the bladder to ensure that the bladder and urethra have not been included in the suture. The needle is then directed across the lower half of the cervix at least 1.2 cm (half an inch) cranial to

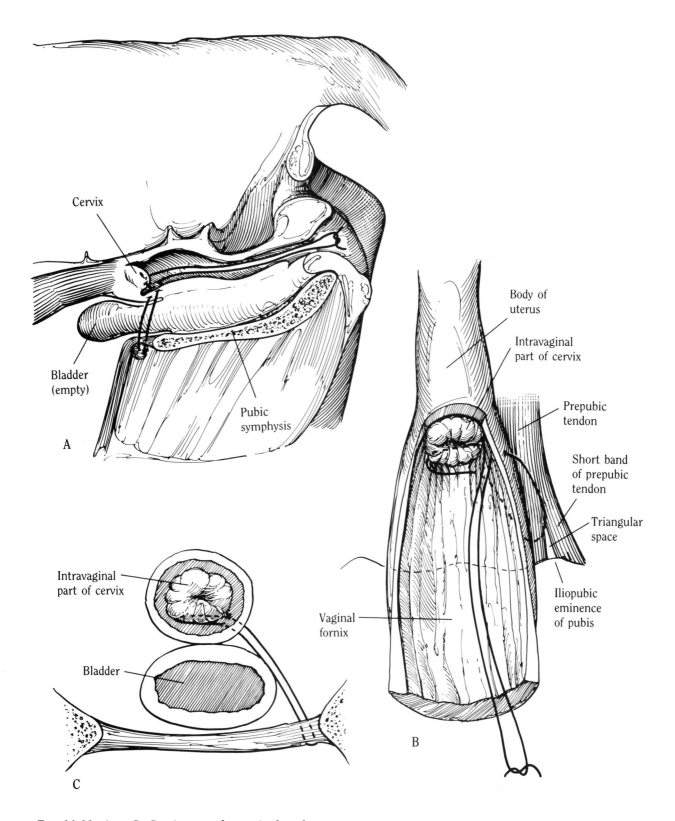

Labels in figure:

Cervix

Bladder
(empty)

A

Pubic
symphysis

Body of
uterus

Intravaginal
part of cervix

Prepubic
tendon

Short band
of prepubic
tendon

Triangular
space

Iliopubic
eminence
of pubis

Vaginal
fornix

B

Intravaginal
part of cervix

Bladder

C

FIG. 14-11. A *to* C, *Cervicopexy for vaginal prolapse.*

the caudal limits of the intravaginal part of the cervix. The suture ends are exteriorized, and the first throws of a surgeon's knot are performed and are then advanced craniad, tight enough to prevent caudal movement of the cervix (Fig. 14-11C).

Postoperative Management

The cow should be given appropriate antibiotic therapy.

Comments

This procedure can be used in cows in which external retention techniques have been unsuccessful. Postoperative tenesmus has been minimal or completely absent with this technique. The suture has remained in position for as long as a year in some cows. In one cow, the suture was still present when the cow was slaughtered (for unrelated reasons) 7 years after repair of the prolapse.[2]

Peritonitis has been associated with this technique when umbilical tape is used, and a suture of less capillarity is recommended. Care must be taken not to deviate too far from the midline when placing the suture through the tendon; otherwise, inadvertent penetration of arteries of the pelvic cavity may result.[2]

References

1. Hudson, R. S.: Genital surgery of the cow. *In* Current Therapy in Theriogenology. Vol. 2. Edited by D. A. Morrow. Philadelphia, W. B. Saunders, 1986, p. 350.

2. Winkler, J. K.: Personal communication, 1987.

3. Winkler, J. K.: Repair of bovine vaginal prolapse by cervical fixation. J. Am. Vet. Med. Assoc., *149*:768, 1966.

15

MISCELLANEOUS
BOVINE
SURGICAL
TECHNIQUES

Digit Amputation

The following are indications for amputation of the bovine digit: severe foot rot unresponsive to antibiotics and complicated by osteomyelitis, abscess formation with osteoarthritis of the distal interphalangeal joint, tenosynovitis, or infectious arthritis; severe phalangeal fractures; and dislocations of the phalangeal joints.[1]

This surgical procedure is indicated to relieve pain and to return the animal to soundness and milk yield, as well as to prevent ascending infection of the limb.

Anesthesia and Surgical Preparation

The animal is usually placed in lateral recumbency by means of ropes and chemical restraint, or it is secured to a surgical table, with the affected claw uppermost. The procedure may be performed with the animal standing, but this is not generally recommended. The limb is clipped from the mid-metacarpal region or midmetatarsal region distad, and the area is prepared surgically prior to administering local anesthesia. The claw and interdigital space are cleared of all fecal material and debris; a scrub brush and hoof knife are useful for this initial preparation. Intravenous local analgesia is the preferred method of local desensitization (see Chap. 2), but regional nerve blocks or a ring block may also be used. Following administration of the local anesthetic, the surgical site is given a final surgical scrub. If the intravenous analgesic technique is not used, a tourniquet (rubber tubing) is applied at this stage. The limb is draped so the foot is exposed, and a sterile glove may be applied over the claw, so it can be handled by the surgeon during surgery.

Additional Instrumentation

This procedure requires an obstetric wire saw or Gigli wire saw.

Surgical Technique

The technique illustrated in Figure 15-1 uses a skin flap and attempted closure. The skin incision is made along the abaxial and axial surface of the coronary band; then vertical incisions are made cranially and caudally (Fig. 15-1A). The skin and subcutaneous tissues are incised to the bone. The skin incision on the axial surface is made first so as not to obscure the surgical field with blood. The skin is then dissected free from the underlying digit, and one attempts to save as much of the skin flap as possible. Alternatively, a circumferential skin incision can be made in a similar plane to the wire cut illustrated in Figure 15-1B and C.

The amputation may be performed in two locations. A low amputation is performed when only the coffin joint and distal phalanx are diseased; this amputation is directed through the middle phalanx. We describe the technique of high amputation, which is used in cases with involvement of the coffin joint, distal phalanx, pastern joint, and middle phalanx. This amputation is directed through the junction of the middle and distal third of the proximal phalanx.

An obstetric saw is placed in the incision in the interdigital space. An assistant is needed for the sawing procedure (Fig. 15-1B). The amputation is commenced with the wire saw directed parallel to the long axis of the limb until the wire is located at the distal end of the proximal phalanx. The saw is directed perpendicular to the long axis of the proximal phalanx to seat the wire in the bone, and then the position of the wire is directed so it is approximately 45° to the long axis of the proximal phalanx (Fig. 15-1C). The sawing motion should not be too rapid because heat necrosis of tissues, including bone, may occur, leading to excessive sloughing during the healing period. Care should be taken to avoid invading the fetlock joint capsule. Once the digit has been removed, excess interdigital adipose tissue and all necrotic tissue, especially that involving the tendons and tendon sheaths, should be dissected sharply from the wound. If the digital artery can be located, it should be ligated.

Some of the skin flap may be sutured down, but when the surgical site is swollen from infection and when some skin necrosis is present in the region, then this is not usually possible. Complete closure is contraindicated because infection will resolve more rapidly if the skin flap is not completely sutured, to allow better ventral drainage (Fig. 15-1D).[2] The value of skin flaps and of any attempt at closure has been questioned.[1] An antibiotic powder is applied to the area and is followed by sterile gauze sponges. A tight bandage is applied to prevent hemorrhage when the tourniquet is removed (Fig. 15-1E), and some form of impervious covering may be indicated.

Postoperative Management

The bandage should be changed 2 to 3 days after surgery. The limb is kept bandaged until the wound has healed. The length of time the wound will need to be bandaged depends on the individual case and to what degree the wound was left open. Some cases of digit amputation may require only 10 to 14 days to heal, whereas others may require several more weeks for the wound to heal by secondary intention.

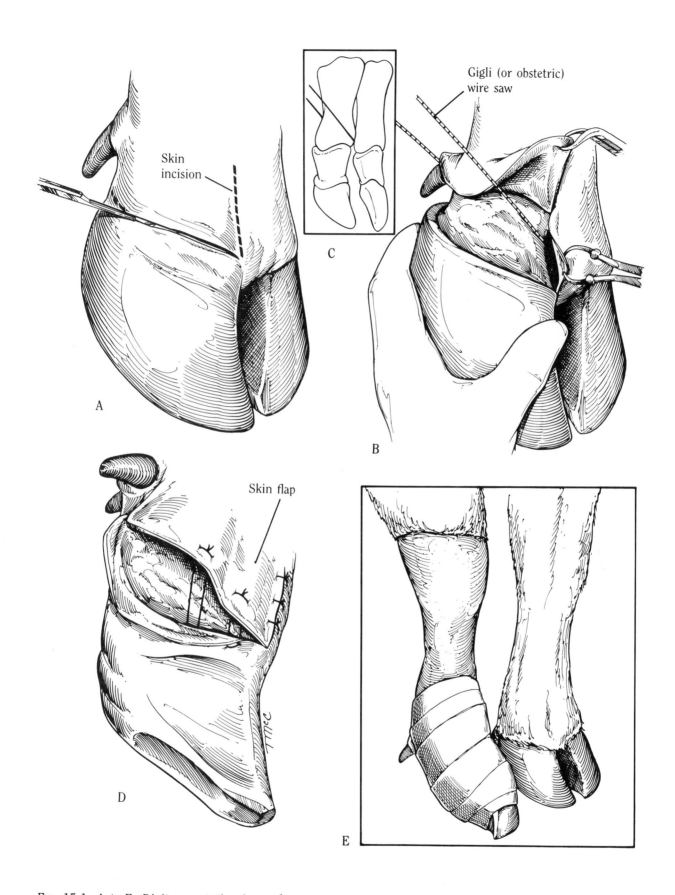

Skin
incision

C

Gigli (or obstetric)
wire saw

A

B

Skin flap

D

E

FIG. 15-1. A to E, *Digit amputation in cattle.*

In the initial stages of healing, the animal should be housed in dry conditions where food and water are easily accessible, to avoid overuse of the remaining digit.

Comments

The following are contraindications for digit amputation: sepsis of the fetlock joint; involvement of both digits of the same foot; and heavy bulls or cows (these animals generally break down the remaining claw). Cows with amputated digits are usually culled sooner than herdmates and have a lower market value.

The same basic technique of digit amputation is applicable to pigs and small ruminants.

References

1. Greenough, P. R., MacCallum, F. J., and Weaver, A. D.: Treatment and control of digital disease. *In* Lameness in Cattle, 2nd Ed. Edited by A. D. Weaver. Philadelphia, J. B. Lippincott, 1981. p. 228.

2. Knight, A. P.: Personal communication, 1980.

Eye Enucleation

Although the operation is called an enucleation of the eye, it is, for all practical purposes, an extirpation because everything within the orbit is generally removed; there is no demand for cosmetic repair as in other species. Enucleation involves the removal of the globe, leaving adipose tissue and muscles, whereas extirpation involves removal of everything within the orbit: globe, muscles, adipose tissue, and lacrimal gland. Extirpation in cattle is indicated for neoplasia (usually squamous cell carcinoma) of the upper and lower eyelids, third eyelid, and cornea that is too extensive to be removed by other, less radical operations such as lid resections, H-plasties, or superficial keratectomies. Septic panophthalmitis, severe trauma beyond repair, and severe trauma with loss of globe contents are also indications for enucleation.

Anesthesia and Surgical Preparation

The animal, which is wearing a halter, should be adequately restrained in a chute and its head secured to one side. Local anesthesia is administered by infiltration of the retrobulbar tissues. The four-point retrobulbar block is performed by injecting through the eyelids, both dorsally and ventrally, and at the medial and lateral canthi (Fig. 15-2*A*). A slightly curved, 8- to 10-cm gauge needle is directed to the apex of the orbit where the nerves emerge from the foramen orbitorotundum. About 40 ml of local anesthetic are injected, divided into 10 ml per site. Exophalmos, corneal anesthesia, and mydriasis indicate a satisfactory retrobulbar block.[1] Other surgeons use the Peterson retrobulbar eye block for this procedure. The four-point retrobulbar technique is quick and easier to administer.

Prior to administering the retrobulbar block, the surgeon clips the hair around the animal's eyes. The surgical site should also be scrubbed prior to the administration of the nerve block. Because this particular surgical procedure is performed for large, necrotic, ocular neoplasms or severe trauma, proper aseptic preparation of the surgical site may be impossible. Generally, draping is not performed for this procedure. If there are large amounts of necrotic, neoplastic tissue, then some of it may be trimmed prior to the surgical scrub.

Surgical Technique

Following surgical preparation, the patient's eyelids are grasped with towel clamps and are closed, to minimize contamination of the surgical field. A recommended alternative is to suture the eyelids together and to leave the suture ends long. Sutures provide a better seal from necrotic debris than towel clamps. Using these methods, the instruments or ends of the sutures can be used to put traction on the eye throughout surgery. A transpalpebral incision is made around the orbit, leaving as much normal tissue as possible (Fig. 15-2*B*). The incision is generally 1 cm from the margin of the eyelid. The ventral incision and subsequent dissection are done first. Sharp or blunt dissection is used for 360° around the orbit continuing down to the caudal aspect of the orbit, but avoiding entrance through the palpebral conjunctiva (Fig. 15-2C). All muscles, adipose tissue, the lacrimal gland, and fascia are removed, along with the eyelids and eyeball. If the indication for enucleation is neoplasia, then one must make sure that all neoplastic tissue is removed. If the eye is enucleated for a non-neoplastic condition, such as irreparable trauma, then the surgeon can afford to leave some of the retrobulbar tissue, to reduce the amount of dead space and intraoperative hemorrhage.

When the optic stalk and its blood supply are reached, a pair of right-angled forceps or a similar instrument is used to grasp the stalk, which is then severed distally (Fig. 15-2D). Following removal of the eye, considerable dead space remains and is virtually impossible to obliterate. The cavity fills with a blood clot that will organize during the healing period and will leave a large depression in the orbit.

Closure consists of a layer of simple interrupted sutures, or a simple continuous suture, in the skin using synthetic nonabsorbable suture material (Fig. 15-2E). Polymerized caprolactam (Vetafil) is used for this closure by most bovine practitioners. Sutures are removed 2 to 3 weeks postoperatively. If infection is present, some of the skin sutures should be removed to permit drainage. Some surgeons prefer to pack the eye with sterile gauze to control hemorrhage and to remove the gauze a day or so after hemorrhage has stopped. Generally, this is not necessary because a tight seal with a skin suture seems to allow pressure to build up within the orbit and to create hemostasis through a tamponade effect. Packing the orbit usually only increases the extent of postoperative management, which may be difficult in field conditions. Packing is indicated in cases of massive, uncontrollable hemorrhage.

Another variation of the enucleation technique is to pack the orbit as soon as the globe and surrounding structures have been removed and to leave the packing in place until the last skin sutures have been tied. The pack is then removed, and the closure is completed. Some surgeons prefer to use an absorbable suture in the skin, to obviate the need for suture removal; this would be useful on the range, where it may be impractical to round up the animal for suture removal.

Postoperative Management

Antibiotics are indicated if sepsis is present. If dehiscence occurs, granulation tissue will generally fill the wound satisfactorily. If healing is delayed, the surgeon may suspect a recurrence of the neoplastic process if it was the original indication for enucleation. Much hemorrhage occurs at the time of surgery, and it may alarm the inexperienced surgeon. We believe that, if the surgery progresses quickly, blood loss will be minimal. For this reason, some surgeons prefer a simple continuous pattern for closure.

Reference

1. Gelatt, K. N., and Titus, R. S.: The special sense organs. *In* A Textbook of Large Animal Surgery. Edited by F. W. Oehme and J. E. Prier. Baltimore, Williams & Wilkins, 1974.

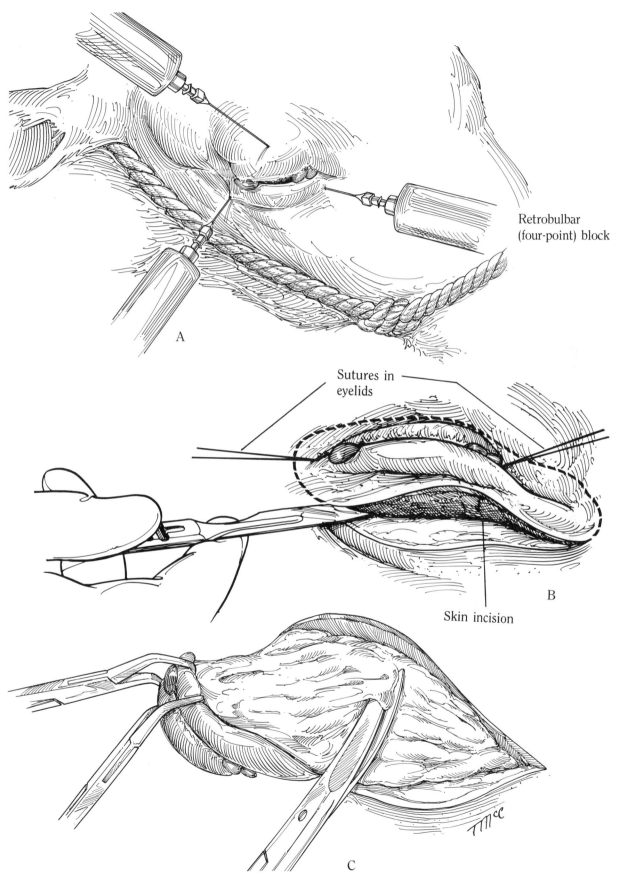

Retrobulbar
(four-point) block

Sutures in
eyelids

Skin incision

A

B

C

FIG. 15-2. A *to* E, *Eye enucleation in cattle.*

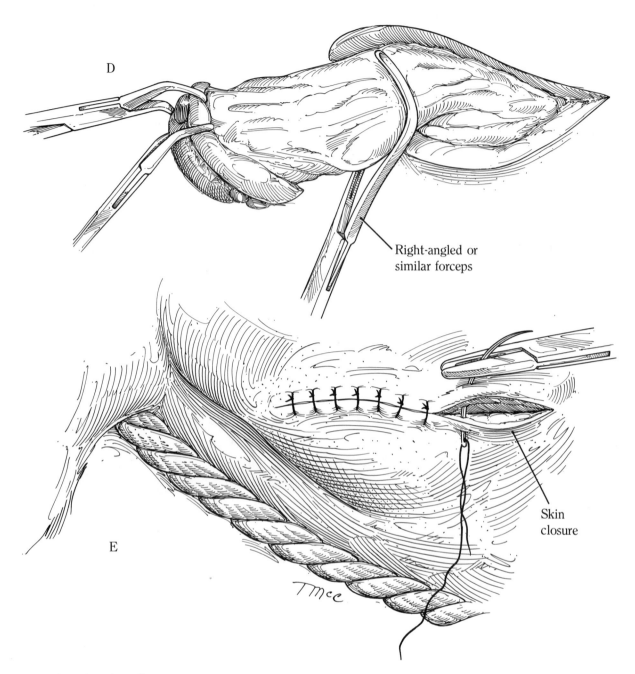

D

Right-angled or
similar forceps

E

Skin
closure

TMcc

FIG. 15-2. *(continued).*

Cosmetic Dehorning

Dehorning is performed in cattle to reduce injuries and carcass damage caused by fighting. Cosmetic dehorning permits closure of the skin over a normal defect created by the amputation of the horn at its base. Ideally, this results in primary-intention healing, a lower incidence of frontal sinusitis, and less hemorrhage. It is generally reserved for show animals and expensive breeding livestock in which postoperative appearance of the poll is important.[1] The method is best suited for cattle under 1 year of age because there may not be enough skin to close the defect after horn removal in older animals.[2]

Anesthesia and Surgical Preparation

The animal is restrained in a squeeze chute with its head secured to one side with a halter. The hair is removed from the poll, the base of the ears, and the face as far as the eyes; the ears are wrapped with adhesive tape and are pulled back out of the way (not illustrated). The area is scrubbed and prepared for cornual nerve block, but it is not draped. A cornual (zygomaticotemporal) nerve block is performed using an 18-gauge, 4- to 5-cm needle. In some of the larger breeds, an 8-cm needle is more satisfactory.[2] The needle is inserted through the skin at a point midway between the lateral canthus of the eye and the base of the horn (Fig. 15-3A). The needle is directed through the frontalis muscle and under the lateral aspect of the temporal portion of the frontal bone. At this point, 5 ml of local anesthetic are injected in a fan-like manner, and another 2 ml are deposited under the skin as the needle is withdrawn. Then the needle is directed subcutaneously toward the base of the horn, and an additional 2 to 3 ml of local anesthetic are deposited below the skin. The injection sites are massaged to disperse the local anesthetic. The block is repeated on the other side of the head. Generally, the head is swung around to the other side of the squeeze chute and is restrained to permit access to the sites that are to be blocked for the contralateral horn. The surgical site is given a final scrub prior to commencing surgery.

Additional Instrumentation

This procedure requires an obstetric wire and handle.

Surgical Technique

An incision is made from the lateral limit of the nuchal eminence (poll) in a lateral direction toward the base of the horn. The incision curves rostroventrad around the base of the horn and along the frontal crest for about 5 to 7 cm. The incision should be no more than 1 cm from the base of the horn. A second incision is begun from a point about 5 to 8 cm from the origin of the first incision, near the nuchal eminence. This incision is carried around the rostral aspect of the horn, about 1 cm from the base, to unite it with the first incision ventrally. The limits of the incisions are illustrated in Figure 15-3B. The incisions are deepened until bone is encountered, and the edges of the incision are undermined using sharp dissection. The rostral incision must be undermined in an area bounded by the ends of the incision (Fig. 15-3B, shaded area). The caudal incision is undermined just enough to allow placement of the wire saw ventrally and deep to the base of the horn on the frontal crest. Care should be taken when the incisions are deepened not to divide the auricular muscles (located caudally and ventrally). Generally, bleeding is controlled by torsion of the cornual artery located rostroventral to the bony stump.

The stump is then removed using either an obstetric wire as a saw or a dehorning saw. The rope securing the head is untied, and the head is swung around to the other side of the chute to facilitate positioning of the wire saw. The saw must seat itself in the frontal bone at an adequate distance from the base of the horn to allow removal of sufficient bone. If this is not done, the approximation of the skin edges will be under excessive tension, and closure may be impossible. If more horn must be removed, the surgeon may use a hammer and chisel, so the cut will be flush with the frontal bone. The remaining horn is removed in an identical manner. Once the horns and attached skin are removed, the head is repositioned in preparation for the closure of the wound.

The surgical sites are flushed with a suitable physiologic solution, such as Ringer's solution, to rinse out any bone dust. Skin closure is usually performed in one layer using a heavy, nonabsorbable material, such as polymerized caprolactam (Vetafil), in a simple continuous pattern (Fig. 15-3C). To assist in hemostasis and reduction of dead space, a roll of gauze is placed over the ventral half of the incision and is anchored by a large horizontal mattress suture in the skin (a stent bandage).

Postoperative Management

The stent bandage is removed 24 to 48 hours postoperatively, and the skin sutures are removed 2 to 3 weeks postoperatively.

Comments

The following are the three most common errors of the inexperienced surgeon: removal of too much skin at the base of the horn that subsequently will be removed with the horn; improper seating of the wire saw at the base of the horn, resulting in a stump of bone; and failure to undermine the skin edges adequately. These errors result in the surgeon's inability to appose the skin edges. If this happens, a varying degree of sinusitis, along with wound healing by secondary intention, is the end result.

References

1. Greenough, P. R.: The integumentary system: skin, hoof, claw and appendages. *In* Textbook of Large Animal Surgery. Edited by F. W. Oehme and J. E. Prier. Baltimore, Williams & Wilkins, 1974.

2. Wallace, C. E.: Cosmetic dehorning. *In* Bovine Medicine and Surgery, 2nd Ed. Vol. II. Edited by H. E. Amstutz. Santa Barbara, CA, American Veterinary Publications, 1980, p. 1240.

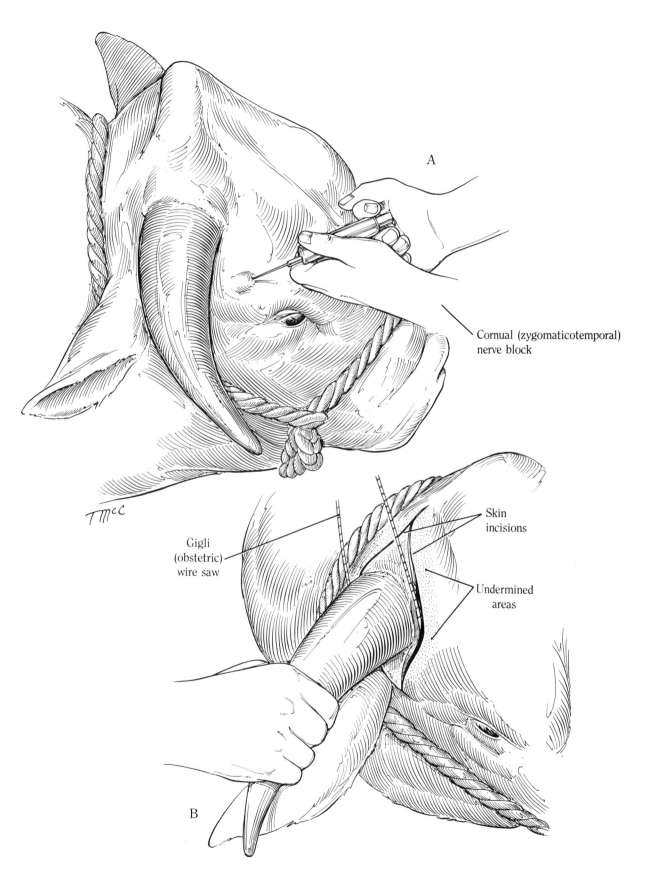

Cornual (zygomaticotemporal)
nerve block

Gigli
(obstetric)
wire saw

Skin
incisions

Undermined
areas

Fig. 15-3. A *to* C, *Cosmetic dehorning in cattle.*

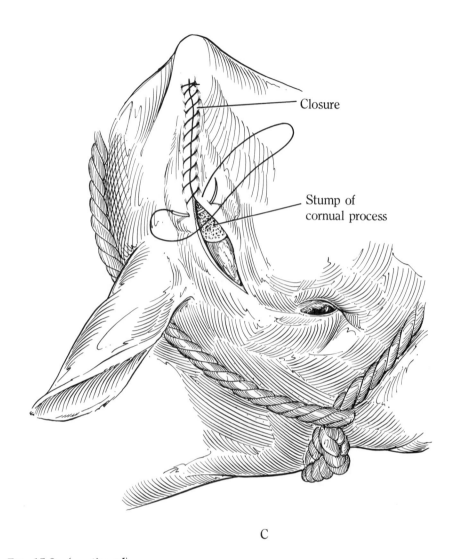

Closure

Stump of
cornual process

C

Fig. 15-3. (continued).

Rib Resection and Pericardiotomy

Rib resection and pericardiotomy in cattle are performed primarily to treat pericarditis resulting from penetration of the pericardial sac by a foreign body from the reticulum (traumatic reticulopericarditis). The foreign object penetrates the reticulum and then the pericardial sac, with resulting pericarditis, chronic pericardial effusion, and constrictive pericarditis. Generally, congestive heart failure due to pericardial and myocardial pathologic changes ensues, along with weight loss, ill thrift, and eventually, death. Drainage is indicated because the process is a closed-cavity infection, similar to an abscess, which seldom responds to antibiotic therapy alone. Drainage using a Foley catheter introduced through a large trocar may be unsuccessful because of fibrin accumulation and pocket formation in the pericardial sac.[2]

Generally, pericardiotomy is considered a salvage operation to "buy time" before the animal can be slaughtered. Although the aim of the surgery may be to allow time for a cow to calve, many cows with pericarditis abort from the stress of the disease process or the stress of the disease combined with surgery. When pericarditis is confirmed by clinical signs or pericardiocentesis, or when rumenotomy gives evidence of pericardial involvement, pericardiotomy is indicated.

Most animals with advanced pericarditis are in poor physical condition and have congestive heart failure, which makes them poor surgical risks. Animals under 5 years of age that can ambulate normally and are relatively normal in body function and condition can usually withstand the operation.[3] The surgery should be performed before the animal's body condition deteriorates to a point where there is no chance for survival. Advanced pregnancy and stress from other diseases hinder success.

Anesthesia and Surgical Preparation

Generally, preoperative antibiotics are indicated. Corynebacterium pyogenes is commonly the offending organism and is usually sensitive to common antibiotics. Mixed bacterial infections from the reticulum may be present, however, and it is preferable to culture the exudate from the pericardium and to obtain specific antibiotic sensitivities. Fluid therapy during and after surgery is beneficial in counteracting the effects of surgical and septic shock.

Because most candidates for pericardiotomy are poor anesthetic risks, the surgery is generally performed with the animal under local anesthesia. Sedation may also be required. General anesthesia should be avoided if possible. The intravenous sedation techniques combined with local anesthesia are generally accompanied by struggling, but they are usually safer in an animal in poor condition.

Prior to casting, a large area over the left thorax and elbow region is clipped. The surgery is performed with the animal placed in right-lateral recumbency, with the aid of casting ropes or a tilt table. If a tilt table is available, it is advantageous to operate at a 30 to 40° tilt, to allow any exudate to drain from the surgical site. This position also seems less stressful than full-lateral recumbency with the animal in the horizontal position. Generally, sedation is commenced prior to placing the patient on the tilt table. Once the patient is positioned, the clipped area over the left ventral chest wall is prepared for aseptic surgery. The left thoracic limb should be pulled craniad to help expose the area over the fifth rib, and local analgesia is instituted by direct infiltration of a local analgesic agent along the incision line (line block).[3] The analgesic solution is infused initially into the subcutaneous space, into the underlying muscle, and onto the surface of the fifth rib. The operating time should be kept to an absolute minimum, to reduce stress on an already compromised patient. The surgical site is given a final scrub, during which time the local anesthetic will be taking effect.

Additional Instrumentation

This procedure requires an obstetric wire saw or Gigli wire saw and handles.

Surgical Technique

The skin incision extends from the costochondral junction to a point 20 cm dorsally on a line over the fifth rib (Fig. 15-4A). The latissimus dorsi and serratus ventralis muscles are incised to expose the rib. The periosteum is incised and is reflected from the rib (Fig. 15-4B). Following exposure of 12 to 14 cm of the fifth rib, a wire saw (Gigli or obstetric) is inserted under the rib with forceps and is positioned at the dorsal commissure of the incision. The rib is transected dorsally and then is grasped and broken at the costochondral junction (Fig. 15-4C). This portion of the rib is discarded. Some surgeons prefer to let the patient stand at this point in the operation before the parietal pleura is opened, to assist drainage.[1] If the animal is restrained on a tilt table, it can be positioned at a steeper angle to aid drainage of exudate. The incision is then continued through the exposed periosteum and parietal pleura for about 12 cm, using a pair of blunt-tipped scissors (Fig. 15-4D).

The initial opening of the pleura should be small because a sudden influx of air may cause respiratory distress. Usually, however, the pericardium is adherent to the parietal pleura, and pneumothorax does not occur. To avoid opening the pleural cavity, some surgeons suture the periosteum, the parietal pleura, and the pericardium together using no. 2 chromic catgut in a simple continuous pattern prior to opening the pleura. If the pericardium is not adherent to the parietal pleura, or if suturing is not performed, leakage of pus into the pleural cavity will result in contamination and pleuritis.[2]

An incision is then made between the suture lines. Once the pericardium is visible, it is opened sufficiently to allow the introduction of the surgeon's hand. A variable amount of pus will escape from the incision. Suction, if available, should be used to aid evacuation of the exudate. The pericardial sac should be explored for a foreign body. Any foreign body should be removed, but often all that is found is a firm fibrous tissue mass in the

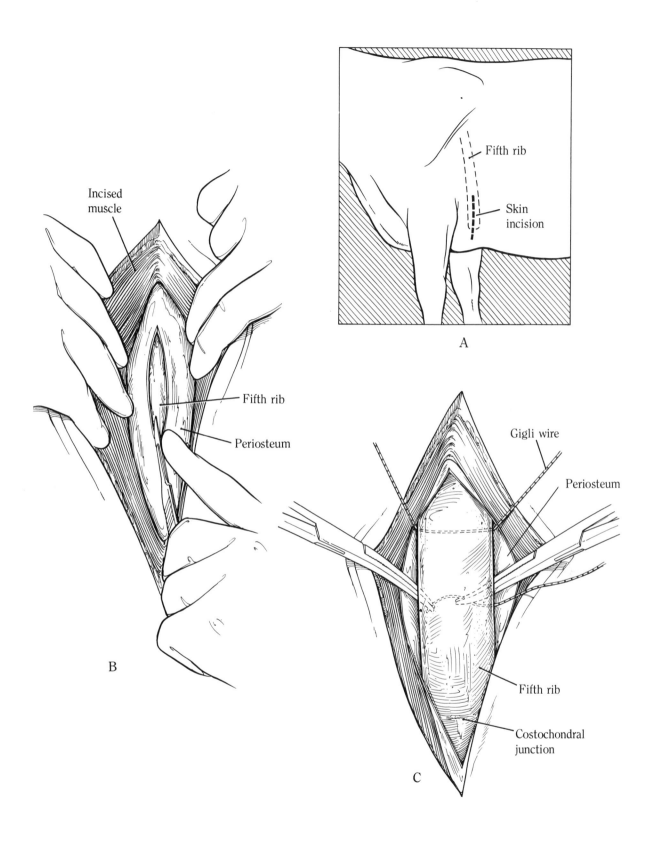

Incised
muscle

Fifth rib

Periosteum

B

Fifth rib

Skin
incision

A

Gigli wire

Periosteum

Fifth rib

Costochondral
junction

C

FIG. 15-4. A *to* E, *Pericardiotomy.*

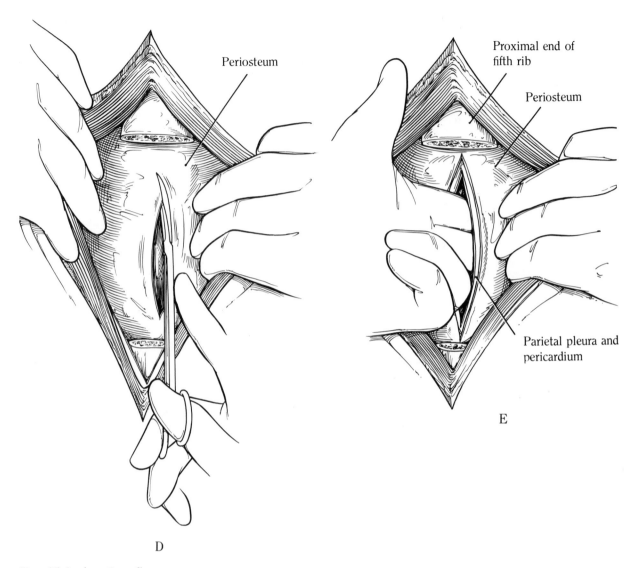

Periosteum

Proximal end of
fifth rib

Periosteum

Parietal pleura and
pericardium

E

D

Fig. 15-4. *(continued).*

caudal aspect of the pericardial sac. As much fibrinous exudate as possible
should be removed (Fig. 15-4E). Adhesions should be broken down gently
at this stage by passing the hand around the heart. It is unwise to proceed
with a dissection that is too extensive, however, for fear of rupturing coronary
vessels.[3] Following drainage, exploration, and the removal of any foreign
object, the cavity is lavaged copiously with warm isotonic electrolyte solution.
The inclusion of antibiotics or antibacterial agents in the lavage solution
is believed to be beneficial. Drains are sometimes indicated if postoperative
flushing is to be done. The wound may be closed or left open to allow
drainage.

Closure consists of simple continuous sutures of no. 2 or 3 chromic
catgut. The parietal pleura, adherent pericardium, and deep periosteal layer
are included in the first row. Periosteum and intercostal musculature are
closed in a second row, and nonabsorbable suture material is used for the

skin closure. No attempt is made to evacuate air from the pleural cavity because normal lung function returns in about 7 to 10 days.[3] If the wound is to be left open, the combined edges of the periosteum, parietal pleura, and pericardium are everted and are sutured to the subcutaneous tissue, to create a pericardial fistula.

Postoperative Management

Postoperative antibiotics are administered. If drains have been placed in the wound, they are flushed daily with a mixed antibiotic-isotonic solution. These treatments are continued until it is judged either that the animal is overcoming the infectious process or that the animal should be sent to slaughter.

Comments

The pericardial sac can also be approached through resection of the sixth rib, rather than the fifth rib. In some cases, a rumenotomy will be indicated if the wire foreign body is still protruding through the reticulum and was not retrieved through the pericardiotomy. The prognosis for traumatic reticulopericarditis is poor. Long-term recovery is unusual because the resulting constrictive pericarditis is generally fatal.

References

1. Horney, F. D.: Surgical drainage of the pericardial sac. Can. Vet. J., *1*:363, 1960.

2. Mason, T. A.: Suppurative pericarditis treated by pericardiotomy in a cow. Vet. Rec., *105*:350, 1979.

3. Noordsy, J. L.: The cardiovascular system. *In* Textbook of Large Animal Surgery. Edited by F. W. Oehme and J. E. Prier. Baltimore, Williams & Wilkins, 1974.

Repair of Teat Lacerations

Teat lacerations are common in dairy cows. Lacerations that do not penetrate the mucosa of the teat generally heal rapidly by secondary intention with the aid of topical medication and bandaging. Teat lacerations that penetrate the mucosa of the teat require suturing to maintain normal teat function for milking and to prevent the development of teat fistulae or acute mastitis and loss of the quarter. As with any lacerations, early attention to the condition improves the success rate.

Anesthesia and Surgical Preparation

The methods of restraint and anesthesia are important in any teat surgery because the repair must be meticulous. A tilt table, ideal for restraint, generally is not available to most practitioners who must deal with teat lacerations in the field. Xylazine hydrochloride (Rompun), although not approved for cattle in the United States, is a useful means of restraining the cow in lateral recumbency for teat surgery. If the cow's disposition is good, teat surgery may be attempted with the cow in the standing position using local anesthesia, but results are more predictable if the cow is tabled or cast and is neither uneasy nor kicking. Local anesthetic injected around the base of the teat (circle or ring block) is the most common technique for anesthesia (Fig. 15-5A). Epinephrine should not be used with the local anesthetic. Topical anesthetic can be infused directly into the teat canal to supplement ring block anesthesia. For topical anesthesia, 2% lidocaine (not procaine) should be used. Epidural anesthesia is an effective alternative for teat surgery (see Chap. 2).

To control hemorrhage and milk flow, a rubber tourniquet may be applied to the base of the teat. Doyen forceps clamped across the base of the teat can also be used successfully. When lacerations involve the base of the teat, suturing has to be performed without the benefit of a tourniquet.

The udder and surrounding teats should be washed thoroughly. Harsh disinfectants should be avoided because they can cause further tissue necrosis if they contact the lacerated tissue. The affected teat can be draped with a slit drape, so it protrudes from the opening in the drape. Once the borders of the laceration have been assessed carefully, a prognosis can usually be given.

Additional Instrumentation

This procedure requires a teat cannula (Larson's teat tube).

Surgical Technique

The wound edges should be freshened to remove any devitalized tissue and foreign material. Debridement is one of the most important procedures in repairing lacerated teats. Hemorrhage should be controlled because blood clots in the lumen of the teat delay healing by making milking painful and difficult for the animal.

The wound edges should be apposed under as little tension as possible. There are many opinions about which layers should be closed and which suture material should be used. Most veterinarians in dairy practice agree that the method should be as simple as possible.

The incidence of fistulae was thought to be higher if the mucosa was penetrated with suture, but if fine suture materials using swaged-on needles are used, the incidence of fistula formation may, in fact, be less. Absorbable suture material as fine as 2-0 to 4-0 is recommended for the mucosal layer, which requires more careful technique and, of course, absolute restraint of the cow. Better results can be expected with the finer suture materials on atraumatic swaged-on needles.

The first layer closed is the mucosa. This layer can be closed in a simple continuous or interrupted pattern (Fig. 15-5A). When the mucosa has been closed, a teat cannula should be inserted through the teat sphincter, and the suture line should be gently probed to check its integrity. The second layer closed should be the submucosa. Again, this layer can be closed in a simple continuous or interrupted pattern and should support the delicate mucosal closure (Fig. 15-5B). The remainder of the teat and the skin are ideally closed with a vertical mattress suture of nonabsorbable material, 0 or 2-0. This suture is placed so the deep bite is adjacent to the previously placed submucosal suture and the superficial layer is shallow (Fig. 15-5 C and D). The tourniquet should be removed following closure of the laceration, and, with gentle hand pressure applied to the teat, the suture line should be checked for milk leakage. Milk in the suture line will almost certainly result in a teat fistula.

Postoperative Management

Traditionally, a self-retaining teat tube, such as a Larson's teat tube, is inserted for about a week. The cap of the tube can be removed to permit the quarter to drain while the other quarters are being milked; this procedure takes advantage of the "let-down" phenomenon at the time of milking, or it can be left off permanently. The teat should not be hand-milked, but regular drainage is necessary to take the pressure off the suture line. If closure has been meticulous, as previously described, then immediate machine-milking appears to have no adverse effects on healing. This alternate post-operative program has worked in both an experimental series and 2 years of clinical experience in which closure as described here was used by one of us (B.L.H.).

Intramammary antibiotics should be infused into the affected teat, and systemic antibiotics should be used as indicated. If the laceration is of some duration, mastitis will be present. This can be verified with the aid of a California Mastitis Test. Bacterial cultures and sensitivity testing are indicated in some cases.

The sutures are removed at about 14 days postoperatively.

Comments

Vertical lacerations have a better prognosis than do horizontal teat wounds because circulation to the wound edges is better. For the same reason, a V-shaped flap attached proximally has a better prognosis than a V-shaped flap attached distally.

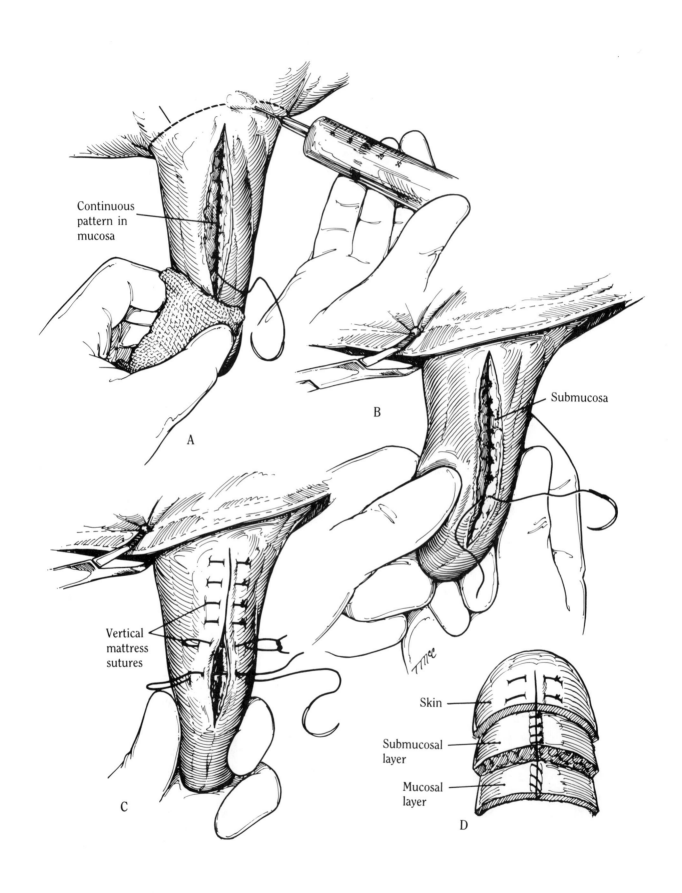

Continuous
pattern in
mucosa

A

B

Submucosa

Vertical
mattress
sutures

C

Skin

Submucosal
layer

Mucosal
layer

D

FIG. 15-5. A *to* D, *Repair of teat laceration.*

16

SURGICAL
TECHNIQUES

Castration of the Piglet

Generally, castration of the piglet is performed to improve the manageability of the herd; it also improves carcass quality because it removes taint. It is preferable to castrate piglets within the first 3 weeks of life. Although generally regarded as poor management, castration of larger pigs is occasionally indicated. The litter of piglets scheduled to be castrated should be clean and in good physical condition; if piglets in a litter are scouring, castration should be postponed. The area where the castration is to be performed should be relatively clean and free of dust. If castration is to be performed in hot weather, it should be done early in the morning.

Anesthesia and Surgical Preparation

For practical reasons, anesthesia is not used for the routine castration of young piglets. Young piglets (less than 3 weeks old) can be restrained by holding their hind legs around the hock. The herdsman should hold the piglet in a vertical position, either against his body or in a clean V-trough. Any evidence of inguinal hernia should be noted at this time, and the inguinal and scrotal areas are scrubbed with a suitable disinfectant (Fig. 16-1A).

Physical restraint of larger pigs is difficult, but this difficulty is overcome by the use of some form of general anesthesia. A practical anesthetic technique that requires a minimum of physical effort and personnel is intratesticular injection of pentobarbitone sodium (see Chap. 2). A 16-gauge needle 4 cm long is inserted below the tail of the epididymis in the upper third of the testis at an angle of 30° from the perpendicular; 300 mg/15 lb bodyweight are injected into each testis. Anesthesia sufficient to permit castration is attained within 10 minutes. That excessive barbiturate is removed with the testes eliminates the chance of overdosage.[1]

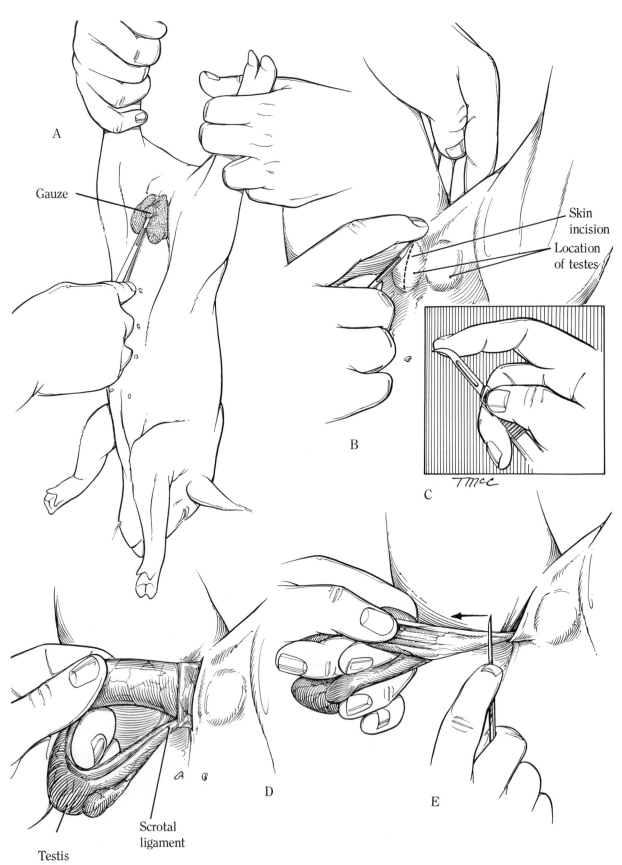

Gauze

Skin
incision

Location
of testes

A

B

C

D

E

Testis

Scrotal
ligament

Fig. 16-1. A *to* E, *Castration of the piglet.*

Additional Instrumentation

This procedure requires no. 12 scalpel blades.

Surgical Technique

By pressing the fingers of the left hand into the animal's scrotum, the testes are pushed craniad into the inguinal area. A longitudinal incision through the skin, subcutaneous tissue, and fascia is made directly over each testis with a no. 12 scalpel blade (Fig. 16-1*B*). (Figure 16-1*C* shows the method of holding the no. 12 scalpel blade and handle). Using blunt dissection with fingers, the surgeon grasps the testis in one hand while applying sufficient traction to break the scrotal ligament; this delivers the tunic-covered testis through the wound (Fig. 16-1*D*). If the incision results in an open vaginal tunic, the tunic should be retrieved immediately to reduce the incidence of scirrhous cord. Traction on the testis is maintained by the left hand while a sterile scalpel blade is used to scrape and sever the tunic and cord structures. The scraping should be performed as proximal as possible on the cord, so the severed end of the cord retracts into the inguinal region. This reduces the chances of infection and scirrhous cord formation. To minimize the chances of accidentally lacerating the piglet in some other area, the scraping should be performed in a direction *away* from the animal (Fig. 16-1*E*). This procedure is repeated on the opposite testis. The resulting incisions are located cranial to the normal position of the testes, to provide adequate ventral drainage. The left-handed operator uses the right hand to press the testis forward and holds the scalpel in his left hand.

Postoperative Management

Some surgeons prefer to dust the surgical site with an antibacterial powder; this is generally unnecessary if piglets can be turned into a clean, dry pen. The piglets should not be allowed into dirty quarters until healing is complete, usually within 5 to 7 days.

Comments

If there is evidence of inguinal-scrotal hernia, then the entire spermatic cord should be transfixed and ligated before it is severed (see the discussion in this chapter of inguinal herniorrhaphy in the piglet).

If intratesticular anesthesia is used to castrate boars, the testes must be disposed of carefully. Ingestion of testes containing residual pentobarbitone by dogs can be fatal.

Reference

1. Henry, D. P.: Anesthesia of boars by intratesticular injection. Aust. Vet. J., *44*:418, 1968.

Inguinal Herniorrhaphy in the Piglet

Frequently, inguinal hernias are discovered in piglets at the time of castration. These hernias generally do not reduce spontaneously, and when the ordinary castration procedure is used, evisceration is a frequent post-castration complication. The economics of hernia repair in the pig should be discussed with the client before surgery is undertaken.

Anesthesia and Surgical Preparation

For practical and economic reasons, no anesthetic is used routinely for small piglets; however, larger pigs require anesthesia similar to that used for castration of large pigs. The pig is restrained in a vertical position by the herdsman or by ropes in a clean V-trough, if the pig is too large. The skin of the inguinal and scrotal areas is scrubbed with a suitable antiseptic.

Surgical Technique

An incision approximately 7 cm long is made through the skin, sub-cutaneous tissues, and fascia over the external inguinal ring (Fig. 16-2A). Extensive hernias may require a larger incision. The testis, spermatic cord, and surrounding fascia are isolated using blunt dissection. Steady traction is exerted on the testis, tunics, and cord, pulling them loose from their attachment in the scrotum (scrotal ligament) (Fig. 16-2B). The freed vaginal tunic should not be incised. By grasping the testis, the surgeon twists the vaginal sac, to return the intestines to the abdomen. Fingers may be used to "milk" the intestines into the abdomen. A pair of Kelly forceps is used to grasp the sac while a transfixation ligature is applied on the proximal end of the cord just distal to the inguinal ring (Fig. 16-2C). Generally, the ligature is of strong, absorbable suture material, such as no. 1 or no. 2 catgut (Fig. 16-2D). At this point, some operators prefer to anchor the hernia sac to the inguinal ring with the ends of the transfixation ligature. The testis and excess spermatic cord are removed (Fig. 16-2E).

The skin incision may be partially closed with absorbable suture material, or it may be left completely open to allow ventral drainage. Because hernias may be hereditary, the bilateral castration of hernia-affected pigs is recommended. Hernias may be bilateral, so one should also transfix the cord of the opposite side, to prevent postoperative herniation.

Postoperative Management

The surgical site may be dusted with a suitable antibacterial powder. This is generally unnecessary if piglets can be turned into a clean, dry pen. The piglets should not be allowed in dirty quarters until healing is complete.

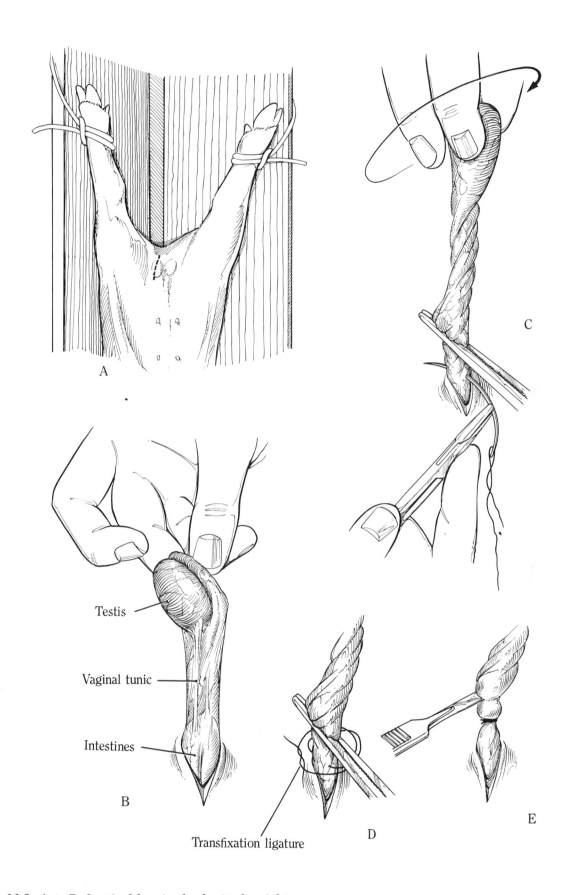

Testis

Vaginal tunic

Intestines

Transfixation ligature

A

B

C

D

E

FIG. 16-2. A *to* E, *Inguinal herniorrhaphy in the piglet.*

Cesarean Section in the Sow

Cesarean section in the sow is indicated for the relief of dystocia. The following are common causes of dystocia: uterine inertia; excessive adipose tissue around the birth canal; relative fetal oversize in small, immature sows; fetal monsters; and malformation of the birth canal due to previous pelvic fractures or injuries during previous parturitions. Cesarean section is also indicated for the production of specific-pathogen-free (SPF) piglets.

The operation is successful if done early in the parturition process; however, the large animal surgeon frequently is presented with an exhausted animal subjected to numerous attempts to remove the piglets manually. Generally, tissue damage to the birth canal is considerable, and emphysematous fetuses may be present in such cases. These sows are frequently in a state of endotoxic shock and are poor risks for surgery.

Anesthesia and Surgical Preparation

The sow is positioned in lateral recumbency, and ropes are tied to its feet if necessary. Adequate restraint is essential, so aseptic technique is not compromised. Once the sow has been placed in either left- or right-lateral recumbency, the surgical site is prepared. Local anesthesia in the form of a line block, an inverted L block, or an epidural block may be administered at this time (alternate sedative and general anesthetic techniques are presented in Chapter 2). Three basic types of incisions are used for cesarean section in sows: the first is a vertical incision, either in the left or right paralumbar fossa and flank region; and the second is a horizontal incision in the ventral paralumbar area about 6 to 8 cm above the well-developed mammary tissue (Fig. 16-3). The third, ventral midline incision, which we do not describe in this chapter, allows access to both uterine horns, but it is awkward to position the sow for this incision.

The surgical site is clipped, but shaving is generally unnecessary. Local anesthetic is administered, depending on which approach is to be used (we prefer the vertical incision). The surgical site is given an additional scrub and is prepared for aseptic surgery in a routine manner.

Surgical Technique

The following technique is for the vertical incision. The surgeon makes a 20-cm vertical skin incision that commences 6 to 8 cm ventral to the transverse processes of the lumbar vertebrae, midway between the last rib and the thigh muscles. The incision is continued through the skin, subcutaneous adipose tissue, muscles of the flank, subperitoneal adipose tissue, and peritoneum. The layer of adipose tissue encountered before peritoneum is generally thick in this species, and the neophyte surgeon may confuse the extensive subperitoneal fat for omentum with adhesions. The abdominal cavity is explored for the bifurcation of the uterus. The surgeon makes a 15- to 20-cm incision through the uterine wall, as close to the body of the

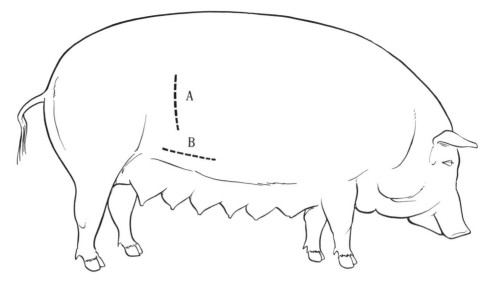

A, B: Location of the skin incisions for cesarean section

FIG. 16-3. *Cesarean section in the sow.*

uterus as possible, being careful not to cut one of the piglets. If the bifurcation can be located, the entire litter can be brought out through one incision. This leaves only one uterine incision to close and decreases surgery time. If this is not possible, an incision is made in each uterine horn close to the bifurcation, and the piglets are removed from each horn separately. If an assistant is present, piglets can be massaged down the uterine lumen toward the incision as the others are removed, but it is generally necessary for the surgeon to reach up into each uterine horn in search of more piglets while pulling the uterine walls up the surgeon's arms as one would pull on the arms of a thick woolen sweater. Great care should be exercised in exposing the ovarian end of each uterine horn. Its attachment is friable in the sow, and if one is not careful, the ovarian artery may be easily torn, possibly resulting in fatal hemorrhage. One should be sure to explore the vaginal canal for remaining piglets, and any loose placentae are removed.

Dead and emphysematous piglets usually have their corresponding placentae detached and are easily removed. Prior to closure of the uterine incisions, any intrauterine medication is administered. The uterus is closed with any of the inverting patterns described in the discussion of bovine cesarean section in Chapter 14. If infection is present, a two-layer closure is recommended.[1] The uterine horns are placed in the abdominal cavity individually, making sure they are not twisted.

The combined muscle and subcutaneous layers are closed as one, using no. 1 or 2 chromic catgut in a simple continuous pattern. The skin is closed with an interlocking pattern using polymerized caprolactam (Vetafil) in a manner similar to closure of the bovine flank.

Postoperative Management

During closure of the uterus and body wall, an assistant should dry the piglets vigorously and should place them in warm surroundings. Once surgery is completed, the sow is moved to a clean, dry pen, and the piglets are placed beside the sow.

Toxic patients should receive pre- and postoperative antibiotics, as well as other forms of supportive therapy for shock, such as intravenous fluids. Oxytocin can aid in contraction of the uterus and in milk let-down.

Reference

1. Hokanson, J. F.: Surgery; female genital tract; experimental and miscellaneous. *In* Diseases of Swine. Edited by H. W. Dunn and A. D. Leman, 4th Ed. Ames, Iowa State University Press, 1975.

17

MISCELLANEOUS
SURGICAL
TECHNIQUES

Dehorning the Mature Goat

The mature goat is dehorned either to reduce the danger to man and other animals or if its horn(s) are broken. Some breed societies require dehorning to register the goat, although flock goats are generally left horned as protection from predators. Dehorning of male goats is sometimes combined with removal of the scent (horn) glands to reduce odor.[1,2] Dehorning may have profound side effects that the goat owner should be aware of: reduction in milk production; impairment of spermatogenesis; sinusitis and myiasis; and loss of social status in the herd. The surgery should be planned to minimize these effects. For prevention of myiasis, the procedure should be reserved for the cooler months.[1]

Anesthesia and Surgical Preparation

As with other ruminants, food should be withheld from the goat for 12 to 24 hours before surgery to avoid ruminal tympany, regurgitation, and possible aspiration pneumonia if general anesthesia is administered.

Goats do not tolerate pain associated with even minor surgical procedures and can die of shock if sufficient analgesia is not provided. Although the exact cause of this shock is not known, it is believed to be a reaction to intense fear or fright from a combination of restraint and pain.[1] All goats should be anesthetized or deeply sedated before dehorning; refer to Chapter 2 for details of anesthetic techniques in goats.

Sedation needs to be supplemented with local analgesia of the horn. Once the goat is recumbent, the head region is clipped and prepared for a cornual nerve block. The cornual branch of the lacrimal nerve is blocked by injecting 2 ml of local anesthetic as close as possible to the caudal ridge of the root of the supraorbital process to a depth of 1 to 1.5 cm. The cornual branch of the infratrochlear nerve is also blocked by injecting 2 ml of local anesthetic at the dorsomedial margin of the orbit. In larger goats, a ring block around the entire base of the horn may be necessary (Fig. 17-1A).

While the anesthesia is taking effect, the area around the horn is prepared for aseptic surgery.

Surgical Technique

The skin is incised 1 cm from the base of the horn. Enough skin must be removed from the caudolateral and caudomedial areas, where scars are likely to occur (Fig. 17-1B). While an assistant supports the goat's head, the surgeon seats an obstetric wire saw or Gigli wire saw in the caudomedial aspect of the incision and removes the horn by directing the saw in a craniolateral direction (Fig. 17-1C). Some surgeons prefer a dehorning saw because it has less tendency to break and is less likely to leave a protuberance in the middle of the horn that may grow back.[1]

In male goats, the scent glands are located at the base of each horn (caudal and medial) and generally are removed during the dehorning procedure. Hemorrhage from the superficial temporal artery can be severe and should be stopped by ligating the artery with 0 chromic catgut or by pulling and twisting it with a hemostat.

When a goat is dehorned correctly, its frontal sinuses are exposed because of the extensive communication between the lumen of the cornual process and the frontal sinus. Dehorning should be performed as aseptically as possible to avoid sinusitis. The head may be bandaged postoperatively to prevent both myiasis and the collection of foreign material in the sinus. Prior to bandaging, a topical antibacterial powder, such as nitrofurazone, is dusted onto the dehorning site (Fig. 17-1D and E). Bandaging is not accepted by everyone. Some surgeons believe that the wound should not be covered and should be allowed to remain dry. If the wound is neglected, myiasis can develop under the bandage, and the consequences may be more serious than if the wound was left open.

Postoperative Management

If the animal's head is bandaged, the first bandage should be changed on the second postoperative day and replaced. The second bandage is left on for an additional 5 to 6 days. After this time, healing is generally sufficient that the bandage can be removed completely.

In the summer, when flies are a problem, prevention of myiasis is important for several more weeks. The goat should be housed in an area free of dust and isolated from dirty surroundings. It is also advisable that the goat not mix with other members of the herd until the wound has healed. Any abnormal odor, purulent nasal discharge, head shaking, or rubbing are often indications of frontal sinusitis, which necessitates removal of the bandage and treatment.

References

1. Bowen, J. S.: Dehorning the mature goat. J. Am. Vet. Med. Assoc., *171*:1249, 1977.

2. Guss, S. B.: Management and Diseases of Dairy Goats. Scottsdale, AZ, Dairy Goat Journal Publishing, 1977.

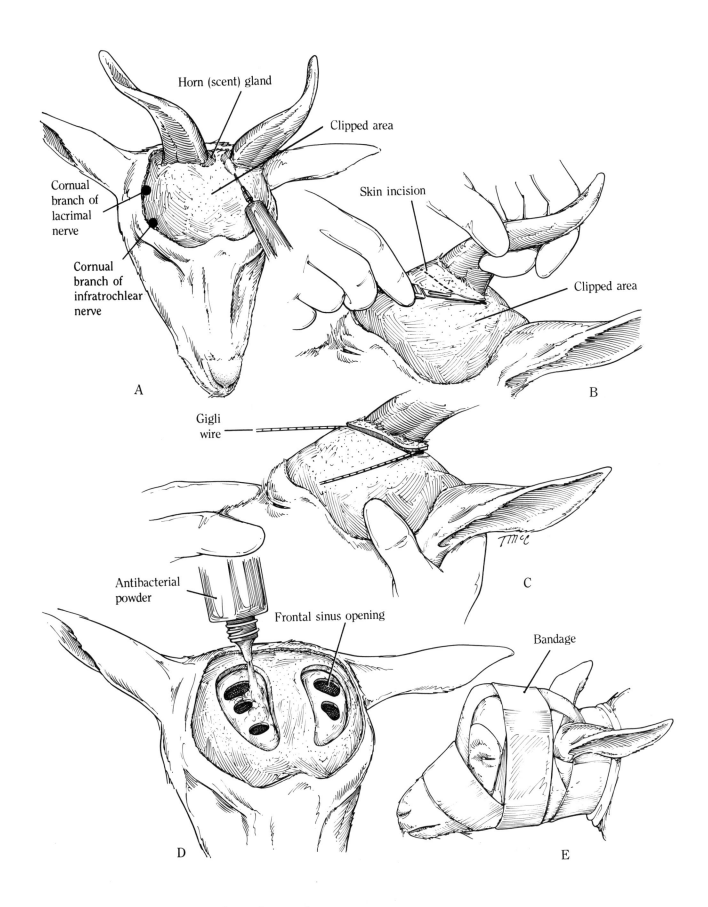

Horn (scent) gland

Clipped area

Cornual branch of lacrimal nerve

Cornual branch of infratrochlear nerve

A

Skin incision

Clipped area

B

Gigli wire

C

Antibacterial powder

Frontal sinus opening

D

Bandage

E

FIG. 17-1. A *to* E, *Dehorning the mature goat.*

Tooth Removal in the Llama

As a management tool to prevent fighting, removal of canine teeth of the llama may be necessary. The other indication for removal of canine teeth is a tooth root abscess. A root abscess may occur secondary to partial removal in which the crown has been amputated and the pulp cavity is exposed. Partial amputation is done to minimize injuries inflicted to other herd members. Infection subsequently migrates down the pulp cavity. Removal of molar teeth is usually to resolve a root abscess. The common causes of root abscesses of the molars are broken teeth. Some abscesses are caused by actinomycosis (resembling "lumpy jaw" in cattle), whereas others are spontaneous, with no apparent cause. Signs of a tooth problem include swelling of the mandible, pain, head shyness, a draining fistula, or impaired mastication. Radiographs of the affected tooth show varying degrees of bone lysis at the tooth root. Animals with chronic cases have radiographic evidence of increased bone density (sclerosis) surrounding the tooth root.

The dentition of the llama is shown in Figure 17-2. The root of the canine follows a caudal direction, a factor important at the time of tooth removal.

Anesthesia and Surgical Preparation

Tooth removal in the llama is performed with the animal under general anesthesia. Xylazine, in combination with local anesthesia, has been used by some surgeons, but we prefer inhalation anesthesia (halothane). The llama is given a guaifenesin-ketamine or guaifenesin-thiamylal combination intravenously to effect, an endotracheal tube is placed, and halothane-oxygen is administered. The llama is positioned in lateral recumbency with the affected tooth uppermost. A mouth speculum, similar to that used in dogs, is positioned to allow the surgeon free access to the incisor teeth or the ability to palpate the affected molar tooth. If a canine tooth is to be removed, the mucosa around the tooth is surgically prepared. If a molar tooth is to be removed, the hair over the surgical site is clipped, and routine surgical preparation is performed. The exact location of the surgical site is determined by the position of the affected molar on radiographs.

Additional Instrumentation

This procedure requires a mouth speculum (canine mouth gag), small mallet, small chisel (approximately quarter-inch width), curette, dental punch, small periosteal elevator, and forceps to grasp the tooth.

Surgical Technique

REMOVAL OF CANINE TEETH

For removal of a canine tooth, a fusiform incision is made through the mucous membrane around the tooth and is extended down to the mandibular

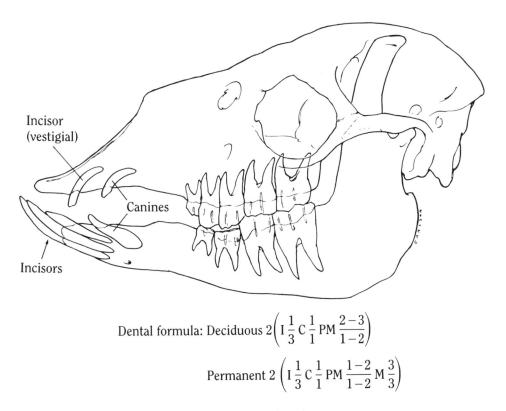

Dental formula: Deciduous $2\left(I\dfrac{1}{3}\,C\dfrac{1}{1}\,PM\dfrac{2-3}{1-2}\right)$

Permanent $2\left(I\dfrac{1}{3}\,C\dfrac{1}{1}\,PM\dfrac{1-2}{1-2}\,M\dfrac{3}{3}\right)$

FIG. 17-2. *Dentition of the llama (Lama glama).*

bone (Fig. 17-3*A* and *B*). A second incision is made directly over the tooth, curving caudad, in the direction of the long axis of the tooth (Fig. 17-3*B*). Using a periosteal elevator, the surgeon reflects the gingiva and periosteum away from the lateral surface of the mandible, in the direction of the tooth root. Similar elevation is performed on the medial side of the tooth extending about an eighth of an inch from the gum-tooth margin. A segment of bone on the lateral side of the tooth is then removed (Fig. 17-3*C*). Periosteum may first be reflected from this region, although we have not found this important. This lateral bone is removed because this is the direction in which the tooth will be extracted. The use of a chisel on the lingual side of the tooth facilitates removal of the tooth. Knowledge of the direction of the canine tooth root is important for atraumatic removal of this tooth. As bone is removed, the tooth should be grasped periodically and moved in a side-to-side motion, to ascertain when it is ready for extraction. Eventually, the tooth can be extracted without risking fracture of the mandible. The alveolus is then curetted, to remove all diseased bone associated with the root abscess (Fig. 17-3*D*). Debris is flushed from the site with sterile saline solution. The gingiva is then apposed over the empty socket using 2-0 polyglactin 910 (Vicryl) or 2-0 polyglycolic acid (Dexon) (Fig. 17-3*E*).

REMOVAL OF MOLAR TEETH

The exact location of the affected tooth is confirmed on the radiographs and by palpation of the crown of the tooth with the fingertips. A straight incision is made directly over the longitudinal axis of the tooth (Fig. 17-3*F*). The periosteum is reflected (optional). The bone lateral to the tooth

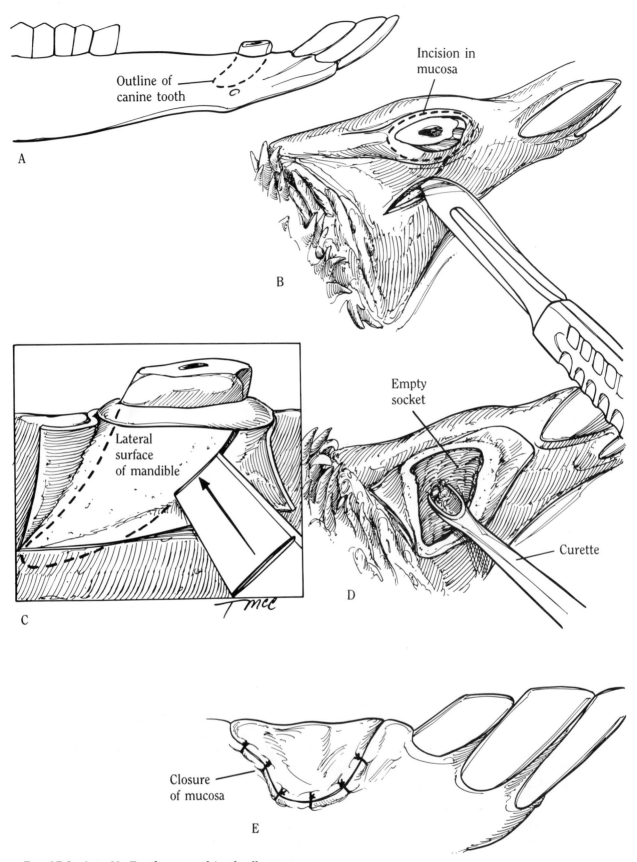

A, Outline of canine tooth

B, Incision in mucosa

C, Lateral surface of mandible

D, Empty socket — Curette

E, Closure of mucosa

Fig. 17-3. A *to* H, *Tooth removal in the llama.*

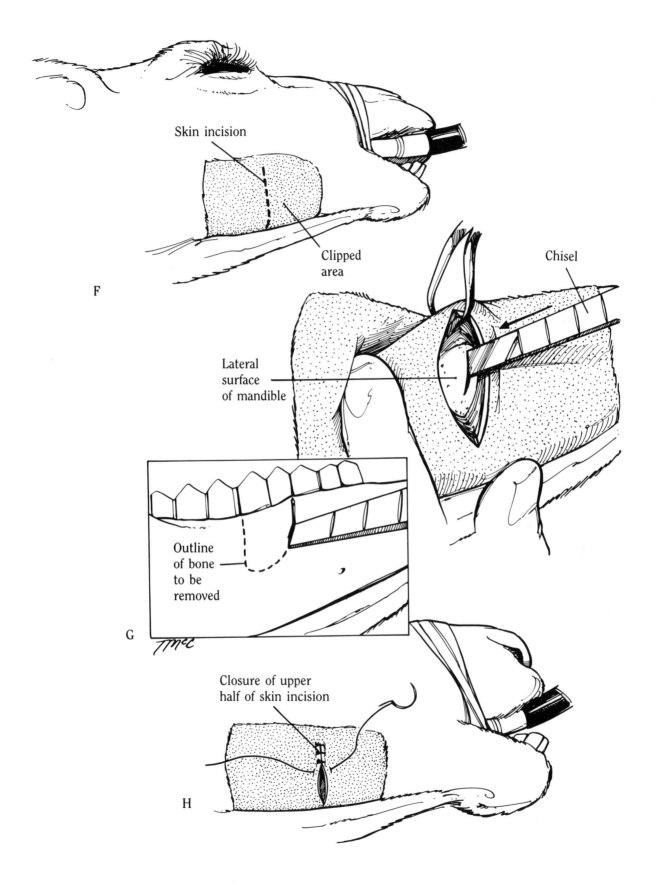

Skin incision

Clipped area

F

Chisel

Lateral surface of mandible

Outline of bone to be removed

G

Closure of upper half of skin incision

H

FIG. 17-3. *(continued)*.

is removed, but the bone immediately ventral to the tooth is preserved (Fig. 17-3G). The tooth should be freed of bone at its rostral and caudal surfaces using a chisel. A dental punch is placed on the tooth root, and with gentle tapping, it seats itself into the root of the tooth. The surgeon should place his fingertips over the crown of the tooth and guide the punch with the other hand. An assistant then delivers the blows to the punch. The surgeon feels the vibrations of the blows transmitted through the tooth to his fingertips. Occasionally, the punch has to be redirected. The tooth gradually loosens, and the blows of the mallet should then become less forceful.

Following repulsion of the tooth, any small fragments of bone or teeth are removed. The alveolus is curetted and is flushed. The ventral half of the incision is left open, to provide ventral drainage of the alveolus. The upper half is closed with simple interrupted sutures with nonabsorbable suture material (Fig. 17-3H).

Postoperative Management

The llama should be placed on antibiotics preoperatively and for approximately a week following surgery. The wound where the canine tooth has been removed usually requires little postoperative care. Following molar extraction, the alveolus can be flushed daily with a mild antiseptic solution or until granulation tissue has begun to fill the defect.

Comments

If the equipment is available, a Hall air drill with the appropriate bur can be used to remove the bone from the lateral surface of the canine tooth. Most important is the position of the canine tooth root within the bone. The tooth root is extensive and follows a marked caudal direction.

We have seen uncomplicated healing after removal of canine and molar teeth. Daily flushing of the alveolus seems to keep food and debris from lodging in the wound in the case of molar teeth. This sort of aftercare can be performed by the owner.

APPENDIX

Proprietary Drugs and Supplies Cited in Text and Their Manufacturers

Acepromazine Maleate Injectable (Ayerst Laboratories)

Barrier Incise Drape (Johnson & Johnson)

Betadine Ointment (Purdue Frederick Company)

Betadine Scrub (Purdue Frederick Company)

Betadine Solution (Purdue Frederick Company)

Braunamid (B. Braun Melsungen A. G., West Germany)

Carbocaine (Breon Laboratories, Inc.)

Chloropent (Fort Dodge Laboratories, Inc.)

Control Release (Ethicon, Inc.)

Dacron (Davis and Geck)

Demerol (Winthrop Laboratories)

Dermalon (Davis and Geck)

Dexon (Davis and Geck)

Ethibond (Ethicon, Inc.)

Ethiflex (Ethicon, Inc.)

Ethilon (Ethicon, Inc.)

Glycodex (Burns-Biotec Laboratories)

Harleco CO$_2$ apparatus (Harleco Company)

Innovar-Vet (Pitman-Moore, Inc.)

Ketalar (Parke-Davis)

KY Jelly (Johnson & Johnson)

Lidocaine Hydrochloride Injection 2% (Vedco, Inc.)

Mag-Chloral Relaxant Solution (Haver-Lockhart)

Mersilene (Ethicon, Inc.)

Normosol-R (Abbott Laboratories)

Nurolon (Ethicon, Inc.)

Pentothal (Abbott Laboratories)

Perivaginal Suture Tape (Jorgensen Laboratories)

Polydek (Deknatel, Inc.)

Polyethylene (Davis and Geck)

Polysal (Cutter Laboratories, Inc.)

Prolene (Ethicon, Inc.)

Promazine Hydrochloride Injection (Fort Dodge Laboratories, Inc.)

Proximate, Skin Stapling Device (Ethicon, Inc.)

Redi-Vacette Perforated Tubing ¼" (64 mm) O.D. (Orthopedic Equipment)

Rompun (Haver-Lockhart)

Special K Needle (Deknatel, Inc.)

Steri-drape (3-M Animal Care Products)

Stiglyn (Pitman-Moore, Inc.)

Stresnil (Pitman-Moore, Inc.)

Supramid (Jensen Salisbury Lab)

Surital (Parke-Davis)

Talwin-V (Winthrop Laboratories)

Telfa Sterile Pads (The Kendall Company)

Tevdek (Deknatel, Inc.)

Ticron (Davis and Geck)

Umbilical Tape (Ethicon, Inc.)

Valium (Hoffman-La Roche Inc.)

Vetafil (Bengen W.S. Jackson Company)

Vicryl (Ethicon, Inc.)

Vi-Drape Adhesive (Parke-Davis)

Water Pik (Teledyne-Water Pik Corporation)

Manufacturers' Addresses, Proprietary Drugs (Generic Names in Parentheses), and Supplies

Abbott Laboratories
North Chicago, Illinois 60064
  Normosol-R
  Pentothal (thiopental sodium)

Ayerst Labs.
Div., American Home Products Corp.
New York, New York 10017
  Acepromazine Maleate Injectable (acetylpromazine maleate)

Bengen W.S. Jackson Company
Washington, D.C. 20014
  Vetafil (polymerized caprolactam)

Breon Laboratories Inc.
Subs., Sterling Drug, Inc.
New York, New York 10016
  Carbocaine (mepivacaine hydrochloride)

Burns-Biotec Laboratories
Div., Chromalloy Pharmaceuticals, Inc.
Omaha, Nebraska 68103
  Glycodex (guaifenesin)

Cutter Laboratories, Inc.
Berkeley, California 94710
  Polysal

Davis and Geck
Div., American Cyanamid Co.
Pearl River, New York 10965
  Dacron
  Dermalon
  Dexon (polyglycolic acid)
  Polyethylene
  Ticron

Deknatel, Inc.
Queens Village
Long Island, New York 11429
  Polydek
  Special K Needle
  Tevdek

Emery Medical Supply Co.
Arvada, Colorado 80002
  General Surgical Instruments

Ethicon, Inc.
Somerville, New Jersey 08876
Control Release
Ethibond
Ethiflex
Ethilon
Mersilene
Nurolon
Prolene (polypropylene)
Proximate, Skin Stapling Device
Umbilical Tape
Vicryl (polyglactin 910)

Fisher Scientific
Richmond, Virginia
Carboy (20 L)

Fort Dodge Laboratories, Inc.
Fort Dodge, Iowa 50501
*Chloropent (chloral hydrate/magnesium
sulfate/pentobarbital sodium)*
Pentobarbitone sodium
*Promazine Hydrochloride Injection
(promazine hydrochloride)*

Harleco Company
Div., American Hospital Supply Company
Gibbstown, New Jersey 08027
Harleco CO_2 apparatus

Haver-Lockhart
Box 390
Shawnee, Kansas 66201
*Mag-Chloral Relaxant Solution (chloral
hydrate/magnesium sulfate)*
Rompun (xylazine hydrochloride)

Hoffman-La Roche Inc.
Nutley, New Jersey 07110
Valium (diazepam)

Jensen Salisbury Lab
Division of Burroughs Wellcome Co.
Kansas City, Missouri 64141
Supramid (polymerized caprolactam)

Johnson & Johnson
Health Care Division
New Brunswick, New Jersey 08903
Barrier Incise Drape
KY Jelly

Jorgensen Laboratories
Loveland, Colorado 80538

Perivaginal Suture Tape
Complete infusion set

The Kendall Company
Health Care Division
Chicago, Illinois 60606
Telfa Sterile Pads

Lane Manufacturing, Inc.
Denver, Colorado 80231
Cole pattern endotracheal tubes

Misdom-Frank and Sklar Instrument
Companies
201 Carter Drive
West Chester, Pennsylvania 19380
General surgical instruments

Orthopedic Equipment
Bourbon, Indiana 46504
*Redi-Vacette Perforated Tubing ¼"
(64 mm) O.D.*

Parke-Davis
Div., Warner-Lambert Co.
Morris Plains, New Jersey 07950
Ketalar (ketamine hydrochloride)
Surital (thiamylal sodium)
Vi-Drape Adhesive

Pitman-Moore, Inc.
Washington Crossing, New Jersey 08560
Innovar-Vet (droperidol/fentanyl citrate)
Stiglyn (neostigmine)
Stresnil (azaperone)

Purdue Frederick Company
Norwalk, Connecticut 06856
Betadine Ointment (povidone-iodine)
Betadine Scrub (povidone-iodine)
Betadine Solution (povidone-iodine)

Teledyne-Water Pik Corporation
Fort Collins, Colorado 80521
Water Pik

3-M Animal Care Products
3-M Center
Medical Products Division
St. Paul, Minnesota 55105
Steri-drape

Vedco Inc.
Omaha, Nebraska 68127

Lidocaine Hydrochloride Injection 2%
(lidocaine hydrochloride)

Winthrop Laboratories

Subs., Sterling Drug, Inc.
New York, New York 10016
Demerol (meperidine hydrochloride)
Talwin-V (pentazocine)

INDEX

Page numbers in *italics* indicate figures; those followed by "t" indicate tables.